RECENT ADVANCES IN ANÆSTHESIA AND ANALGESIA

RECENT ADVANCES IN ANÆSTHESIA AND ANALGESIA

(INCLUDING OXYGEN THERAPY)

BY

C. LANGTON HEWER

M.B., B.S.(Lond), M.R.C.P.(Lond)., F.F.A.R.C.S.

*Senior Anœsthetist, St. Bartholomew's Hospital, St. Andrew's Hospital, Dollis Hill
Consultant Anœsthetist, The Luton & Dunstable Hospital, Mid-Herts, West-Herts
& Harpenden Hospitals.
Formerly
Member of the Board of Faculty of Anœsthetists.
Examiner in Anæsthesia to the Royal College of Physicians of London & to the
Royal College of Surgeons of England.
Senior Anæsthetist to the Queen's Hospital for Children.
Anæsthetist to the Brompton Chest Hospital.
Anœsthetic Specialist, R.A.M.C.*

SEVENTH EDITION

WITH 169 ILLUSTRATIONS

THE BLAKISTON COMPANY

NEW YORK

1953

First Edition	.	.	1932
Second Edition	.	.	1937
Third Edition	.	.	1939
Fourth Edition	.	.	1943
Fifth Edition	.	.	1944
	Reprinted		1946
Sixth Edition	.	.	1948
Seventh Edition	.	.	1953

Printed in Great Britain

PREFACE TO THE SEVENTH EDITION

DURING the five years which have elapsed since the publication
of the sixth edition of this book, the most dramatic development in
anæsthesia has been the introduction of induced hypotension with
the object of minimizing blood loss during operation. A new
chapter has accordingly been inserted dealing with this innovation.
It will be found that there are several discrepancies relating to
induced hypotension on the one hand and resuscitation on the other.
No attempt has been made to reconcile these, as the whole question
is still in a fluid state, but at the time of writing it is quite obvious
that the original enthusiasm for the hypotension method has waned,
and it appears practically certain that in the near future it will be
confined to a very limited sphere. The arrangement of the rest of
the book has been unaltered but many chapters have been practically
re-written.

It is usually held that the collection and re-publication of other
peoples' views is the lowest form of literary activity, and the writer
has tried to avoid this stigma by giving his own opinions where
possible, but it is doubtful whether, at the present time, any one
individual is in a position to pronounce upon all types of anæsthetic
problems ; the writer certainly makes no such claim. The truly
general anæsthetist is becoming as rare as the truly general surgeon.

It will be found that fresh information has been given upon the
following subjects amongst others :

the risks of pre-operative glucose by mouth,
effects of anæsthesia on the peripheral circulation,
method of automatic control of depth of narcosis by electrical
impulses from the brain,
use of mucates of alkaloids for prolonged effects,
a device to measure continuously the oxygen saturation of
arterial blood during narcosis (the oximeter),
cyclobutane, a homologue of cyclopropane,
a new type of plastic artificial airway,
international colour code for gas cylinders,
automatic warning devices when using incorrect gases,
properties of lesser known anæsthetic ethers,
isopropyl chloride (proponesin),
a new one-handed nasal spray,
a wide-bore tapered tracheal tube,
an apparatus to detect an explosive gas mixture,
an apparatus to detect dangerous static charges,
a new short-acting barbiturate (surital),
a non-clotting intravenous needle (Gordh's),

treatment of inadvertent intra-arterial injection of thiopentone,
a new long-acting relaxant, the dimethyl ether of d-tubocurarine iodide (D.M.E.),
two medium-action relaxants, gallamine triethiodide (flaxedil) and decamethonium-iodide (C.10),
two short-acting relaxants, succinycholine and brevidil,
two new local analgesics, lucaine and xylocaine,
use of the " spreading factor " (hyaluronidase) in local analgesia and in subcutaneous infusions,
the physiology of refrigerated tissues,
a needle-less injector for analgesic solutions (the hypospray),
stellate ganglion block,
dangers of caudal block and therapeutic uses of fractional caudal block,
elimination of drugs injected intrathecally,
total spinal block,
a new theory for the causation of sixth nerve palsy after spinal analgesia,
arteriotomy for inducing hypotension,
two ganglion-blocking drugs, pentamethonium and hexa-methonium,
the application of negative pressure to limbs to produce hypotension,
two plasma substitutes, dextran and plasmosan,
distinction between adrenaline and *nor*-adrenaline,
the Crutchfield caliper in cranial surgery,
oxygen inflator for sphygmomanometer cuffs,
two types of dental cartridge syringe,
anæsthetic adapter for bronchoscope,
bipod support for Davis gag,
anæsthesia for cardiac, catheterization, and angiocardiography,
observations on the Trendelenburg position,
automatic nitrous oxide-oxygen apparatus for use in labour,
electrical stimulation of phrenic nerve in neonatal asphyxia,
design of anæsthetic rooms and post-operative recovery rooms,
the " nerve gases ".

Of the 169 figures, 52 are new, and I should like to thank the various firms and individuals for the loan of blocks. If any acknowledgment of works quoted has been inadvertently omitted, I would express regret to the authors.

Once again it is my pleasure to thank the publishers for their unfailing courtesy in bringing out this edition.

C. LANGTON HEWER.

against an increased peripheral resistance and bleeding from cut surfaces tends to be diminished.[17]

Carbohydrate Metabolism and Ketosis

The administration of any of the more toxic anæsthetics for an appreciable time and the injection of local analgesics diminish the **alkali reserve** of the blood, the greatest decrease being at the end of a long anæsthesia. The normal is rapidly regained during the recovery stage[20] and is hastened by the administration of carbon dioxide-oxygen mixtures (Yandell Henderson).

If the lowering of alkalinity be permitted experimentally to go too far, the kidneys eventually cease to function.[21] For these reasons the administration of large quantities of sodium bicarbonate before operation was considered good practice, but recently it has been shown that the accompanying ketosis is the important factor, and much better results are obtained by giving glucose.[22] This is especially important if chloroform or bromethol is to be used. Barley sugar is perhaps the most palatable form in which to give the drug, and it could, before the war, be obtained with an 85 per cent. content of pure glucose. It should not, however, be given within a few hours before operation (see below). The striking effects of insulin given with glucose in diabetes suggested that it might be of equal service in post-operative ketosis, and this has been borne out by experience. It has been shown that an increase in **blood sugar** (due to the mobilization of glycogen from the liver) occurs during and after operations performed under chloroform, di-ethyl ether,[23] di-vinyl ether,[24] cyclopropane,[25] as well as basal narcotics such as bromethol and local and spinal analgesia.[26]

It is thought by some physiologists that di-ethyl ether, at any rate, produces hyperglycæmia in two distinct ways. The initial glucose mobilization is held to be due to a direct stimulation action on the production of adrenaline, while a secondary rise dependent upon the depth of anæsthesia is due to an unknown mechanism interfering with carbohydrate metabolism.[27] In any event, hyperglycæmia due to anæsthetics is diminished if a preliminary injection of insulin has been given.[28] Premedication with the barbiturates also reduces the hyperglycæmia due to ether and other anæsthetics but the exact mechanism is obscure.[29]

Sugar tolerance is diminished after general and local anæsthesia, but this effect can also be prevented by the pre-operative administration of insulin.[23]

It has been suggested that prolonged narcotization with

chloroform or ether might be beneficial in carcinoma by combating the alkalosis which is present in this condition. The retrogression of growths, which is not uncommon following exploratory operations, may possibly be explained by the acidosis induced by the anæsthesia.[30] Recent cancer research seems to confirm the value of diminishing the alkali reserve.

The diagnosis of **ketosis** before or after anæsthesia is usually made by a urine analysis, but delay in obtaining a specimen may occur. Since it has been shown that the acetone contents of the blood and alveolar air are proportional,[31] a modified Roth technique can be used for determining rapidly the acetone content of the breath. 2 to 3 c.cm. of Scott-Wilson solution are placed in a special blow-tube and the patient is asked to blow through it six times. If the solution remains clear, acetone is absent, while the degree of cloudiness is proportional to the amount of acetone present. The solution is made in the following way : A cooled solution of 180 g. sodium hydroxide in 600 c.cm. water is added to 10 g. mercuric cyanide dissolved in 600 c.cm. water. The mixture is stirred and $2 \cdot 9$ g. silver nitrate dissolved in 400 c.cm. water are added. A clear solution results which is ready for use.[32]

The chief clinical manifestations of ketosis are hyperpnœa, hot, dry skin, furred tongue, a feeling of lassitude and nausea and vomiting.

Anæsthesia in Diabetes

Both anæsthesia and operative trauma may cause grave metabolic upset in diabetics, and prior to the advent of insulin a major surgical operation was a hazardous procedure. At the present time, however, it can be said that, provided the disease is adequately controlled, a diabetic has practically a normal risk. The usual preparation for such a patient is to omit the meal and insulin before the operation and to substitute 50 g. of glucose in lemonade with 25 units of soluble insulin two hours before operation. Recently, however, grave doubts have been thrown on the safety of giving glucose by mouth before operation, several deaths from regurgitation having been reported. Water passes rapidly into the duodenum, but hypertonic glucose solution prolongs the emptying time of the stomach.[95] In some animals the solution has to be diluted in the stomach until it is isotonic before it passes into the duodenum.[96] This may be the explanation for these unfortunate occurrences and it would seem wise to discontinue the practice of giving oral glucose before operation. If it is essential, it should be given as an intravenous drip. The type of anæsthesia or analgesia used will naturally vary with the operation, but there is no doubt that chloroform and di-ethyl ether should be avoided. The post-operative treatment will depend on the amount of sugar and ketone bodies present in the urine.

Diabetes which is only discovered immediately before an urgent operation presents a different problem. If ketonuria is absent, the preparation just described will suffice, but if ketones are present in any quantity, an intravenous infusion of 10 per cent. glucose in saline at the rate of 1 pint per hour should be given with 50 units of insulin for every 50 g. glucose until the urine test for ketones is negative. It is not essential to have blood-sugar estimations performed in cases of emergency.[33]

It is worth noting that if a diabetic patient does not return to consciousness within a normal time after the cessation of an anæsthetic, hypoglycæmia is probably present and intravenous glucose should be given.[34]

Effects of Anæsthetics on Pancreas and Adrenals

There is some evidence to show that general and local anæsthetics stimulate the adrenal bodies to produce a hypersecretion of adrenaline.[23] This apparently causes some condition in the body associated with acetonuria, which is the prime factor accounting for the diminished efficiency of the pancreas resulting in the lowered sugar tolerance.[37] The reaction which follows such stimulation may play some part in the production of shock (q.v.).

Effects of Anæsthesia on Gastro-Intestinal Tract

It appears from experimental work on animals that anæsthesia usually depresses gastric tone and motility, presumably from sympathetic stimulation.[35] Light cyclopropane narcosis is an exception to this rule.[36] The depth of narcosis has more effect than the agent used, but premedication with morphine, anoxia, and rough handling all increase the time taken by the stomach to recover its normal condition. It is rather surprising that spinal analgesia also depresses gastric tone and motility. It is possible that these observations have some bearing on the rare but serious complication of acute dilatation of the stomach.[38]

The same remarks apply to the small intestine except that in this case a high spinal block *increases* the tone and motility.[39] Other drugs used during anæsthesia such as adrenaline, ephedrine, neosynephrine and atropine decrease intestinal tone and movements, the first three from sympathetic stimulation. Morphine arrests intestinal propulsion by causing spasm of the musculature[40] but pitressin,[41] on the other hand, increases intestinal movements.

The effects of curare on intestinal movements are considered in Chapter XI.

Effects of Anæsthetics on the Liver

The liver has so many diverse functions that many tests have been devised to measure them. Until recently, dye-retention tests were considered the most reliable for estimating the effects of anæsthetics. For example, bromsulphalein can be injected intravenously and the liver should be able to remove it completely from the blood within a given time.[42]

Using these tests, it has been shown in mammals that nitrous oxide, ethylene and cyclopropane produce no impairment of liver function if the oxygen supply is adequate.[43] Di-vinyl ether produces a slight effect, but di-ethyl causes a distinct impairment of function, often lasting for more than twenty-four hours.[11] Chloroform may cause grave and prolonged changes. Half an hour's chloroform anæsthesia can produce impairment of function lasting for eight days, while two hours' anæsthesia has inflicted injury lasting for no less than six weeks. The clinical condition in man of **delayed chloroform poisoning** has, of course, long been recognized, and confirms these findings. This condition has been observed after only 4 drachms of the drug had been inhaled.[44] A more sensitive assessment of hepatic damage known as the cephalin flocculation test[45] was first described in 1938. The principle of the reaction is that the serum of patients suffering from parenchymatous hepatic lesions causes flocculation in cephalin-cholesterol emulsions. This test offers advantages over previous ones in specificity, sensitivity and ease of application. When applied to anæsthetics, it seems clear that trichlorethylene, di-ethyl ether and chloroform cause progressively more hepatic damage in that order.[46] No impairment of function could be found after intravenous procaine. Liver cells which are laden with glycogen are more resistant to toxic agents including anæsthetics. The usual practice of giving glucose before operation should ensure that this condition is present but, as noted above, oral glucose should not be given for some hours owing to the risk of regurgitation. Some physiologists hold that the liver converts lactic acid more easily than glucose into glycogen and consequently recommend the administration of sodium lactate.[47]

It has been proved that the administration of excess oxygen with a normally toxic volatile anæsthetic greatly minimizes liver damage.[49]

Conversely, it has been shown that anoxia increases liver damage and can even cause changes by itself. For example, in dogs exposed for two hours to an atmosphere of 15 per cent. oxygen and 85 per cent. nitrogen, 28 per cent. showed signs of definite hepatic damage.[49]

During anæsthesia, phosphoric acid appears to leave the muscles and to remain in the liver until the resumption of normal kidney function, when it is redistributed and partly excreted.[50]

The effects of anæsthetics on the liver are also considered under the individual drugs (q.v.), whilst the precautions to be observed in jaundiced patients are mentioned in Chapter XXIII.

Effects of Anæsthetics on the Heart

Heart failure during anæsthesia can occur from (i) reflex effects acting on the neuromuscular mechanism, and (ii) failure of the cardiac muscle itself from acute anoxia[30] ; this subject is discussed in Chapters VII and XVII.

Electrocardiographic Changes. During narcosis with all the volatile agents, but especially with chloroform, trichlorethylene and cyclopropane, a great variety of transient E.C.G. changes have been noted. It is probable that most of these are of little practical

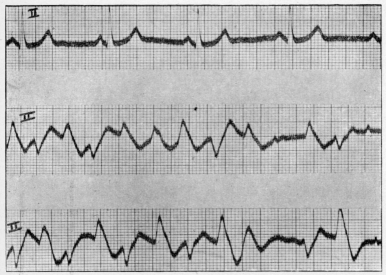

Fig. 1. E.C.G. showing *a* normal sinus rhythm before induction, *b* and *c* multifocal ventricular tachycardia at 19 and 20 minutes respectively after induction of inhalation anæsthesia. (Barnes & Ives, *Pro. Roy. Soc. Med.*)

significance with the exception of multifocal ventricular tachycardia. It has been shown[51] that in the case of chloroform this type of arrhythmia may be the precursor of ventricular fibrillation—e.g. if adrenaline is injected—and this is one of the mechanisms of primary cardiac failure which is such a tragic possibility with this drug. In the case of cyclopropane and trichlorethylene, however, although multifocal ventricular tachycardia has been demonstrated in about 10 per cent. of administrations with each drug,[52] primary cardiac failure is exceedingly rare so that too much importance should not be attached to this change in the E.C.G. if chloroform is not being used.

In some thoracic units it is now customary to take continuous E.C.G. observations during cardiac operations. Some instruments provide a luminous image on a dark background while others provide a continuous record on a tape, e.g. the Elmquist system.

The question of anæsthetizing patients with **morbus cordis** frequently arises. A compensated lesion is no disability for operations of moderate severity provided that cardiac poisons, such as chloroform, are avoided, and that anoxia and hypotension are not allowed to occur. When compensation is incomplete, however, or if anginal pain has occurred, greater care is necessary, the safest general anæsthetic under such risks probably being ether and oxygen.

Various **cardiac and respiratory efficiency tests** have been devised to evaluate the operative risk : for example, *Moot's formula* states that $\dfrac{\text{pulse pressure}}{\text{diastolic pressure}} = \frac{1}{2}$ or 50 per cent. in normal patients, and the degree of deviation from this figure is an indication of the risk involved. If it is below 25 per cent. or above 75 per cent. the operative risk is extremely high.[53]

Barach's Index is obtained by multiplying the systolic (S.P.) and diastolic (D.P.) pressures by the pulse rate (P.R.) and adding the results together. Thus Barach's Index = (S.P. × P.R.) + (D.P. × P.R.). The normal limits are put at 13,000 to 20,000, between which the patient is operable. These figures depend upon the energy expended by the heart per minute.

A recent investigation of Barach's and Moot's formulæ was made in patients moribund from cardiac failure, and in no less than 62 per cent. the results were misleading. One patient was " operable " by both formulæ fifteen minutes before death.[54]

The *Crampton test* appears to be the most reliable guide at present known to a patient's general condition and has been adopted as the standard for disqualification from athletics by the Amateur

Athletic Association of America. The test consists in taking the pulse rate and systolic blood pressure lying down. The patient then stands for two minutes and the readings are again taken. The " Crampton value " is estimated from the table on p. 10. On this scale, 100 is theoretical perfection, 75 is good and below 65 is poor. In extremely bad risks the figure may fall below zero.

The main disadvantage of the Crampton test is that it is inapplicable to bedridden patients.

Probably the most reliable rough and ready means of estimating cardiac and respiratory efficiency is the *breath-holding test of Sebrasez*. While resting in bed the patient takes one deep inspiration, then closes his mouth, pinches his nose and holds his breath for as long as possible. Any time exceeding twenty-five seconds is normal but less than fifteen seconds is taken to indicate marked reduction of cardiac and respiratory reserve.[55]

The *vital capacity* can be measured by a volumetric spirometer and if lowered is said to increase the gravity of the prognosis after severe operations, when taken in conjunction with other pre-operative tests.[56] On the other hand the vital capacity may be misleading because the rate of taking the maximum breath is not recorded, e.g. in asthma the main difficulty is the retardation of the rate of respiratory exchange.[97] Incidentally if there is reason to believe that appreciable bronchospasm exists, it is always worth trying the effect of making the patient inhale a vaporized bronchodilator.

In certain congenital heart lesions and in some forms of shock, etc., there is an excess of red corpuscles in the blood leading to an increase in viscosity and in the work of the heart. If excessive, cyanosis of the head, neck and shoulders develops and this should be regarded seriously. It is now considered that a *hæmatocrit value* [volume of red cells compared to that of blood] of over 50 per cent. renders a patient a very poor subject for general anæsthesia.[98]

One must assume that at the present time it is impossible to assess a patient's condition accurately by mathematics, and each case must be considered on its merits in the light of the anæsthetist's previous experience. There is no doubt that, if time permits, every patient suffering from severe morbus cordis should have preliminary treatment with digitalis or other drugs in order to get the heart into as efficient a state as possible before operation.

Contrary to some previous views, it is now held that **high blood pressure,** even in extreme degrees, unaccompanied by myocardial

HEART RATE Increase per Minute on Standing / Decrease on Standing	Blood Pressure Increase in Mm. of Mercury on Standing.									Decrease in Mm. of Mercury on Standing										
	16-15	14-13	12-11	10-9	8-7	7-5	4-3	2-1	0	1-2	3-4	5 6	7-8	9-10	11-12	13-14	15-16	17-18	19-20	21-22	23-24
8-12	130	125	120	115	110	105	100	95	90	85	80	75	70	65	60	55	50	45	40	35	30
4- 8	125	120	115	110	105	100	95	90	85	80	75	70	65	60	55	50	45	40	35	30	25
0- 4	120	115	110	105	100	95	90	85	80	75	70	65	60	55	50	45	40	35	30	25	20
0- 4	115	110	105	100	95	90	85	80	75	70	65	60	55	50	45	40	35	30	25	20	15
5- 8	110	105	100	95	90	85	80	75	70	65	60	55	50	45	40	35	30	25	20	15	10
9-12	105	100	95	90	85	80	75	70	65	60	55	50	45	40	35	30	25	20	15	10	5
13-16	100	95	90	85	80	75	70	65	60	55	50	45	40	35	30	25	20	15	10	5	0
17-20	95	90	85	80	75	70	65	60	55	50	45	40	35	30	25	20	15	10	5	0	—5
21-24	90	85	80	75	70	65	60	55	50	45	40	35	30	25	20	15	10	5	0	—5	—10
25-28	85	80	75	70	65	60	55	50	45	40	35	30	25	20	15	10	5	0	—5	—10	—15
29-32	80	75	70	65	60	55	50	45	40	35	30	25	20	15	10	5	0	—5	—10	—15	—20
33-36	75	70	65	60	55	50	45	40	35	30	25	20	15	10	5	0	—5	—10	—15	—20	—25
37-40	70	65	60	55	50	45	40	35	30	25	20	15	10	5	0	—5	—10	—15	—20	—25	—30
41-44	65	60	55	50	45	40	35	30	25	20	15	10	5	0	—5	—10	—15	—20	—25	—30	—35
45-48	60	55	50	45	40	35	30	25	20	15	10	5	0	—5	—10	—15	—20	—25	—30	—35	—40
49-52	55	50	45	40	35	30	25	20	15	10	5	0	—5	—10	—15	—20	—25	—30	—35	—40	—45
53-56	50	45	40	35	30	25	20	15	10	5	0	—5	—10	—15	—20	—25	—30	—35	—40	—45	—50
57-60	45	40	35	30	25	20	15	10	5	0	—5	—10	—15	—20	—25	—30	—35	—40	—45	—50	—55
61-64	40	35	30	25	20	15	10	5	0	—5	—10	—15	—20	—25	—30	—35	—40	—45	—50	—55	—60
65-68	35	30	25	20	15	10	5	0	—5	—10	—15	—20	—25	—30	—35	—40	—45	—50	—55	—60	—65
69-72	30	25	20	15	10	5	0	—5	—10	—15	—20	—25	—30	—35	—40	—45	—50	—55	—60	—65	—70
73-76	25	20	15	10	5	0	—5	—10	—15	—20	—25	—30	—35	—40	—45	—50	—55	—60	—65	—70	—75
77-80	20	15	10	5	0	—5	—10	—15	—20	—25	—30	—35	—40	—45	—50	—55	—60	—65	—70	—75	—80

or renal insufficiency, diabetes, or hyperthyroidism, adds only slightly to the operative risk,[57] while **low blood pressure,** uncomplicated by jaundice, diabetes, syphilis or Addison's disease, indicates an exceptionally good risk.[58]

The whole question of anæsthesia in relation to cardio-vascular affections has been discussed in various papers to which the reader is referred for fuller details.[59]

The current theory of blood-pressure maintenance and methods of control are discussed in Chapters XV, XVI and XVII.

Effects of Anæsthesia on the Peripheral Circulation

The peripheral circulation has been studied during operations performed under various types of general anæsthesia by means of plethysmographs fitted to the calf, foot and hand. It has been found that the blood flow through the limbs is usually increased considerably during the induction of anæsthesia and for some time afterwards. As the blood pressure is relatively unaffected, this change must be due to vasodilatation produced either by the action of the anæsthetic drug on the vasomotor centre or directly on the blood vessel walls or both.[99]

At a later stage in severe operations, decreased flow, due to vasoconstriction occurs and this must be regarded as a compensatory mechanism and precedes the onset of shock.[100]

Further observations have recently shown that there are coincidental and reciprocal changes in the blood flow in the limbs and lower bowel under general anæsthesia, i.e. as the flow increases in the limbs so it decreases in the rectum.[101]

Effects of Anæsthetics on the Kidneys and Urine

Chloroform and ether anæsthesia, if prolonged, tend towards *oliguria* or actual *anuria*, especially if any renal dysfunction is present.[1] Bromethol and the barbiturates also reduce the urinary output temporarily, but this is soon made up if the kidneys are undamaged.[60]

Albuminuria practically always occurs after the prolonged administration of ether and in about 20 per cent. of patients anæsthetized with chloroform. Some changes in the renal cells apparently occur.[61]

Acetonuria has been demonstrated in 67 per cent. of patients operated upon under all forms of general anæsthesia, and in no less than 85 per cent. under local analgesia.[62] It can often be prevented by the pre-operative injection of insulin.[23]

The *blood urea* usually shows a moderate rise after ether anæsthesia, but it seems doubtful whether this is due to any toxic effect on the kidneys.[63] Minnitt, however, holds that the increase is due to the action of the drug on the renal cells, and has demonstrated that no such effect occurs with nitrous oxide and oxygen.[64]

Effects of Anæsthetics on the Nervous System

The nervous system is of special interest to the anæsthetist, and is the one upon which anæsthetics have their main action. As we have very incomplete knowledge of the normal physiology of the central nervous system it is not surprising that there are many theories of the way in which general anæsthetics act upon it. There is little profit in pursuing these but the leisured and speculative reader is referred to the textbook entitled " Anesthesia " by J. T. Gwathmey where he will find nineteen theories discussed at some length.

Nervous tissue appears to have a selective affinity for anæsthetics circulating in the blood stream, and chloroform at any rate is found in greater proportion per unit weight in the brain and spinal cord than in any other tissues of dogs killed by an overdose of this drug (Nicloux). As much as $551 \cdot 5$ mg. of chloroform has been found in 1,000 g. of brain tissue. A similar result has been obtained with rabbits under the influence of bromethol.[65] The "minute-volume " blood supply of brain cells is greater than that of other tissue cells so that a greater proportion of anæsthetic would naturally be found there in the early stage of anæsthesia. It occurs, however, at all periods of narcosis, and this is due to the fact that nerve tissue is particularly rich in lipoids and that these probably combine with the anæsthetic agent. (The lipoid content of brain and nerve tissue is between 12 and 15 per cent. of the total weight, while that of liver and muscle is from 7 to 8 per cent.)

In order to act as narcotics, drugs must be water-soluble as well as lipoid-soluble for transport to the nerve cells to occur. The ratio of solubility per given amount of lipoids to that of an equal volume of water is called the oil/water ratio and the higher the value of this ratio, the greater the potency of the drug. This is known as the Overton-Meyer theory and although exceptions to the rule occur, most narcotics follow it.

The order in which the different parts of the central nervous system are affected by volatile anæsthetics is the reverse of that of their development, the highly specialized cortical area being put out of action first and the vital medullary centres last. If this were not the case death would of course ensue before the establishment of anæsthesia. The peripheral nerves are affected hardly at all by general anæsthetics, and consequently traumatic stimulation from the area of operation is constantly occurring, and while it is not perceived by the patient, owing to the suspension of function of the sensory area in the cortex, yet it can cause serious reflex effects through the spinal cord and medulla. The realization of these facts cause Crile to advance his " anoci-association " method which is discussed later. The reason why anæsthetic drugs should select the cortical cells for their main action seems to lie in the high rate at which these cells use oxygen. It has been established that nervous tissue as a whole metabolizes more rapidly than other tissues.[66] The nature of the actual biochemical reactions which occur during cerebral metabolism has been the subject of much discussion. By comparing the composition of carotid and internal jugular blood and measuring the cerebral blood flow and also by studying isolated brain tissue it seems probable that the main change is the oxidation of glucose and lactic acid in the presence of the enzyme vitamin B_1.[67] It has been estimated that the basal oxygen requirements of the brain demand 1,400 c.cm. of blood per minute and that at rest the brain receives one-third of the ventricular output although it represents only 2 per cent. of the body weight.[68] Direct experiments on the oxygen consumption of different types or nerve cells are both difficult to perform and inconclusive in their results, but the rates at which the different types of cell die when deprived of oxygen have been determined in animals, the approximate figures being :[69]

The cerebrum, small pyramidal cells—eight minutes.

The cerebellum, Purkinje cells—thirteen minutes.

The medullary centres—twenty to thirty minutes.

The spinal cord—forty-five to sixty minutes.

The sympathetic ganglia—three to three and a half hours.

It appears reasonable to infer that the rate of oxygen consumption is in the same order and that cortical cells have a higher metabolic rate than the others. If then the oxygen percentage is reduced in the body as a whole the cortical cells will be affected first and consciousness lost, and by adjustment of the oxygen percentage at that exact level the other cells of the body should have sufficient oxygen to function normally; in other words general anæsthesia will be established. It would appear from this reasoning that by merely cutting down the oxygen supply in air we could obtain anæsthesia, but we know that in practice asphyxia results, although it is sometimes possible to produce brief periods of anæsthesia. The reason for this appears to lie partly in the question of solubility of the gases in blood.[1] Nitrogen is almost insoluble, but if we substitute a soluble but non-toxic gas our aim might be attained. Nitrous oxide is such a gas, being more than a hundred times as soluble in blood plasma as oxygen. It is also thought by most workers that nitrous oxide itself has a slight anæsthetic effect and when absorbed by lipoids causes a slight diminution in cell oxidation possibly by inhibiting one of the enzymes concerned. This would account for the fact that under certain conditions (e.g. severe shock or anæmia) it is sometimes possible to produce anæsthesia with a higher percentage of oxygen than is present in atmospheric air, e.g. 75 per cent. N_2O and 25 per cent. O_2. (See also Chapter III.) In practice anæsthesia is rapidly produced by the inhalation of nitrous oxide-oxygen mixtures. It can be maintained for a very considerable time without ill-effects (forty-eight hours in animals)[70] and recovery time is practically equal to that of induction. It would seem reasonable to conclude, therefore, that nitrous oxide acts chiefly in a physical way by limiting the oxygen supply to the cells of the cerebral cortex but some workers do not admit this. It is clear that solubility in blood must play some part in the narcotic effect of gases as it has recently been shown that krypton has practically no effect and xenon about the same as ethylene, although their oil/water ratios are about the same and higher than that of ethylene. Solubility is the only obvious physical difference.[93] Chloroform, on the other hand, probably enters cells containing lipoids through the cell membrane and temporarily poisons such cells, thus diminishing their powers of using oxygen for their normal function of oxidizing carbohydrates, i.e. it produces a histotoxic anoxia. It is thought by some that the cell activity is reduced to the sole function of oxidizing succinic acid which supplies the minimal amount of energy compatible with the life of the cell. This is assumed to have a " saving action " in preventing permanent injury from the narcotic drug.[94] An ingenious theory supposes that this lessened carbohydrate oxidation diminishes the amount of available acetylcholine and thus prevents the transmission of impulses at synapses in the central nervous system.[71] It is thought that the actual change inside the cells is a reversible coagulation of the proteins.[72] " Gelatinization " possibly gives a better indication of the process which has been studied in various plasmodia and has been demonstrated in conditions of heat, cold and electrical current, as well as by exposure to narcotic

The Common Inhalation Anæsthetics and their Properties

Anæsthetic Agent.	Chemical Formula.	Boiling point (C.)	Vapour Density.	Toxicity.	Degree of Muscular Relaxation Obtainable.	Rate of Elimination.	Inflammability.
Nitrous oxide	N_2O	$-150°$	1·5	Practically nil apart from anoxia	Practically nil apart from adequate pre-medication	Practically equal to that of its absorption	−
Cyclopropane	H_2C-CH_2 $\vee$ CH_2	$-35°$	1·5	Slight apart from respiratory depression and cardiac arrhythmias	Variable	Rapid	+
Ethyl chloride	C_2H_5Cl	$+21·5°$	2·2	Slight	Variable	Rapid	+
Di-vinyl ether	$O{<}{C_2H_3 \atop C_2H_2}$	$+28·3°$	2·4	Moderate	Variable	Rapid	+
Di-ethyl ether	$O{<}{C_2H_5 \atop C_2H}$	$+34·6°$	2·6	Moderate. Irritant to respiratory passages	Good	Slow	+
Chloroform	$CHCl$	$+61°$	4·0	High, particularly to cardiac mechanism and to liver	Very good	Very slow	−
Trichlor-ethylene	$C\,Cl_2\text{-}CHCl$	$+87°$	4·5	Slight apart from tachypnœa	Poor	Slow	−

agents.[73] The process can also be demonstrated *in vitro* in yeast cells and in an albumin solution in the presence of an electrolyte. There is also some evidence to show that anæsthetized cells tend to lose water.[74] It is obvious, therefore, that toxic changes must be produced temporarily, not only in the cortical cells, but in others rich in lipoids. These may progress to permanent damage as in the acute yellow atrophy of the liver occurring in delayed chloroform poisoning, which has already been mentioned. The remaining volatile anæsthetics can be fitted in between the innocuous nitrous oxide and the toxic chloroform. It will be noticed that the same order holds good for the boiling points, vapour densities, toxicity, degree of muscular relaxation and rates of elimination. Trichlor-ethylene is somewhat of an exception to this rule as although it comes at the end of the table on its physical properties, it is much less toxic than chloroform.

If the higher centres are very active (as in the case of an excited patient), a higher concentration of the anæsthetic drug will be required to inhibit function. The value of pre-operative sedation can thus be clearly seen.[75]

Electrical Changes in Central Nervous System

It has been recognized for some time that active animal tissues are electro-negative and inactive tissue electro-positive. During rest, sleep and general anæsthesia the cerebral cortex becomes

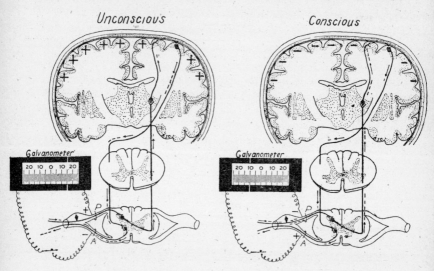

Fig. 2. The diagram marked " unconscious " shows that the motor anterior roots of the cord carry more negative charges away from the brain during anæsthesia than are brought in over the sensory posterior roots, resulting in a loss of negative charges, thereby causing the brain cortex to become electro-positive in deep anæsthesia. The diagram marked " conscious " shows the reverse to be true in the conscious state, namely, that the posterior sensory roots carry more negative charges to the brain in the conscious animal than are carried away by the anterior motor roots, resulting in a gain of negative charges, thereby rendering the brain cortex electro-negative in the conscious animal. (From *Anesth. & Anal.*, 1941, Mar.-Apr., p. 99 (after Burge).)

electro-positive, and the ingenious suggestion has been made that the struggling of the second stage of anæsthesia is due to the excess of negative charges (or nerve impulses) leaving the brain and passing out over the motor nerves to the muscles.[76] The suggested paths of electric currents can be followed by reference to Fig. 2.

The introduction of the **electro-encephalograph** has advanced our knowledge of the electrical changes which occur in the brain. If electrodes are applied to the head, one being over the occipital region, it can be demonstrated that rhythmic discharges occur which can be amplified and recorded by an oscillograph.[77] In the absence of visual activity, two types of waves are recognized. The α waves are predominant and have a frequency of about 10 per second while

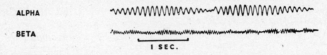

FIG. 3. Normal Electro-encephalogram.

the β waves are smaller in amplitude with a frequency of from 17 to 30 per second. Deep anæsthesia produced by any means usually suppresses the α rhythm, and attempts have been made to control automatically the depth of anæsthesia during an operation by an electronic device termed a " servo-anæsthetizer " connected on the one hand to an electro-encephalograph and on the other to either a gas-oxygen machine or to an intravenous drip depending on the technique of narcosis employed.[78] The principle on which the device works is that the fluctuating electrical potentials of the brain are amplified and made to charge a condenser, the rate of charge being proportional to the number and amplitude of the waves in a given time. At a predetermined voltage, the condenser discharges, actuating a relay which pushes forward the plunger of an intravenous syringe or controls a regulator on a vaporizer.

Since it has been shown that changes in potential occur during anæsthesia, attempts have been made to produce anæsthesia by electric currents, the first successful experiment probably being that of d'Arsonval in 1890. Both local and general anæsthesia can be produced in animals by a direct current of about 30 volts, interrupted at the rate of 4,000 to 5,000 times per minute, and the vessels on the surface of the brain can be constricted or dilated according to the type of current employed.[74] If local analgesia is to be produced, both anode and cathode are applied to the relevant nerve trunk. The relationship of electrical potential to activity can easily be studied in the goldfish and the current which it generates on moving can be measured by a galvanometer connected to electrodes at each end of the glass cylinder in the water of which it is swimming.[79]

If, however, the conditions are reversed and a 2 milliamp. direct current of 110 volts is passed through the water in which the goldfish is swimming, the head of the fish is drawn towards the positive electrode. The animal remains quiescent and apparently deeply anæsthetized. If the current is cut off, the fish immediately resumes its activity, while if reversal of the current is effected, the fish swims towards the other electrode and again becomes quiescent.[80]

About 1900, Professor Stéphane Leduc produced " electrical sleep " in France, by a unidirectional pulse current and tried it on himself.   In 1907, the Parisian surgeon Tuffier actually performed an operation on a patient made unconscious by this means,[81] but subsequent investigations showed that dangerous convulsions and coma might ensue.   Since that time **electrical convulsion therapy** has been developed for the treatment of certain types of mental disorders. 600 milliamp. currents of 90 to 145 volts passed through the head for $0 \cdot 1$ to $0 \cdot 2$ seconds produce instantaneous loss of consciousness accompanied by sudden contraction of the extensor muscles of the spine and often by flexion of the hips and elbows.   A latent period of a few seconds relaxation is then followed by violent clonic spasms.[82]   In practice the violence of the convulsions is now mitigated by the injection of a relaxant drug such as succinylcholine as fractures were not uncommon (see Chapter XI).   Even with such currents as avoid the possibility of convulsions, the subject is complicated by the existence of a **" nightmare state ",** in which the patient cannot move and appears to be deeply anæsthetized, although actually he retains consciousness.   Respiration is sometimes inhibited during the nightmare state, and an instance is recorded of a patient who knew that he could not breathe voluntarily and dreaded lest artificial respiration should be abandoned.[83]

More recent experiments with vertebrate animals show that carefully controlled currents of 10 volts and from 2 to 10 milliamperes, interrupted from 100 to 120 times per second, can produce a tranquil narcosis with muscular relaxation for a considerable time with no apparent after-effects.   The cathode is applied to the head and the anode to the back near the tail of the animal.

So-called **" electronarcosis "** or **" electrocoma "** is tending to replace convulsive therapy in schizophrenia, the current being rapidly raised from zero to about 200 ma. and kept at this level for about 5 minutes.   A generalized tonic contraction continues throughout this period and although the patient is relatively quiescent and unconscious the state is unsuitable for surgical work to be carried out.   It is possible, however, that future research will result in a suitable type of current for this purpose.

Secondary Saturation

If nitrous oxide anæsthesia is pushed without oxygen or with insufficient oxygen to maintain life, a point is reached where the pupil becomes fixed and dilated and respiration slows down and finally ceases. If at this point, or immediately before it, the lungs are inflated with a high percentage of oxygen, natural respiration is re-established, the pupil contracts, the colour returns to normal and it is possible to continue a pure nitrous oxide-oxygen anæsthesia with a very considerable degree of muscular relaxation. The whole process may have to be repeated.[84] This method still has some vogue in America, but the general opinion in this country is that it throws considerable strain on the right side of the heart : in any case it should not be attempted by an inexperienced anæsthetist or without a machine capable of inflating the lungs instantly with oxygen under pressure. It seems probable that the cerebral changes which have been described in America after pure N_2O—O_2 anæsthesia are due to the anoxia which is inseparable from the practice of secondary saturation (see Chapter III).

Muscular Relaxation

Muscle tone is probably due to a slow asynchronous discharge from anterior horn cells producing a partial tetanus.[77] Abolition of this tone or muscular relaxation is necessary for the satisfactory performance of many operations. It may be brought about by the anæsthetist in three ways[85] :

(1) In the deeper planes of general narcosis using either volatile or intravenous drugs. The exact mechanism is doubtful but appears to be associated with depression of the anterior horn cells in the spinal cord.

(2) Individual muscles or groups of muscles can be temporarily isolated from their nerve supply either by single or multiple nerve blocking with local analgesic drugs.

(3) Impulses travelling along motor nerves can be blocked at the myoneural junctions by a drug such as curare (q.v.).

Effects of Anæsthetics on Respiratory System

The effects of the volatile anæsthetics on the respiration are described in all text-books under the various planes of narcosis, the most obvious feature being progressive intercostal paralysis as anæsthesia deepens until purely diaphragmatic breathing becomes established. Further " pushing " of the drug leads to apnœa presumably from poisoning of the respiratory centre. Before this occurs, short jerky inspirations may be observed accompanied by a "**tracheal tug**". This usually takes place under deep ether anæsthesia and is almost certainly due to paralysis of the sternocostal fibres of the diaphragm while the crural ones still contract and pull on the roots of the lungs and bronchial tree during inspiration.

It is easy to describe these effects but extremely difficult to explain their mechanism, as the physiology of normal respiration is by no means perfectly understood.

The Hering-Breur reflex has been known for some time and consists of two parts : expansion of the chest inhibiting further activity of the respiratory muscles and collapse of the chest initiating respiratory efforts. Until recently it has been thought that the whole reflex could be explained on the basis of one set of afferent or stretch-fibres from the pulmonary alveoli up the vagi to the respiratory centre. It is now almost certain that a second set of fibres running from the small blood vessels in the lungs to the vagi are responsible for the deflation-reflex.[86] From animal experiments it appears that all the volatile anæsthetics sensitize the stretch-reflexes and can thus cause shallow respiration. The deflation-reflexes, on the other hand, are affected differently. For example, ether first stimulates and then paralyses them while trichlorethylene (q.v.) causes stimulation throughout so that in deep narcosis the respiration rate rises with this drug.

Apart from the Hering-Breur reflex, pulmonary ventilation is proportional to the metabolic rate and varies with the slightest change in the H-ion concentration of the blood. Again, increased blood pressure in the aortic arch and carotid sinus reflexly produces a reduction both in the rate and depth of respiration and vice versa. It is also usually held that chemo-receptors in the carotid body are susceptible to diminished oxygen tension in the blood and cause increased depth of respiration. In man, at any rate, this mechanism may not avert death from anoxia during a period of acapnia (see Chapter IV). Even if the respiratory centre is cut off entirely from afferent impulses from the lungs, circulatory system and higher centres it still possesses an inherent periodicity and slow regular breathing will continue.[77]

The effects of surgical stimuli on the rate, type and rhythm of respiration have been fully described in a recent important paper to which the reader is referred for full particulars.[87]

Respiration in the New-born

The essential difference between respiration in adults and infants is that in the latter case breathing is mainly abdominal and diaphragmatic with very little thoracic movement. In order to compensate for the small volume of tidal air (about 19 c.cm.) and vital capacity (about 170 c.cm.) the rate is high. For 24 hours after birth, air progressively enters the gastro-intestinal tract so that extrusion of the hollow viscera tends to occur when the abdomen is open.[88] Furthermore in infants muscle tone is relatively absent and acapnia occurs with great rapidity—factors which make for the rapid induction and easy maintenance of controlled respiration (see below) without the use of muscle relaxants.[89]

Controlled Respiration

This involves abolishing natural respiratory movements and substituting intermittent positive pressure either by some modification of Frenkner's spiropulsator or more simply by rhythmic compression of the rebreathing bag of a closed-circuit apparatus.[90] (see Chapter V). Natural respiration can be stopped by (1) paralysing the respiratory centre by " overdosage " with a depressant drug, such as cyclopropane, (2) paralysing the myoneural junctions with curare or other peripheral relaxant, (3) lowering the CO_2 tension in the blood by hyperventilation with the patient breathing through an absorber or some such device as an Oxford vaporizer, or (4) a combination of methods. The first and second techniques cause central or peripheral respiratory paralysis respectively by what was once termed " overdosage " and must not be used if the drugs involved cause circulatory depression at the same plane at which breathing stops. For example, it is unjustifiable with chloroform or the barbiturates.[91] The third method is the only one which can strictly be termed " controlled respiration ". It is physiologically sound but may be difficult in practice so that the fourth is commonly employed. Controlled respiration is chiefly useful in thoracic and abdominal surgery (q.v.).

The irritating effects of the volatile anæsthetic on the lungs and respiratory passages are discussed in Chapter XXV.

Elimination of Volatile Anæsthetics

The bulk of inhalational anæsthetic drugs are eliminated through the *lungs*, e.g. 87 per cent. of di-ethyl ether,[74] but it has been shown recently that an appreciable amount of gas diffuses through the *skin* during anæsthesia. This partly accounts for the fact that small volumes of gas must be added to the inhaled mixture during total rebreathing anæsthesia with carbon dioxide absorption. The estimated figures for different gases in milligrams per hour per square centimetre of body surface are[92] :

Nitrous oxide	..	..	..	..	0·04
Ethylene	..	..	..	..	0·001
Carbon dioxide		..	..	..	0·007

It is possible that traces of ether and chloroform are oxidized by the *liver* and the resulting products excreted by the kidneys.[75]

References

1. McMechan, F. H. *Brit. Med. Jour.*, 1926, Dec. 11, pp. 1107 *et seq.*
2. Dahle, M. *Norsk. Mag. f. Laeg.*, 1931, Dec., p. 1319.
3. Borsotti. *Arch. Ital. di Chir.*, 1932, Mar., p. 229.
4. Bourne, W. *Yale Jour. Biol. & Med.*, 1938, Dec., p. 149.
5. Harkins, H. N. *Anesth. & Anal.*, 1942, Sept.-Oct., p. 273.
6. Sachs, L. *Anesth. & Anal.*, 1939, March-April, p. 101.
7. Goldschmidt, S., *et al.* *Jour. Amer. Med. Ass.*, 1934, **102**, p. 21.
8. Hamburger and Ewing. *Jour. Amer. Med. Ass.*, 1908.
9. Hesper. *Arch. of Surg.*, 1933, May, p. 909.
10. Searles, P. W. *Jour. Amer. Med. Ass.*, 1939, Sept. 2, p. 906.
11. Borgström, S. *Acta. Chir. Scand.*, 1943, **89**, No. 1, p. 68.
12. Graham. *Jour. Amer. Med. Ass.*, 1911.
13. Bloor, W. R. *Physiol. Rev.*, 1922, **2**, p. 92.
14. Mahler, A. *Jour. Biol. Chem.*, 1926, **69**, p. 653.
15 and 16. Marenzi, A. D., and Gerschman, R. (Paris), 1932 and 1934.
17. Featherstone, H. W. *Brit. Med. Jour.*, 1937, July 31, p. 224.
18. Buckmaster and Gardner. *Jour. of Physiol.*, **41**, p. 246.
19. Hesper. *Arch. of Surg.*, 1933, May, p. 909.
20. Lawrence, R. D. *Pro. Roy. Soc. Med.* (An. Sec.), 1929, Feb. 1.
21. MacNider, W. de B. *Pro. Amer. Ass. Anesth.*, 1919, June.
22. Maclean, H. *Pro. Roy. Soc. Med.* (An. Sec.), 1926, Dec. 10.
23. Minnitt, R. J. *Pro. Roy. Soc. Med.* (An. Sec.), 1932, Dec. 2.
24. Goldman, V. *Brit. Med. Jour.*, 1937, Dec. 25, p. 1267.
25. Pratt, C. L. G. *Pro. Roy. Soc. Med.* (An. Sec.), 1938, Oct. 1.
26. { Widenhorn, H. *Anesth. & Anal.*, 1932, March-April.
    { Thoresen. *Norsk. Mag. f. Laeg.*, 1932, May, p. 499.
27. Pratt, C. L. G. *Pro. Roy. Soc. Med.* (An. Sec.), 1938, April 1.
28. Lamare, J. P. *Brit. Med. Jour.*, 1932, Sept. 24, p. 52.
29. David, N. A., *et al.* *Anesth. & Anal.*, 1948, Jan.-Feb., p. 25.
30. Benner, R. W. *Anesth. & Anal.*, 1935, Sept.-Oct., p. 205.
31. Widmark. *Jour. Biochem.*, 1920, **14**, p. 379.
32. Lorman, P. H. *Anesth. & Anal.*, 1938, Nov.-Dec., p. 316.
33. Hunter, J. B., and Himsworth, H. P. *Pro. Roy. Soc. Med.* (Comb. Mtg.) 1939, Feb. 1.
34. Graham, G. *Pro. Roy. Soc. Med.* (An. Sec.), 1945, May 4.
35. Knoefel, P. K. *Anesth. & Anal.*, 1936, **15**, p. 137.
36. Burstein, C. L. *Pro. Soc. Exper. Biol. & Med.*, 1938, **38**, p. 530.
37. Southwood, A. R. *Med. Jour. Austral.*, 1923, Nov. 3, p. 460.
38. Johnson and Mann. *Surgery*, 1942, **12**, p. 599.
39. Golden, R. F., and Mann, F. C. *Anesthesiology*, 1943, Nov., p. 577.
40. { Slaughter, D., and Lacky, R. W. *Pro. Soc. Exper. Biol. & Med.*, 1940, **45**, p. 8.
    { Vaughan Williams and Streeten. *Brit. Jour. Pharmacol.*, 1950, **5**, p. 584.

41. DALE, H. H. *Biochem. Jour.*, 1909, **4**, p. 427.
42. ROSENTHAL, S. M., and WHITE, E. C. *Jour. Amer. Med. Ass.*, 1925, **84**, p. 1112.
43. ROSENTHAL, S. M., and BOURNE, W. *Anesth. & Anal.*, 1928, Sept.-Oct.
44. TODD, T. F. *Lancet*, 1934, Sept. 15, p. 597.
45. HANGER, F. M. *Trans. Ass. Amer. Phys.*, 1938, liii., p. 148.
46. ARMSTRONG, D. M. *Anæsthesia*, 1947, Apr., p. 45.
47. OTTENBERG, R. *Jour. Amer. Med. Ass.*, 1935, **104**, p. 1681.
48. BOURNE, W. *Amer. Jour. Surg.*, 1936, Dec., p. 486.
49. GOLDSCHMIDT, RAYDIN and LUCKE. *Jour. Pharmac.*, 1937, Jan., p. 1.
50. BOURNE, W., and STEHLE, R. L. *Jour. Biol. Chem.*, 1924, **60**, No. 1, p. 17.
51. { LEVY, A. G. *Heart*, 1913, **5**, p. 299.
{ HILL, I. G. W. *Lancet*, 1932, i, p. 1139.
52. { KURTZ, C. M., *et al. Jour. Amer. Med. Ass.*, 1936, **106**, p. 434.
{ BARNES, C. G., and IVES, J. *Pro. Roy. Soc. Med.* (An. Sec.), 1944, May 5.
53. MOOTS, C. N. *Brit. Jour. Anæsth.*, **4**, p. 51.
54. SYKES, W. S. *Anesth. & Anal.*, 1934, May-June, p. 99.
55. WOODBRIDGE, P. D. *Amer. Jour. Surg.*, 1936, Dec., p. 410.
56. LASSEN, H. K., *et al. Acta. Chir. Scand.*, 1938, **81**, p. 343.
57. McQUISTON, J. S., and ALLEN, E. V. *Collected Papers, Mayo Clinic*, 1932, p. 467.
58. McQUISTON, J. S. *Jour. Iowa State Med. Soc.*, 1935, July, p. 331.
59. { GOODALL, J. S. *Pro. Roy. Soc. Med.* (An. Sec.), 1923, Feb. 2.
{ LAKIN, C. E. *Pro. Roy. Soc. Med.* (An. Sec.), 1926, March 5.
{ PRICE, F. W. *Brit. Med. Jour.*, 1926, Nov. 13, p. 879.
{ HAYWARD, G. W. *Anæsthesia*, 1952, Apr., p. 67.
60. WEBBER, H. N. *Med. World*, 1933, May 19, p. 240.
61. STEPHEN, F. *Brit. Jour. Anæsth.*, 1929, **6**, p. 194.
62. SCHULZE, F. *Zentralb. f. Chir.*, 1924, **51**, p. 2688.
63. SHACKLE, J. W. *Jour. Clin. Med.*, 1932, Oct., p. 138.
64. MINNITT, R. J. *Brit. Jour. Anæsth.*, 1933, July, p. 160.
65. GETTLER, A. O., and BLUME, H. *Arch. of Path.*, 1931, June.
66. PARKER, G. H. *Jour. Gen. Physiol.*, 1925, Nov. 20.
67. { HOLMES. " The Metabolism of Living Tissue," 1937.
{ PAGE. " The Chemistry of the Brain," 1937.
68. ROSSEN, R., *et al. Arch. Neurol. Psychiat.*, 1943, **50**, p. 510.
69. MACLEOD. *Physiol. & Biochem. in Modern Med.*, 6th edit.
70. HEIDBRINK. *Pro. Florida Dental Anesth. Soc.*, 1924, Dec.
71. MACINTOSH, R. R., and PRATT, C. L. G. *Brit. Med. Jour.*, 1938, Oct. 1, p. 695.
72. BANCROFT, W. D. *Anesth. & Anal.*, 1932, **11**, No. 3, p. 49.
73. SEIFRIZ, W. *Anesthesiology*, 1950, Jan., p. 24.
74. BARBOUR, H. C. *Amer. Jour. Surg.*, 1936, Dec., pp. 438 and 441.
75. FEATHERSTONE, H. W. *Brit. Med. Jour.*, 1937, July 31, p. 224.
76. BURGE, W. E. *Anesth. & Anal.* { 1936, Mar.-Apr., p. 53.
{ 1940, Mar.-Apr., p. 102.
{ 1941, Mar.-Apr., p. 99.
77. WRIGHT, S. " Applied Physiology," 7th edit.
78. Annotation. *Brit. Med. Jour.*, 1950, Sept. 16, p. 667.
79. BOURNE, W. *Yale Jour. Biol. & Med.*, 1938, Dec., p. 149.
80. BURGE, W. E., *et al. Anesth. & Anal.*, 1936, Nov.-Dec., p. 261.
81. PATERSON, A. S. and MILLIGAN, W. I. *Lancet*, 1947, Aug. 9, p. 198.
82. SHEPLEY, W. H., and McGREGOR, J. S. *Brit. Med. Jour.*, 1939, Dec. 30, p. 1269.
83. HUME, C. W., *Lancet*, 1934, Dec. 15, p. 1370.
84. McKESSON, E. I. *Pro. Roy. Soc. Med.* (An. Sec.), 1926, July 15.
85. HEWER, C. L. Lecture delivered at Roy. Coll. Surg., 1946, Mar. 28.

86. WHITTERIDGE, D. M., and BÜLBRING, E. $\begin{cases} Jour.\ Pharmacol.,\ 1944,\ \textbf{81},\ \text{p. 340.} \\ Brit.\ Med.\ Bull.,\ 1946,\ \text{Vol. 4,}\ \textbf{2},\ \text{p. 85.} \end{cases}$

87. MORTON, H. J. Y. *Anœsthesia*, 1950, July, p. 112.

88. Annotation. *Brit. Med. Jour.*, 1950, Dec. 23, p. 1433.

89. REES, G. J. *Brit. Med. Jour.*, 1950, Dec. 23, p. 1419.

90. NOSWORTHY, M. D. *Pro. Roy. Soc. Med.* (An. Sec.), 1941, Apr. 4 and 1940, Dec. 4.

91. HEWER, C. L. *Lancet*, 1946, Apr. 20, p. 591.

92. ORCUTT, F. S., and WATERS, R. M. *Anesth. & Anal.*, 1933, Jan.-Feb., p. 45.

93. $\begin{cases} \text{CULLEN, S. C., and GROSS, E. C.}\ Science,\ 1951,\ \textbf{113},\ \text{p. 580.} \\ \text{JONES, H. B. \ ``Medical Physics,''}\ \textbf{2},\ \text{Chicago, 1950.} \end{cases}$

94. QUASTEL, J. H. Various papers.

95. MORTON, H. J. V. and WYLIE, W. D. *Anœsthesia*, 1951, Oct., p. 190.

96. GAIN, E. A., *et al.* *Canad. Med. Ass. Jour.*, 1951, **64**, p. 32.

97. TOVELL, R. M. *Ann. Roy. Coll. Surg.*, 1951, Dec., p. 383.

98. BARBOUR, C. M. *Anesthesiology*, 1950, **11**, p. 155.

99. CUSHHY, A. R. *Textbook of Pharmacol. & Therap.*, 9th edit. London. Churchill.

100. LYNN, R. P., and SHACKMAN, R. *Brit. Med. Jour.*, 1951, Aug. 11, p. 333.

101. SHACKMAN, R., and GRABER, I. G. *Brit. Med. Jour.*, 1952, June 14, p. 1284.

CHAPTER II

PREMEDICATION

Sedation—Synergism—Basal Narcosis—Paraldehyde—Bromethol—Trichlorethanol—Barbiturates (Long- Medium- and Short-action)—Choice of Technique.

DRUGS are given before operation (1) to diminish the secretion
of saliva and mucus caused by general anæsthetics and (2) to render
the patient drowsy, amnesic or actually unconscious in bed.

Atropine has been used for many years to check the excessive
secretion of mucus caused by ether. It also tends to stimulate
respiration and may have some protective action against primary
cardiac failure due to chloroform (q.v.). Since atropine tends to
raise the metabolic rate, it should seldom be used alone and it is
definitely contra-indicated in such conditions as thyrotoxicosis. It
is also best avoided under tropical conditions as it interferes with
the normal heat-regulating mechanism of the body.

Sedation

Morphine was isolated from the alkaloids of opium as long ago as
1806 by Sertürner. Morphine, or alkaloids akin to it, is usually
the basis of sedative mixtures given before operation. Some
patients complain of nausea or vomiting after morphia, and it
is said that such preparations as **omnopon** (**pantopon** in America)
or **opoidine** (**alopan, papaveretum**) are less likely to cause these
troubles. **Dilaudid** (**di-hydromorphine**) has considerable vogue in
America and is about ten times as potent as morphine. Although
morphine is usually given *hypodermically* about three-quarters of
an hour before operation, it can be injected in a diluted solution
intravenously, if an immediate effect is required. The initial adult
dose is about gr. $\frac{1}{24}$ and a pause of thirty seconds is allowed for
the response to be judged. The injection is then continued slowly
until the desired effect is obtained.[1] This is a good method of
premedication if the operation is to be performed under local
analgesia, or if the patient is shocked or cold as in air-raid or battle
casualties. In such cases it has been found that the first and
subsequent doses of hypodermic morphine may not be absorbed
owing to the impaired circulation, but that when resuscitation is
carried out signs of morphine overdose may appear.

Pethidine (see Chapter XXIV) is tending to replace morphine for premedication in Great Britain on account of the general feeling that post-operative nausea and vomiting are thereby appreciably diminished. From his own observation the author agrees with this conclusion. 100 mg. pethidine are approximately equal to $\frac{1}{3}$ gr. omnopon.

Scopolamine (hyoscine) is commonly combined with morphine or pethidine in order to add an amnesic action and an inhibitory effect on the secretion of saliva and mucus. The variable results following injections of scopolamine can be explained by the fact that the commercial product contains four alkaloids, viz. :

(a) A lævo-rotatory alkaloid which has a sedative and amnesic effect.

(b) A dextro-rotatory alkaloid which has a stimulant or excitant effect.

(c and d) Two isomeric alkaloids with variable effects.

It is therefore important to be certain in premedication that the scopolamine used contains the pure lævo-rotatory alkaloid alone.[2]

Until recently *children* have not been given morphine and scopolamine to any great extent, but a dosage table has now been worked out which takes into consideration the basal metabolic rate as well as the weight of the child. It must be remembered that the B.M.R. rises from birth till six years, declines to twelve, rises again during puberty and then falls throughout the remaining years of life. The following dosage table has been calculated[3] :

Age yr.	Average Weight st. lb.		Morphine gr.	+Scopolamine gr.
$\frac{6}{12}$ - 1		18$\frac{1}{2}$	1/60	1/900
1- 2		22	1/40	1/600
2- 4	2	2$\frac{3}{4}$	1/32	1/600
4- 8	3	0	1/20	1/450
8-12	4	5$\frac{1}{2}$	1/16	1/450
12-16	6	6	1/12	1/300

Elderly patients may be very susceptible to scopolamine and as a rule it is inadvisable to give the drug in extreme old age.

Many anæsthetists prefer to add a small dose of atropine to morphine and scopolamine as this not only aids the " drying-up " effect of the mixture but tends to counteract the respiratory depression caused by the two other drugs. This tends to shorten the induction period of inhalation anæsthesia. The well-known preparations known as " **Hyoscine Compounds A and B** " contain these three drugs.

It is said that if the **mucates of morphine and atropine** are substituted for the more usual sulphate or tartrate, a much more prolonged effect is obtained.[4]   For example, an injection of morphine mucate gr. $\frac{1}{4}$ and atropine mucate gr. $\frac{1}{75}$ has a peak effect in about one and a half hours and a noticeable effect for at least eight hours. This facilitates the premedication of patients in long operating lists where the timing may go badly astray.   The mucates are available under the trade name of " hyperduric." alkaloids.

In Italy, a combination of drugs known as **" preanest "** has attained great popularity.   This fluid, which can be injected either intramuscularly or intravenously, is said to contain " bromidrates of the total alkaloids of opium, scopolamine bromidrate and hypertonic sodium bromide ".[5]

Rectal alcohol has been tried in America with good results as a pre- and post-operative sedative.   Wine, usually port, in doses of 100 to 300 c.cm. is given beforehand and 1 pint is put into an enema can after operation and kept at the level of the patient's rectum. It is said that excellent sedation without intoxication is seen with this procedure.[6]

Synergism

The first attempt to render a patient actually unconscious in bed before inhalation anæsthesia was made by Gwathmey in 1913 with his rectal oil-ether solution.   Some years afterwards he developed his synergistic method of using multiple drugs which is based on Burgi's hypothesis.[7]   This states that " drugs having the same pharmacological action summarize their therapeutic effect when given together, but drugs of different pharmacological actions increase their activity markedly more than the sum of their action when given separately ".   Thus preliminary narcotic drugs mutually reinforce each other and also the general anæsthetic following, so that it may be possible to secure adequate relaxation with a combination of drugs and nitrous oxide-oxygen alone, or with an amount of ether quite inadequate by itself.[8]   It cannot be said however, that the synergistic theory is universally accepted by pharmacologists, and, indeed, it has recently been shown that in animals the simultaneous exhibition of magnesium sulphate and ether results in a simple summation of anæsthetic and toxic effects.[9] This is directly contrary to previous statements.   Gwathmey worked out many formulæ of drug combinations, one of his rectal injections containing no less than ten ingredients, including morphine sulphate, hyoscine hydrobromide, magnesium sulphate, ether, paraldehyde and alcohol.   These complicated techniques have tended to fall out of use since it has been found that single

drugs can be given safely in sufficient dosage to produce unconsciousness without surgical anæsthesia. Such drugs have been
given the name of basal narcotics, and they thus lie midway between
preliminary hypnotics, such as morphine and scopolamine, on the
one hand, and anæsthetics, such as chloroform and ether, on the
other.

Basal Narcosis

Advantages. The advantages of basal narcosis are : (1) The
absence of any apprehension by the patient ; in fact, very nervous
people need not even be told when the operation is to take place.
Secondary advantages accruing from the absence of fear are that
there is no excess of adrenaline in the circulation which predisposes
to ventricular fibrillation, and the metabolic rate is lowered, a
factor of great importance if nitrous oxide and oxygen is to be
administered.[92]   (ii) Less general anæsthetic is necessary.
(iii) There is less after-pain.   (iv) There is less vomiting.

Disadvantages. The disadvantages are : (i) Most methods of
administration take some time and involve some calculation of
dosage, that is, no routine dosage is possible.   (ii) More nursing
care is necessary after operation.   (iii) The diminished or absent
reflexes after operation may be disadvantageous in certain cases.
(iv) Great care is necessary to avoid cumulative effects with other
sedative drugs : several fatalities have occurred from this cause.

Basal Narcotics in General Use. The basal narcotics in general
use are : (1) paraldehyde ; (2) bromethol ; (3) the barbiturates.

Methods of Administration. Administration may be (i) by
mouth ; (ii) intramuscularly ; (iii) intravenously ; and (iv) per
rectum.

Paraldehyde

Paraldehyde is a polymer of acetaldehyde with the formula
$C_6H_{12}O_3$. It is colourless liquid with an unpleasant smell and
was introduced into therapeutics as a narcotic by Cervello in 1884.[10]

Advantages. Paraldehyde is probably the safest basal narcotic
known and in normal dosage produces little respiratory or circulatory
depression.

Disadvantages. Since paraldehyde is excreted partly through
the lungs, the patient's breath smells for some time and this may
prove offensive to those about him although he himself rarely
complains. It is worth noting that if a closed-circuit technique is
used for the subsequent inhalation anæsthesia, the paraldehyde
concentration can be built up in the respiratory passages to a point

where irritation occurs as evidenced by laryngeal spasm or coughing. Cases of paraldehyde idiosyncrasy are not unknown, one man of twenty weighing 123 lb. nearly succumbing to 4 drachms of the drug given per rectum.[11]

Dosage and Methods of Administration. Paraldehyde is used in a 10 per cent. solution in water and is run into the *rectum* slowly at blood heat. The usual dose is 1 drachm of pure paraldehyde per stone body weight if the patient weighs under 8 stone. Thus 8 drachms can be regarded as the usual adult dose, which it is rarely necessary to exceed. This represents about 12 oz. of solution.[12]

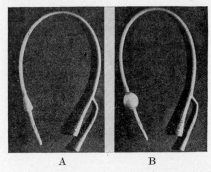

FIG. 4. Rectal catheter before (A) and after (B) distension of the bulb. (Ingraham and Campbell, *Annals of Surgery*.)

The smaller dosage of 0·5 drachms paraldehyde per stone, preceded (in adults) by morphia gr. $\frac{1}{4}$ and scopolamine gr. $\frac{1}{100}$, has been recommended, but in this case there is a marked fall in blood pressure and some respiratory depression.[13] This technique appears to the writer unwise.

Paraldehyde is given about three-quarters of an hour before operation, the patient being in the semi-prone position to aid retention of the enema. Retention enemas should always be given with the patient lying on his left side as a larger area of absorptive gut is available.[14] The method is extremely useful for nervous children who need never see the surgeon or anæsthetist or indeed know that they have had an operation.[15] If the child is very uncöoperative the special catheter shown in Fig. 4 aids retention. This is inserted so that the deflated balloon lies just inside the internal sphincter. 6 to 10 c.cm. of water are injected to inflate the balloon and the narcotic solution is then run in.[16] When the catheter for a retention enema is once in position, the buttocks should be tightly strapped together with adhesive plaster. Expulsion then becomes almost impossible.

Paraldehyde has also been used *intravenously* as a basal narcotic in doses of from 0·1 to 0·2 c.cm. of the pure drug per kg. body weight in a 2 to 5 per cent. solution[17] but at the present time it is mainly used by this route as an anti-convulsant.[18]

The pharmacological antidotes to over-dosage with paraldehyde are said to be picrotoxin and camphor.[19]

Bromethol
(Avertin, Ethobrome, " E. 107 ", Rectanol, and Tribromethanol)

Bromethol is the official designation for tribromethylalcohol. Its formula is CBr_3CH_2OH. It was first produced in 1923 by Willstätter and Duisberg by the reduction of bromal by yeast. It was first used in anæsthesia by F. Eicholtz in 1926. Bromethol is a white crystalline solid having a melting-point of 80° C. and is soluble with difficulty up to 3·5 per cent. in water at 40° C. For the sake of convenience "bromethol fluid" is now generally used ; this is a solution of bromethol in amylene hydrate. It is a clear liquid, 1 c.cm. of which contains 1 g. of bromethol. Since amylene hydrate is volatile, bottles of bromethol fluid should be kept tightly stoppered. In this connection it is interesting to recall that amylene itself has been used as an anæsthetic, a series of 238 administrations being reported in 1857 by Snow.[20]

Advantages. The main advantages of bromethol over paraldehyde are (1) that it is practically odourless, and (2) that induction and recovery are usually quiet, with no excitement.

Dosage. The adult rectal dose for basal narcosis varies from 0·09 to 0·12 g. per kilogramme body weight, except in obstetrics (q.v.). As a rule the higher the patient's basal metabolic rate, the greater will be the necessary dose. When bromethol was first introduced it was claimed to be an anæsthetic, but it was soon recognized that if given to adults in doses sufficiently large to produce anæsthesia it was unsafe.[21]

It has recently been shown, however, that children tolerate the drug better than adults, and, if given in doses of 0·175 g. per kilogramme, combined with morphine, scopolamine and a field block, no additional anæsthesia is required in about 75 per cent. of cases. This method should be used with great caution and never employed in very young or cachectic children.[22] In order to produce basal narcosis only, in children from two to ten years of age, a dosage of about 0·125 g. per kilogramme is required.[23]

An abbreviated dosage table of " bromethol fluid ", calculated on the basis of 0·1 g. per kilogramme body weight, is appended.

Preparation and Testing of Solution. The solution is made up to 2·5 per cent. by vigorous shaking in warm distilled water. The usual test for impurities is the addition of a few drops of Congo Red. The colour must remain orange-red, any tendency towards

Dosage Table for Bromethol Fluid

St.	lb.	Bromethol fluid in c.cm.	Dist. water. to—c.cm.	St.	lb.	Bromethol fluid in c.cm.	Dist. water. to—c.cm.
2	0	1·3	51	8	0	5·1	203
2	4	1·4	58	8	4	5·3	210
2	8	1·6	65	8	8	5·4	218
2	12	1·8	72	8	12	5·6	225
3	0	1·9	76	9	0	5·7	228
3	4	2·1	83	9	4	5·9	236
3	8	2·3	90	9	8	6·1	243
3	12	2·4	98	9	12	6·2	250
4	0	2·5	101	10	0	6·3	254
4	4	2·7	109	10	4	6·5	261
4	8	2·9	116	10	8	6·7	263
4	12	3·1	123	10	12	6·9	276
5	0	3·2	127	11	0	7·0	279
5	4	3·3	134	11	4	7·2	286
5	8	3·5	141	11	8	7·3	294
5	12	3·6	145	11	12	7·5	301
6	0	3·8	152	12	0	7·6	305
6	4	4·0	160	12	4	7·8	312
6	8	4·2	167	12	8	8·0	319
6	12	4·3	174	12	12	8·2	326
7	0	4·4	178	13	0	8·2	330
7	4	4·6	185	14	0	8·9	356
7	8	4·8	192	15	0	9·5	381
7	12	5·0	199				

blue indicating the presence of hydrobromic acid which, with dibromvinyl alcohol, is a decomposition product ($CBr_3CH_2OH \rightarrow HBr + CBr_2CHOH$). The latter may decompose further into dibromacetaldehyde, which is extremely irritant to rectal mucosa ($CBr_2CHOH \rightarrow CHBr_2CHO$). A more delicate test is to transfer 3 c.cm. of the bromethol solution to a clean test tube and cool. An equal volume of the distilled water used for the preparation is then placed in a second test tube and 2 drops of " Universal Indicator B.D.H." are added to each. The colour of both solutions should be the same (greenish-yellow), any change to orange or red indicating decomposition.[24]

Since the drug only remains in solution at about 90° F., it should be freshly prepared and administered before the liquid has time to cool. If it is necessary to keep the solution warm for some hours in a thermos flask, re-distilled water should be used.

Method of Administration. Bromethol is given *per rectum* in exactly the same way as paraldehyde (q.v.), and the patient gradually lapses into unconsciousness. Some anæsthetists give bromethol in divided doses, judging the supplementary dose by the patient's reaction to the initial one.[25] An experience of over 2,000 administrations has not convinced the author that any material advantage is gained by this procedure. It is possible to give bromethol *intravenously*, with a continuous drip of a 1 per cent. solution, but this technique has not made much headway.[26]

It is a good practice to give glucose as a routine before bromethol.[27]

Effects. Bromethol is rapidly absorbed from the rectal mucosa, the maximum concentration in the blood (6 to 9 mg. per cent.) being attained in thirty minutes. On reaching the liver, it loses its toxicity by association with glycuronic acid, and is finally excreted by the kidneys,[28] elimination being practically complete in forty-eight hours.[29] No traces of bromides are found in the fæces or in the expired air.

During basal narcosis the *blood pressure* falls. In a series of 314 administrations the average fall in systolic pressure was 28 mm. Hg in women and 19 mm. in men.[30] In spite of this the *venous oxygen* remains within normal limits as opposed to the condition of true shock.[31] *Electrocardiographic tracings* show few and slight changes, it being generally thought that bromethol in normal doses does not injure the sound human heart.[32] On the other hand, a case suspiciously like ventricular fibrillation has been reported.[33] The drug causes a moderate drop in the *alkali reserve* and a rise in the *blood sugar*, both usually returning to normal in about twenty-four hours.[34] There is a tendency to acidosis and acetonuria.[35] Bromethol also depresses the *respiratory centre* and lowers *body temperature*.[36] Some divergence of opinion has existed over the action of the drug on the *liver*. This is normally slight, but it has been established that cases of jaundice[37] and even of acute yellow atrophy resembling those of delayed chloroform poisoning have occurred in animals[38] and in man.[39]

To certain patients bromethol appears to have an extremely low toxicity. For example, a case has been reported in which it was given on twenty-two occasions within ten weeks for painful dressings without obvious ill-effects.[40] Some observers have found that repeated administrations lead to a *tolerance* for the drug so that the dose has to be increased.[41]

Local toxic effects are rare with properly prepared solutions of bromethol, but transient diarrhœa may occur,[30] and fatal colitis has been reported.[42]

Indications. There is some evidence to show that bromethol and thyroxin are antagonistic drugs,[43] and it is patients with toxic goitre with high basal metabolic rates who feel the greatest benefit from the drug. The technique for thyroidectomy is discussed in Chapter XXI and that for obstetrics in Chapter XXIV.

Bromethol followed by a light general anæsthesia appears slightly to diminish pulmonary complications in lower abdominal operations,[44] but the reverse is probable for procedures affecting the stomach and gall-bladder.[45] Patients suffering from asthma and bronchitis, however, generally do well with bromethol, as it has no irritant effect on the respiratory passages. The drug has also been used successfully in cranial surgery (q.v.) and has been introduced into the Tropics, where it has greatly reduced the difficulties attending ether anæsthesia.[46] Some surgeons have found bromethol of great value for ophthalmic operations as the conjunctiva becomes pale and hæmorrhage is greatly reduced. The technique may usefully be combined with local analgesia in this type of surgery.[47]

Therapeutic Use. Bromethol has been used in medicine for the treatment of such conditions as chorea,[48] angina,[49] asthma,[50] the delirium of pneumonia,[51] and of acute alcoholism,[47] the spasms of strychnine poisoning[52] and of tetanus, one case being recorded in which the patient was kept in bromethol narcosis for five days continuously.[53]

Contra-indications. Bromethol is contra-indicated (i) in patients with very low basal metabolic rates : they do not readily eliminate the drug ; (ii) in patients in whom brisk reflexes are required immediately after operation (unless the drug is washed out of the rectum just before the patient is transferred to the theatre)[54] ; (iii) in patients with abnormally low blood pressures ; (iv) when other methods or drugs that lower blood pressure or depress respiration will be used ; (v) in operations in the region of the rectum or anus or where there is inflammation in these areas ; (vi) in nephritis, jaundice and gross disease of the liver.[55]

Antidotes. The most obvious results of bromethol over-dosage are profound respiratory depression and a low blood pressure. These effects can be treated with inhalation of a carbon dioxide-oxygen mixture. It has been established that the administration of ephedrine interrupts or shortens bromethol narcosis so that this drug can be used, to some extent, as an antidote.[56] It has also been shown that high rectal irrigation with warm hypertonic sodium thiosulphate solution is of great use in combating collapse from the administration of bromethol,[57] as is the intravenous injection of the " analeptic " drugs mentioned later in this chapter for over-dosage with the barbiturates. Benzedrine sulphate (about 20 mg. in adults) given intravenously immediately after the termination of the operation shortens the subsequent period of unconsciousness but also unfortunately seems to increase the incidence of vomiting.[58]

Trichlorethanol

Trichlorethanol (ethapon) or trichlorethylalcohol has the formula CCl_3CH_2OH, so that it is the same compound as bromethol with the three bromine atoms in the molecule replaced by chlorine. It is a heavy colourless liquid with a boiling point of 151° C. and a specific gravity of 1·5, so that each cubic centimetre contains 1·5 g. by weight. The drug is soluble in 30 times its volume of water, but has generally been used in 40 times its volume, the average rectal dose being from 0·08 to 0·01 g. per kilogramme body weight.

The chief advantages of trichlorethanol are its stability in solution (no testing with indicators being necessary), the small volume of fluid necessary to be retained in the rectum and the greater margin of safety between the minimal anæsthetic dose and the minimal lethal dose than is the case with bromethol.[59] Exhaustive tests in animals proved very satisfactory ; respiratory depression being less than with bromethol and no obvious pathological changes in the vital organs being observed. On the other hand, extra systoles were occasionally noted.[60]

When given as a basal narcotic in man, trichlorethanol has proved disappointing. The results are more variable than with bromethol and two fatalities, apparently from primary cardiac failure, appear to render the use of this drug unjustifiable.[61]

Barbituric Acid Derivatives

The barbituric acid derivatives have the following grouping in their chemical formulæ :

$$CO \overset{NH-CO}{\underset{NH-CO}{\diagup \diagdown}} C\diagup$$

They can be divided into three groups by their duration of action, but a certain amount of overlapping occurs.

The long-acting barbiturates are used in medicine as sedatives, hypnotics and anti-convulsants (e.g. in the treatment of epilepsy). Some of the commoner drugs are :

Allonal (allyl-isopropyl barbituric acid with amidopyrin).*
Alurate (sodium allyl, isopropyl barbiturate).
Cibalgin (dial with amidopyrin).
Delvinal (ethyl-l-methyl, butyl barbituric acid).
Dial or **Allobarbitone** (B.P.C.) (diallyl barbituric acid).
Di-dial (dial with ethyl morphine).
Fenemal (phenobarbital sodium or sodium phenyl-ethyl barbiturate).
Gardenal or **Luminal** (phenobarbital or phenyl-ethyl barbituric acid).
Garoin (phenobarbital and phenytoin sodium).
Ipral (sodium ethyl-isopropyl barbiturate).
Medinal or **Sodium barbital** (sodium di-ethyl barbiturate).
Neonal (*n*-butyl ethyl barbituric acid).
Nostal (isopropyl, bromallyl barbituric acid).
Numal (allyl-isopropyl barbituric acid).
Phanodorm or **Cyclobarbital** (cyclo-hexenyl-ethyl barbituric acid).
Phemitone or **Prominal** (n-methyl ethyl phenobarbital).
Rutonal (phenyl, methyl barbituric acid).
Sandoptal (allyl, isobutyl barbituric acid).
Sonalgin (butobarbital, codeine phosphate and phenacetin).
Theogardenal or **Theominal** (phenyl-ethyl barbituric acid with theobromine).
Veronal or **Barbital** (di-ethyl barbituric acid).
Veramon (di-ethyl barbituric acid with amidopyrin).

These drugs are usually given by mouth, but in psychiatry the rectal, intramuscular and intravenous routes are also used. Very prolonged narcosis has been attempted, but in spite of the partial protection of glucose and insulin against subsequent ketosis, the method remains a dangerous one.[62] The long-acting barbiturates have been used to some extent for premedication, but the compounds with a less prolonged effect are more suitable.

It will be noticed that some of the proprietary mixtures listed above contain amidopyrin. It is now recognized that in susceptible patients very small doses of this drug can cause agranulocytosis.

It has been found that of the second group of " medium " barbiturates, those best adapted for basal narcosis have (*a*) an asymmetric carbon atom, and (*b*) the " Nebenthau factor ", i.e. the grouping—$N = C(OH)$—.

* It is understood that Allonal now does not contain amidopyrin.

The commonest barbituric acid compounds which have been used as basal narcotics are :

Somnifene (Somnifaine), consisting of a water-glycerine-alcohol solution of the diethylamine salts of di-ethyl barbituric acid and allyl-isopropyl barbituric acid. This drug has been used to some extent in France as an *intravenous* basal narcotic. The main disadvantage was frequent excitement. Somnifene has more recently been employed intramuscularly in this country in doses of 2 c.cm. in combination with morphine, scopolamine and atropine.[63]

Sodium amytal (sodium iso-amyl ethyl barbiturate) was first described in 1923[64] and used as an *intravenous* basal narcotic by Zerfas of Indianapolis in 1928.[65] It is a white powder, 1 g. of which is dissolved in 10 c.cm. of distilled water. Not more than thirty minutes should elapse between preparation and use. The injection is made at a rate not exceeding 1 c.cm. per minute, and is stopped when the patient just loses consciousness.

The same solution can be used *intramuscularly*, and this technique has been employed extensively in psychiatry.[66] Sodium amytal can also be given *by mouth* in the form of green capsules containing 3 gr. of the drug. At the height of its popularity a usual pre-operative technique for an adult was 3 gr. the night before, and 6 to 9 gr. two hours before operation. The oral method has been used in eclampsia combined with intravenous hypertonic glucose,[67] but a fatal case of anuria after delivery has been reported.[68] Sodium amytal by mouth has also been used extensively in labour, but the extreme restlessness which frequently occurs (in 56 per cent. of cases according to one observer) is a great disadvantage.[69]

Nembutal (Pentobarbital sodium) is sodium ethyl-methyl-butyl barbiturate. It has tended to replace sodium amytal as a basal narcotic, as it usually causes less restlessness after operation.[70] Nembutal is given *intravenously* in a fresh 10 per cent. solution in the same way as sodium amytal. The drug can also be obtained in yellow capsules for *oral administration*, each capsule containing either gr. $\frac{1}{2}$, $\frac{3}{4}$ or $1\frac{1}{2}$. The usual adult dose is from 3 to $4\frac{1}{2}$ gr. one and a half hours before operation.

In no circumstances must nembutal be given both orally and intravenously to the same patient as a cumulative effect can be obtained and fatalities have occurred from this practice. Nembutal has been used *rectally* in 2-gr. suppositories for young children, the average dose being slightly under 1 gr. per year. The suppository should be given about three hours before operation.[71] In animals, nembutal has been used for full surgical anæsthesia, a usual veterinary practice being a dose of $\frac{1}{5}$ gr. per pound body weight, given by the *intraperitoneal* route in dogs and cats.[72]

Premedication, carried out in man with nembutal to the stage of basal narcosis, appears to be a reasonably safe procedure. An investigation carried out upon 1,000 consecutive cases at a general hospital showed no serious after-effects attributable to the drug.[73] As regards the safety margin of the drug, the ratio of the minimal lethal dose to the narcotic dose is stated to be $2 \cdot 4$.[74]

In therapeutics both intravenous and oral nembutal have been successfully used over prolonged periods in the treatment of tetanic convulsions.[75]

Skin reactions occasionally follow the administration of nembutal. These are usually urticarial in nature, but in rare instances may progress to the formation of bullæ and necrosis.[76] Prolonged administration of nembutal occasionally results in liver damage which may prove fatal.[77]

Pernocton (**Pernoston** in America) is sodium 2^y butyl-β-bromallyl barbiturate, and thus contains a bromine atom. Pernocton has been used extensively in Germany since 1927.[78] Its advantage over sodium amytal and nembutal is that it is stable in solution so that no mixing or dilution is necessary. Furthermore, it is given in a 10 per cent. solution and as the usual dose is about 3 c.cm. the induction time is shorter at the standard intravenous rate of 1 c.cm. per minute.[27] Since this solution is hypertonic with a pH of $9 \cdot 5$, it has been suggested that the slower rate of $0 \cdot 75$ c.cm. per minute is safer.[79] If the patient is not asleep a dosage of 1 c.cm. per $12 \cdot 5$ kg. body weight should never be exceeded.[80] Post-operative restlessness and excitement seem to be considerably less frequent with pernocton than with the other barbiturates. In one series of 1,200 administrations severe excitement was only seen in four patients.[81] The drug has been given frequently to drug addicts over a considerable time without obvious ill-effects. Pernocton causes a small rise in blood sugar, but no hæmolysis or other changes in blood chemistry have been observed.[79]

Rectidon (**Sigmodal**) is sodium 2^y amyl-β-bromallyl barbiturate and is thus the homologue of pernocton. The drug is supplied in a 10 per cent. solution ready for use. The *rectal administration* of this compound has been tried extensively on the Continent and is said to be particularly satisfactory for children.[82] The average dosage is :

Up to one year	..	..	..	1 c.cm.
One to three years	..	..	..	1 to 2 c.cm.
Three to six years	..	..	..	2 to 3 c.cm.
Six to ten years	..	..	..	3 to 4 c.cm.
Ten to fourteen years		..	..	4 to 5 c.cm.

In obstetrics, rectidon has been used in doses of 0·12 c.cm. per kilogramme body weight up to a maximum of 9 c.cm. The full effect does not, however, last much longer than one hour.[83]

Sodium Soneryl (Butobarbital sodium). Sodium soneryl, or sodium butyl-ethyl barbiturate, is usually administered *by mouth* in white capsules containing 0·15 g. (2¼ gr.). The average pre-operative dose is based on body weight as follows :

90 to 115 lb.	..	..	..	3 capsules.
120 to 145 lb.	..	..	..	4 ,,
150 to 175 lb.	..	..	..	5 ,,

Sodium soneryl given in this way is said to have a more constant effect than oral nembutal. The safety margin of the two drugs is about the same.[71] Patients frequently remain somnolent for twenty-four hours or more after operation.[84] Sodium soneryl has been combined with syrup of chloral to mitigate the pains of labour.[85] The *intravenous* route has also been tried, using a 5 per cent. solution of sodium soneryl, the average dose being 1 cg. per kilogramme body weight.[86]

Hebaral sodium, or sodium hexyl-ethyl barbiturate, is usually given *by mouth* in purple capsules each containing 0·2 g. (3 g.). The usual pre-operative adult dose is two to three capsules. The drug has a high theoretical safety-margin, the minimal lethal dose in animals being four times the narcotic dose. Recovery has ensued from a dose of no less than 90 gr.[87]

Seconal, or sodium propyl methyl carbinyl allyl barbiturate, is put up in scarlet capsules for oral administration, each containing 0·1 g. (1½ gr.). The usual pre-operative adult dose is two to three capsules, which should be given not longer than an hour before operation.[88]

Pentothal acid (Thionembutal) is ethyl (1-methyl-butyl) thio barbituric acid. The average adult dose is 8 gr. (four capsules) three hours before operation in an alkaline mixture. If necessary the dose can be repeated after an interval of one hour.[89]

The third group consists of short-acting barbiturates, the commonest of which are :

Eunarcon (sodium-c-c-isopropyl-β-bromallyl-N-methyl barbiturate).

Soluble hexobarbitone Evipan sodium (sodium N-methyl-c-c-cyclo-hexenyl methyl barbiturate).

Kemithal sodium (sodium-5-cyclohexenyl-5-allyl-2-thio barbiturate).

Narconumal (1-methyl-5-5-allyl-isopropyl barbituric acid).

Soluble thiopentone or **Pentothal sodium** (sodium ethyl (1-methyl-butyl) thio barbiturate).

Surital sodium (**thioquinal barbitone**) (sodium 5-allyl-5 [1-methyl butyl]-2-thiobarbiturate).

Venesetic (sodium iso-amyl-ethyl thio barbiturate).

These drugs can be given *intravenously* to the stage of basal narcosis, but must be followed by inhalation anæsthesia within a few minutes, or the patient will recover consciousness. The reason for this is that a rapid single-dose injection causes a high concentration of the drug in the brain from the large carotid circulation. If the injection is stopped at the moment of unconsciousness, redistribution occurs throughout all the body tissues and the cerebral concentration will fall below the level necessary for narcosis even prior to any elimination. Some prolongation of effect can be obtained by a slower injection, in which case the concentration of the drug will be approximately the same in all tissues and elimination from the body must begin before consciousness is regained. Even then, after a short time, the superimposed anæsthesia will have to be relied upon alone. For these reasons, the short-acting barbiturates are inferior to the second group for true basal narcosis produced in bed some time before operation. These compounds are mainly used to avoid an inhalation induction and for complete intravenous anæsthesia and are discussed more fully in Chapter X.

The *intramuscular* route has been attempted with the object of obtaining a more prolonged effect, but the irritating nature of the drugs has discouraged the practice. A fatal case of gas-gangrene has been reported following intramuscular hexobarbitone, but the drug cannot be held directly responsible for this catastrophe.[90]

The *rectal* administration of the short-acting barbiturates has met with more success. In the case of hexobarbitone a 10 per cent. solution is used with a dosage of 0·2 c.cm. per pound body weight (=44 mg. per kilogramme).[91] The small volume of fluid required is a definite advantage over bromethol and paraldehyde, while even if the patient is not rendered quite unconscious, it is said that amnesia is usually complete.[92] It may be possible to perform investigations such as cystoscopy without any supplementary anæsthesia.[93] This technique has also been used therapeutically in the treatment of acute and chronic alcoholism.[94] Rectal thiopentone is said to be followed by less respiratory depression and less muscular twitching and spasm than hexobarbitone.[95] The average rectal dose is given as 1 g. per 50 lb. body weight dissolved in 1 oz. of distilled water. (This works out as the same dose per weight as that given for rectal hexobarbitone.) Half this dosage is recommended in the case of rectal narconumal.[96]

The *oral* route is not much used except in the case of soluble thiopentone, which seems of service in obstetric analgesia (q.v.).

The effects of the barbiturates are extremely variable. In a study of 1,000 cases it was found that the most resistant individual required four times the dose of the least resistant one (McNalis). Again, it has been found that the coloured native races are more susceptible to the effects of barbiturates than Europeans.[97] This illustrates well the impossibility of ensuring full basal narcosis with any method of calculating the oral or rectal dose, and shows that the only rational technique is by intravenous injection until consciousness is just lost.

All the barbiturates appear to give some protection against the toxic effects of cocaine and its substitutes, and this is a definite advantage if a local analgesia is to be incorporated in the combined technique.[98] The immediate and remote effects of the barbiturates on the body are discussed under intravenous anæsthesia (q.v.).

Elimination of the barbiturates is not yet completely understood. Experiments on partially hepatectomized or completely nephrectomized rats would seem to show that the routes of elimination can be classified under four headings[99] :

(1) Detoxication mainly in the kidney, e.g. barbital and phenobarbital.

(2) Detoxication mainly in the liver, e.g. alurate, amytal, hexobarbitone, ipral, nembutal, nostal and seconal.

(3) Detoxication equally in the kidney and liver, e.g. delvinal, dial, neonal and phanodorm.

(4) Detoxication in tissues generally, e.g. thiopentone.

It is, however, a mistake to attach too great importance to any one set of experiments as animals differ greatly in their reaction to barbiturates (e.g. thiopentone is extremely toxic to the liver in mice), and it is unlikely that the classification given above applies exactly to man. From direct observation of the effects of the intravenous barbiturates in the human subject, however, it is certain that grossly impaired liver and renal function (e.g. after extensive burns) delays recovery and in extreme cases the narcosis merges into death.[101] This fact has been made use of in the humanitarian treatment of obviously fatal and painful burns (see also Chapter X).

Overdosage is usually characterized by intense respiratory and circulatory depression, and is best treated by assisted or artificial respiration with oxygen or a 95 per cent. oxygen, 5 per cent. CO_2 mixture, a head-down position and by the intravenous injection of such analeptic drugs as nikethamide, leptazol and picrotoxin,[100] the initial dose for adults being about 10 c.cm., 2 c.cm. and 3 mg. respectively. It is doubtful whether any true antagonistic effect exists and it is now thought that stimulation of the respiratory centre constitutes the chief beneficial effect.[101] Good results have also been obtained with icoral[102] and strychnine.[103] Recently disodium succinate hexahydrate in doses of from 1 g. to 3 g. in a 30 per cent. solution has been tried and is said to be a powerful respiratory stimulant in barbiturate overdosage without the side-effects of most analeptics. Repeated lumbar puncture is also said to be good practice in barbiturate poisoning, as some of the drug is excreted into the cerebrospinal fluid.[104]

Choice of Premedication Technique

From the foregoing remarks it will be realized that the anæsthetist now has a very wide range of methods and drugs for premedication, and to give some guide, the author's choice of technique will now be given. It is not, of course, suggested that other combinations of drugs do not give equally good results. The doses are computed for patients in reasonably fit condition.

Age in years.	Drugs and Dosage.	Hours before Operation.
0 to 6/12	Atropine gr. 1/200 hypo	3/4
6/12 to 1	Atropine gr. 1/150 hypo	3/4
1 to 2	{ Atropine gr. 1/100 hypo	3/4
	Seconal gr. 3/4 by mouth	1 1/2
2 to 4	{ Scopolamine gr. 1/400 hypo	3/4
	Seconal gr. 0·6 per stone body weight by mouth. [Max. gr. 3 1/2]	1 1/2
4 to 10	{ Scopolamine gr. 1/300 hypo	3/4
	Seconal gr. 0·6 per stone body weight by mouth. [Max. gr. 3 1/2]	1 1/2
10 to 16	{ Scopolamine gr. 1/200 hypo	3/4
	Seconal gr. 0·6 per stone body weight by mouth. [Max. gr. 3 1/2]	1 1/2

Age in years.	Drugs and Dosage.	Hours before Operation.
16 to 60	{ Pethidine 100 mg. Scopolamine gr. 1/150 } hypo	1
60 to 70	{ Pethidine 100 mg. Atropine gr. 1/100 } hypo	1
70+	{ Pethidine 50 mg. Atropine gr. 1/100 } hypo	1

Particulars as to full basal narcosis in bed will be found under Anæsthesia for Thyroid Surgery.

References

1. BETLACH, C. J. *Pro. Mayo Clin.*, 1937, Nov. 17, p. 733.
2. ABEL, A. L. *Post-Grad. Med. Jour.*, 1937, Dec., p. 437.
3. BAKER, A. H. L., and CHIVERS, E. M. *Lancet*, 1941, Feb. 8, p. 171.
4. ASQUITH, E., and THOMAS, E. *Lancet*, 1948, Dec. 11, p. 930.
5. GIRODANENGO, G. *Anesth. & Anal.*, 1939, Sept.-Oct., p. 251.
6. SORESI, A. L. *Medical Record*, 1935, May 1.
7. { ROWBOTHAM, S. *Pro. Roy. Soc. Med.* (An. Sec.), 1928, Dec. BURGI. *Die Arzneikombinationen, Berlin.*
8. { MEYER and GOTTLIEB. " Pharmacology," p. 42. DONOVAN, E. P., and GWATHMEY, J. T. *Brit. Jour. Anœsth.*, **1**, p. 8.
9. SHACKELLAND, L. F., and BLUMENTHAL, R. R. *Anesth. & Anal.*, 1933, May-June.
10. CERVELLO, V. *Arch. Ital. de Biol.*, 1884, **6**, p. 113.
11. BROWN, G. *Brit. Jour. Anœsth.*, 1935, Oct., p. 25.
12. STEWART, J. D. *Brit. Med. Jour.*, 1932, Dec. 24, p. 1139.
13. GARRETT, B. B., and GUTTERIDGE, E. *Med. Jour. Australia*, 1933, July 8, p. 46.
14. STAMM, W. *Zentralb. f. Chir.*, 1931, 25.
15. { SINGTON, H. *Pro. Roy. Soc. Med.* (An. Sec.), 1929, May. ROWBOTHAM, S. *Brit. Med. Jour.*, 1931, Oct. 17, p. 693.
16. INGRAHAM, F. D., and CAMPBELL, J. B. *Ann. Surg.*, 1940, Mar., p. 501.
17. NITZESCUE, I., *et al.* *Presse Méd.*, 1934, **42**, p. 331.
18. DE ELIO, *et al.* *Rev. clin. esp.*, 1948, **30**, p. 289.
19. WHIGHAM, J. R. M. *Lancet*, 1934, July 28, p. 191.
20. SNOW. *Med. Times & Gazette*, 1857, Jan. 17, p. 60.
21. BLOMFIELD, J., and SHIPWAY, F. *Pro. Roy. Soc. Med.* (An. Sec.), 1929, Nov.
22. BOYD, J. *Brit. Med. Jour.*, 1935, June 1, p. 1120.
23. PERMAN, E. *Nord. med. Tidskr.*, 1935, p. 2089.
24. ASHWORTH, H. K. *Brit. Med. Jour.*, 1933, Sept. 9, p. 489.
25. LEWIS, I. N. *Brit. Jour. Anœsth.*, **8**, No. 1, p. 3.
26. { SEBENING, W. *Anesth. & Anal.*, 1932, **11**, No. 4, p. 160. FEATHERSTONE, H. W. *Brit. Med. Jour.*, 1934, Feb. 23, p. 323 ; and MACINTOSH, R. R., 1943, Personal Communication.
27. GRAHAM, R. S. A. *New Zealand Med. Jour.*, 1932, Apr., p. 80.
28. RIEUNAL, G., and BONSIRVEN, A. *Brux. Med.*, 1933, Jan. 25, p. 938.
29. WATTER, L. *Anesth. & Anal.*, 1933, Nov.-Dec., p. 250.
30. GOLDSCHMIDT, E. F., and HUNT, A. H. *Amer. Jour. Surg.*, 1932, Jan.
31. MADDOX, K. *Brit. Jour. Anœsth.*, 1934, July, p. 143.
32. NORRIS, L. D., and STEVENS, A. H. *Anesth. & Anal.*, 1936, Nov.-Dec., p. 268.
33. BEECHER, H. K. *Jour. Amer. Med. Ass.*, 1938, July 9, p. 122.
34. WIDENHORN, H. *Anesth. & Anal.*, 1932, Mar.-Apr.
35. UNTI, O. *Ann. Paul. de Med. & Cir.*, 1935, Oct., p. 345.

36. BOURNE, W. *Canad. Med. Ass. Jour.*, 1932, Nov., p. 515.
37. HILL, B. P. *Brit. Med. Jour.*, 1938, Aug. 13, p. 348.
38. HARE, T., and WRIGHT, J. G. *Pro. Roy. Soc. Med.* (Comp. Med. Sec.), 1931, Apr. 22.
39. GREELEY, H. *Med. Times and Long Island Med. Jour.*, 1933, Feb., p. 38.
  RUGE, E. *Zentralb. f. Chir.*, 1932, Sept. 24.
40. McKIM, L. H., and BOURNE, W. *Canad. Med. Ass. Jour.*, 1933, Feb., p. 149.
41. WOOD, P. M., *et al. Amer. Jour. Surg.*, 1936, Dec., p. 599.
42. WYMER, I. *Schmerz, Narkose, Anæsthesie*, 1931, April, p. 19.
43. PYBRAM. *Zentralb. f. Chir.*, 1929, Dec. 14, p. 3138.
  CARLTON, H. *Pro. Roy. Soc. Med.* (An. Sec.), 1929, Nov.
44. YOUNG, J. *Brit. Med. Jour.*, 1931, Dec. 5, p. 1026.
  SHAW, W. F., and ASHWORTH, H. K. *Brit. Med. Jour.*, 1931, Dec. 19, p. 1156.
45. HEWER, C. L. *Brit. Med. Jour.*, 1930, Nov. 29.
46. BARNSLEY, A. *Malayan Med. Jour.*, 1932, March, p. 1.
47. WOOD, P. M., *et al. Amer. Jour. Surg.*, 1936, Dec., p. 599.
48. MAGILL, I. W. *Lancet*, 1931, Jan. 10, p. 74.
49. BERNHEIM, B. N., *et al. Ann. Surg.*, 1934, Mar., p. 550.
50. FUCHS. *Jour. Allergy*, 1937, **8**, No. 4, p. 340.
51. BULLOWA, J. *Med. Clinics of N. America*, 1933, July.
52. STALBERG, *et al. Jour. Amer. Med. Ass.*, 1933, July 8, p. 102.
53. STARLINGER, F. *Klin. Woch.*, 1932, No. 22.
54. HARRIS, T. A. B. *Brit. Jour. Anæsth.*, 1939, July, p. 133.
55. HURST, A. *Guy's Hosp. Gaz.*, 1939, Nov. 14, p. 365.
56. RAGINSKGI, B. B., and BOURNE, W. *Anesth. & Anal.*, 1932, **11**, No. 1, p.33.
57. BOLLIGER, A. *Med. Jour. Australia*, 1932, Jan. 23, p. 125.
58. BOYD, J. *Brit. Med. Jour.*, 1940, May 4, p. 729.
59. MARCOTTE, R. J., *et al. Anesth. & Anal.*, 1940, Mar.-Apr., p. 88.
60. MOLITOR, H. *Anesth. & Anal.*, 1938, Sept.-Oct., p. 258.
61. WOOD, D. A. *Anesth. & Anal.*, 1938, Sept.-Oct., p. 252.
  HEWER, C. L., and BELFRAGE, D. *Lancet*, 1938, Dec. 3, p. 1291.
62. QUASTEL, J. H., and STRÖM-OLSEN, R. *Lancet*, 1933, Mar. 4, p. 464.
63. LEAK, W. N. *Brit. Med. Jour.*, 1939, Dec. 9, p. 1162.
64. PAGE. *Jour. Lab. and Clin. Med.*, 1923, **9**, p. 194.
65. ZERFAS, L. C., and McCALLUM, J. T. C. *Jour. Indiana Med. Ass.*, 1929, 22, p. 47.
66. BLECKWENN, W. J. *Jour. Amer. Med. Ass.*, 1930, **95**, p. 1168.
67. HAMBLEN, E. C., *et al. Amer. Jour. Obst. and Gyn.*, 1932, **22**, p. 590.
68. WATT, G. L. *Canad. Med. Ass. Jour.*, 1932, July, p. 53.
69. SWENDSON, J. T. *Minnesota Medicine*, 1932, Dec.
70. MAGILL, I. W. *Lancet*, 1931, Jan. 10, p. 74.
71. JARMAN, R. *Brit. Med. Jour.*, 1936, Feb. 1, p. 236.
72. WRIGHT, J. G. *Pro. Roy. Soc. Med.*, (Comp. Med. Sec.), 1933, Jan. 25.
73. BOYD, A. M. *St. Barts. Hosp. Rep.*, 1932, p. 283.
74. MUTCH, N. *Brit. Med. Jour.*, 1934, Feb. 24, p. 331.
75. O'FARRELL, P. T. *Brit. Med. Jour.*, 1938, Aug. 13, p. 348.
76. MAILER, R. *Lancet*, 1933, Nov. 25, p. 1205.
77. CAMERON, C. R. *Pro. Roy. Soc. Med.* (An. Sec.), 1938, Dec. 2.
78. PFEILER, R. *Schmerz, Narkose, Anæsthesie*, Dec.,1931-Jan., 1932, p. 273.
79. MATTERS, R. F. *Med. Jour. Austral.*, 1931, Nov. 21, p. 650.
80. SCHLAEPPER, K., and VAN ESS, J. *Anesth. & Anal.*, 1934, July-Aug., p. 170.
81. FRIEDLANDER. *Amer. Jour. Surg.*, 1931, Mar. 11, p. 485.
82. MÜNDTRATH, H. *Münch. Med. Woch.*, 1934, Dec. 13, p. 1934.

83. BRAMMER, H.   *Schmerz, Narkose, Anœsthesie*, 1935, Jan., p. 45.
84. DESPLAS, B., and CHEVILLON, G.   *Paris Méd.*, 1933, July 15, p. 77.
85. *Rep. Med. Res. Counc.*, 1934-35.
86. DESPLAS, B., and CHEVILLON, G.   *Bull. et Mem. Soc. Nat. de Chir.*, 1934, Mar. 31, p. 519.
87. KENDRICK, A. I.   *Brit. Med. Jour.*, 1936, Dec. 12, p. 1196.
88. SWANSON, E. E.   *Pro. Soc. Exper. Biol. and Med.*, 1935, **32,** p. 1563.
89. HORSLEY, J. S.   *Brit. Jour. Anœsth.*, 1938, Oct., p. 1.
90. HARRIS, D. P.   *Brit. Jour. Anœsth.*, 1937, Apr., p. 130.
91. GWATHMEY, J. T.   *Amer. Jour. Surg.*, 1936, June, p. 411.
92. HARRISON, J. H., and DUNPHY, J. E.   *New Eng. Jour. Med.*, 1938, Jan. 6, p. 10.
93. GRANT, *et al.*   *Jour. Urol.*, 1939, Aug., p. 204.
94. McNELLIS, P. J.   *Anesth. & Anal.*, 1937, July-Aug., p. 195.
95. WEINSTEIN, M. L.   *Anesth. & Anal.*, 1939, July-Aug., p. 221.
96. HUNTER, H. K.   *Brit. Jour. Anœsth.*, 1941, July, p. 167.
97. ASHWORTH, H. K.   *Pro. Roy. Soc. Med.* (An. Sec.), 1946, Feb. 1.
98. BROWN, G.   *Med. Jour. Austral.*, 1932, Oct. 8, p. 437.
99. MASSON, G. M. C., and BELAND, E.   *Anesthesiology*, 1945, Sept., p. 483.
100. SLOT, G.   *Brit. Med. Jour.*, 1940, May 25, p. 849.
101. BURSTEIN, C. L., and ROVENSTINE, E. A.   *Anesth. and Anal.*, 1937, May-June, p. 151.
102. FRANK, H.   *Deut. Med. Woch.*, 1933, May 19, p. 764.
103. HAGGARD and GREENBERG.   *Jour. Amer. Med. Ass.*, 1932, **98,** p. 1133.

CHAPTER III

NITROUS OXIDE AND THE HYDROCARBON GASES

Nitrous Oxide — Ethylene — Acetylene — Methyl Acetylene — Propylene —
Cyclopropane and its Derivatives — Cyclobutane.

NITROUS OXIDE

THE mode of action of this gas has already been described in
Chapter I, but from time to time patients exhibit curious symptoms
during inhalation and suspicion has fallen upon the quality of the
gas supplied. An investigation of this subject has been made,
and it has been established that (*a*) the gas at present supplied by
manufacturers in Great Britain is of high quality and rarely contains
any impurity other than nitrogen ; (*b*) some nitrous oxide supplied
in another country almost certainly contained nitric oxide which
is highly toxic ; and (*c*) the gas first delivered from a cylinder is that
most likely to give rise to unpleasant symptoms and is that which
contains most impurities.[1] For example, it has been found that
if the nitrous oxide in a cylinder contains an average of 2 per cent.
nitrogen, the gas first delivered (i.e. from the gaseous phase) will
contain 8 per cent. nitrogen. Since the U.S.P. allows up to 5 per
cent. nitrogen,[2] it will be seen that the gas first delivered may be
quite unsuitable for anæsthesia.

The usual commercial process of making nitrous oxide is by
heating ammonium nitrate in a metal retort to 250° C. (NH_4NO_3
$\rightarrow N_2O + 2H_2O$). The resulting gases (consisting chiefly of steam
and nitrous oxide) are passed through suitable purifying towers
and dried. When compressed into cylinders, the gas liquefies and
the amount present can only be measured by weighing (50 gallons
of gas weigh 15 oz.). The pressure, about 650 lb. per sq. in., or
40 atmospheres, remains constant as long as any liquid is left in
the cylinders. The water content of the gas should not exceed
0·005 per cent.[48]

Cyanosis. Since nitrous oxide is the weakest anæsthetic gas,
it must be used in the greatest concentration and some cyanosis
may be present. Confusion still exists in the minds of certain
anæsthetists and surgeons as to the distinction between cyanosis
and anoxæmia (or anoxic anoxia). It has been estimated that
cyanosis first becomes recognizable when the absolute amount of

reduced hæmoglobin in the blood reaches 5 g. per c.cm.[3] The
total amount of hæmoglobin will vary with each individual patient,
and consequently the relationship between cyanosis and anoxæmia
will also vary.

In the subjoined chart (Fig. 5) it is assumed that nitrous oxide
is mixed with enough oxygen (about 9 per cent.) to oxygenate rather
less than two-thirds of the circulating hæmoglobin. A normal
patient A has approximately 15 g. of Hb per cent. of which about
6 g. are reduced so that he will be slightly cyanosed without being
anoxæmic. A slightly anæmic patient B will not show cyanosis

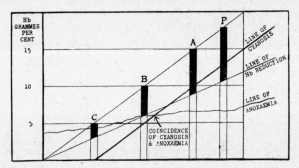

Fig. 5. Chart showing degrees of cyanosis and anoxæmia in four
patients having the same mixture of N_2O—O_2. Shaded columns
represent reduced Hb and unshaded oxyhæmoglobin. (After
R. L. Wynne.)

although anoxæmia is present, while a very anæmic patient C with
a total hæmoglobin of only 5 g. per cent. can never become cyanosed.
At the opposite extreme a plethoric patient P is markedly cyanosed
without any anoxæmia.[4] It is therefore obvious that the significance
of cyanosis will vary with the individual patient and that a cyanosed
plethoric man may be in a much more satisfactory condition than
a pale anæmic girl. Adequate premedication lowers the metabolic
rate and so facilitates NO_2—O_2 anæsthesia without anoxæmia.

In a recent careful investigation[55] involving 339 unpremedicated
patients, it was found that only 3·6 per cent. could be rendered
quiet with fair muscular relaxation within three minutes of inhaling
pure nitrous oxide with an atmospheric percentage of oxygen
(21 per cent.). If the oxygen was reduced to between 15 and
20 per cent. the percentage of satisfactory anæsthesias rose to
27·5. Samples of the gases in the right main bronchus (approxi-
mating to alveolar gases) of a patient inhaling this mixture gave

an oxygen tension of 65 mm. Hg corresponding to 87 per cent. saturation of arterial blood. If satisfactory narcosis cannot be obtained with this mixture it seems best to add a volatile supplement such as ether or trichlorethylene. In the case of the latter drug, it was found that post-operative vomiting was not appreciably increased.

Cyanosis may be due to causes other than an excess of reduced hæmoglobin, e.g. methæmoglobinæmia. The anæsthetist is most likely to meet this condition in patients with infected wounds who have been treated with massive doses of a sulphonamide. These patients have only a proportion of their total hæmoglobin available and their cyanosis is not relieved by the inhalation of oxygen. Before the induction of anæsthesia, intravenous methylene-blue should be given, the ideal dose being $0 \cdot 5$ mg. per kilogramme body weight. In patients too ill to weigh, the average male adult dose is 20 mg. or 2 c.cm. of a 1 per cent. solution of methylene blue.[5]

The types of cyanosis so far considered are of *central* origin but *peripheral* cyanosis may occur from a sluggish local circulation. In this case there may be excessive removal of oxygen by the tissues from the relatively stagnant blood as shown by blueness of the tips of the fingers and toes and ears while the rest of the skin may be quite pink.

A device known as an **oximeter** has been invented to measure the oxygen saturation of arterial blood by mechanical means.[6] This ingenious apparatus has an ear unit fitting over the pinna with an electric bulb in front and a photo-electric cell behind. The heat of the bulb dilates the vessels so that the blood contained in them equals arterial blood in oxygen content. Oxyhæmoglobin transmits red light more easily than does reduced hæmoglobin so that the amount of light passed through the ear can be measured by a galvanometer connected to the photo-electric cell. From this reading the oxygen saturation of arterial blood can be calculated within an error of from 3 to 7 per cent. This device might be of considerable use during anæsthesia as it is obviously more reliable than visual appreciation of cyanosis which often has to be made under difficult conditions.

Effects on Cerebral Cortex. In America, several series of late cerebral complications have been reported following pure NO_2—O_2 anæsthesia. Muscular tremors, rigidity and hyperpyrexia were noted, while post-mortem examination of fatal cases showed extensive damage to the cortex and basal ganglia. Some workers have thought that the gas itself may have a toxic action on the parenchyma while others think that anoxia may be the cause of the trouble.[7] It should be remembered that pure NO_2—O_2 was used extensively in America even for major surgery, sometimes with the " secondary saturation " technique (q.v.). It seems probable that gross anoxia for a considerable time was not very uncommon and this may account for the absence of such reported cases in Great Britain where the toxicity of oxygen lack is perhaps more fully appreciated.

General Analgesia.   Sub-anæsthetic concentrations of nitrous oxide produce general analgesia, the technique of which is described elsewhere.   Besides being extremely useful for various painful procedures and minor operations, narco-analysis is now being carried out under this type of analgesia.[8]

ETHYLENE

Ethylene, or **olefiant gas,** is an unsaturated hydrocarbon having the formula C_2H_4, and is slightly lighter than air (density $0 \cdot 975$).   It was first prepared by Ingenhauss in 1779 and its narcotic action is said to have been discovered by Simpson and investigated by Nunelly of Leeds, but it is doubtful whether these early workers ever anæsthetized patients with it.   In 1920 it was observed that ethylene dissolved in pure ether alters the anæsthetic effect of the latter,[9] and this led to a thorough investigation of the effects of the pure gas, which was carried out mainly in America by Luckhardt, Carter, Easson Brown and others.

Ethylene, like many other organic compounds, differs in its chemically pure and its commercial forms.   When the gas is freshly prepared in the laboratory from phosphoric acid and ethyl alcohol it possesses a faint but rather pleasant ethereal smell.   The commercial gas compressed in cylinders has a strong garlic-like smell, strongly reminiscent of acetylene and definitely unpleasant. This must be due either to some chemical change or to the presence of impurities.   As a matter of fact, the induction of anæsthesia is so rapid with ethylene that the odour is only perceived by the patient for a few breaths and thereafter is chiefly annoying to the anæsthetist and other occupants of the theatre.   Even this can be eliminated by using a closed-circuit machine.   Ethylene being an endothermic gas might conceivably explode spontaneously under pressure, as does acetylene,[10] but up to the present no such catastrophe has occurred from the ordinary 60-atmospheres compression used in storage cylinders.   Since the gas is not liquefied at this pressure a cylinder which would contain 200 gallons of nitrous oxide will only contain about 150 gallons of ethylene, a point to bear in mind when calculating the probable time of anæsthesia. Ethylene can be used in the same way and with the same apparatus as nitrous oxide, the main differences being (i) the induction time is shorter ; (ii) slightly more oxygen can be used (about 20 per cent. as a rule) ; (iii) there is increased vascularity of tissues and secretion of saliva and mucus ; (iv) there is better muscular relaxation ; (v) there is sometimes distressing nausea after anæsthesia and occasional vomiting ; (vi) ethylene is inflammable in the pure state and explosive when mixed in certain proportions with air or oxygen, the force of the explosion sometimes being terrific. The upper and lower limits of explosive mixtures are (i) with air 3·05 per cent. to 28·5 per cent. ; (ii) with oxygen 3·1 per cent. to 79·9 per cent.[11] It is thus unsafe to use the gas with any form of cautery (see Chapter IX). In America there have been twenty explosions involving five deaths in 1,005,375 administrations of ethylene.[12]

The use of this gas has now been given up entirely in Great Britain, but it still has a limited vogue in America.

ACETYLENE

It was observed that acetylene produced anæsthesia in animals as long ago as 1895,[13] but the pharmacological action of the gas was only worked out comparatively recently by Wieland, since when it has been extensively used in anæsthesia in combination with oxygen, under the name **Narcylen,** in Germany, and to a lesser extent in America. Acetylene resembles ethylene in most respects, but must be stored in cylinders containing acetone to avoid spontaneous explosion. Commercial acetylene must not be used for anæsthesia owing to such impurities as phosphine and sulphur. Absolutely pure acetylene has, like ethylene, a faint ethereal odour,[14] but as it is impossible to produce it at reasonable cost the smell is disguised by pine essence. Most characteristics of ethylene are possessed by acetylene, the main differences lying in the oxygen percentage possible. This lies in the region of 50 per cent., so that cyanosis should never occur in any circumstances.[15] The induction of anæsthesia and recovery are alike rapid with acetylene, as has been explained by the findings of blood analyses in rabbits. In five minutes after the induction of anæsthesia 88 per cent. saturation is reached, and in seventeen minutes saturation is complete. In one minute after discontinuing the administration 85 per cent. of the gas has been eliminated, and in twenty minutes none is demonstrable in the blood.[16] Similar precautions against fire and explosion must be taken as with ethylene,[17] one such disaster having actually occurred.[18] The limits of explosibility are from $2 \cdot 8$ per cent. to 50 per cent. acetylene in air and from 3 per cent. to 90 per cent. in oxygen.[19]

Methyl acetylene is more potent than acetylene, 10-15 per cent. being equivalent to 40 per cent. acetylene. Unfortunately it is toxic and clonic convulsive movements accompany anæsthesia.[20]

PROPYLENE

Propylene, the second member of the simple olefine series, with the formula C_3H_6, is an inflammable gas, its explosive limits being from $2 \cdot 2$ per cent. to 9 per cent. propylene in air and from 2 per cent. to 20 per cent. in oxygen.[19] It acts in a way similar to ethylene and acetylene, although only 30 per cent. with oxygen produces unconsciousness.[21] Anæsthesia is said to supervene after an average of only eight respirations, but excessive salivation is sometimes a troublesome feature.[22]

Propylene appears to be a satisfactory anæsthetic in animals,[23] but has as yet not been given an extensive trial in man, owing to a doubt as to its action on the heart rhythm.[24] There is, however, no change in the character of the average electrocardiogram.

CYCLOPROPANE (TRIMETHYLENE)

Cyclopropane is the isomer of propylene and was first prepared in 1882 by Freund,[25] who also demonstrated its cyclic structure :

$$H_2C \Big\langle \begin{array}{c} CH_2 \\ | \\ CH_2 \end{array}$$

Preparation and Cost. Cyclopropane is prepared from the reduction of trimethylene bromide by metallic zinc in alcoholic solution. A new method of preparation is now being developed whereby cyclopropane is obtained by chlorination of the propane present in natural gas. This exists in practically unlimited quantities in parts of America and it is anticipated that the process will lead to a material reduction in cost.[26] The gas is compressed into cylinders and liquefies at a pressure of 75 lb. per square inch. A 100-gallon nitrous cylinder will contain about $62\frac{1}{2}$ gallons of cyclopropane.[27] For occasional use the gas can also be obtained in small containers resembling " sparklets ", which each hold 2 or 6 gallons. Owing to the comparatively low cylinder pressure it is unnecessary to use reducing valves, and in any case no valves incorporating rubber fittings should be employed as pure cyclopropane under pressure rapidly deteriorates rubber.

The fact that the flow rate of cyclopropane is usually controlled solely by a large handwheel on the cylinder without an additional needle valve on the flowmeter constitutes a potential danger. The gas may be inadvertently turned on by someone brushing against the hand wheel and the concentration can then rapidly rise in the breathing circuit with disastrous results.[56]

At the time of writing, the price of the gas in the United Kingdom is 2s. 8d. per gallon.

Properties. Cyclopropane is a colourless gas with a characteristic odour. It is heavier than air, having a density of 1·46. One ounce of the gas is equivalent to about 4·29 gallons. The gas is practically insoluble in water, but extremely soluble in lipoids, 1 c.cm. of olive oil dissolving 103·5 c.cm. of cyclopropane[28] and the oil-water ratio being 34·3. When pure, the gas burns in air and when mixed with oxygen, air or nitrous oxide is explosive within the following limits :

In *air*	3% to 8·5%	cyclopropane.
In *oxygen*	2·5% to 50%	,,
In *nitrous oxide* ..	3% to 28%	,,

The maximum violence of explosion is obtained with 18·2 per cent. cyclopropane in oxygen.[29] It has been estimated that during 1939, 74 cyclopropane explosions occurred in the United States with 13 fatalities.[30]

Impurities. Commercial cyclopropane contains up to 3 per cent. propylene which in the opinion of competent experts is not a dangerous contamination.[31]

Action. Cyclopropane resembles ether in its effects as an anæsthetic except that respiratory depression replaces stimulation and that irritation to the respiratory passages is absent. Tuberculous monkeys have been subjected to prolonged cyclopropane anæsthesia without ill-effects.[32] On the other hand, bronchospasm and laryngospasm occasionally occur. In general it can be said that cyclopropane stimulates the parasympathetic.

As regards the cardio-vascular system, normal electrocardiograph tracings have been obtained in animals up to the point where respiratory arrest occurs from overdosage. As will be seen later, this is not always the case in man. The systolic blood pressure is said to rise, within limits, as the concentration of the gas, and this, accompanied by an increased peripheral blood-flow due to vasodilatation,[33] is presumably the cause of the capillary oozing from wounds which is usually greater than with other forms of general anæsthesia. Waters, however, considers that the rise in blood pressure is not due to the action of the cyclopropane, but to other factors such as a rise in CO_2 concentration.[34]   There is stated to be no alteration in the coagulation time of the blood.[35]   The effect on the pulse varies, but bradycardia is common and arrhythmia sometimes occurs, which disappears if a few breaths of pure oxygen are administered.   Pulse irregularities also tend to cease in deep anæsthesia so that there appears to be a band in the narcosis planes where arrhythmia may occur.   The nature of the irregularities seems to be ventricular extrasystoles.[36]   From experimental work in animals, it seems possible that preliminary medication with a barbiturate instead of morphine may minimize cardiac irregularities due to cyclopropane.[37]   The author, however, has been unable to find much difference between the two types of premedication.   A temporary change-over to ether, on the other hand, may permanently re-establish a regular pulse.[38]   In dogs under light anæsthesia the injection of intravenous adrenaline does not cause ventricular fibrillation, but this does occur if the narcosis is deep.[34]   Procaine appears to give some protection against this event and the intra-cardiac injection of this drug resuscitated 66 per cent. of animals in ventricular fibrillation.[39]   (See also under " electrocardiographic changes " in Chapter I.)   Primary cardiac failure, although rare, has occurred, in man, from cyclopropane.[40]   It must therefore be concluded that very rarely the cardiac effects of the gas simulate those of chloroform.   For this reason, the popularity of cyclopropane has decreased in the past few years.

There has been no evidence to date of damage to the liver or kidneys.[24]   The output of urine is lessened during anæsthesia with a corresponding increase afterwards as is the case with ethylene and ether.

Muscular relaxation is usually good, although cyclopropane does not interfere with the contractions of the gravid uterus.[41] Owing to depression of the respiratory centre, breathing sometimes ceases before anæsthesia has become deep enough for complete relaxation.   In this event, rhythmic squeezing of the rebreathing bag will produce sufficient interchange of gases for adequate oxygenation of the blood (see " Controlled Respiration ").   If it is desired to re-establish spontaneous respiration at once, the CO_2 absorber should be temporarily by-passed and the gas further diluted with oxygen.   A curious idea still exists in some quarters that, owing to the high oxygen concentration obtaining during cyclopropane narcosis, a patient can be left indefinitely in a state of apnœa. It is obvious that asphyxia must occur eventually if there is no respiratory exchange, and fatalities have actually occurred from this cause. It is considered by some anæsthetists that if adequate relaxation cannot be obtained by reasonable dosage of cyclopropane, an adjuvant such as ether or curare should be added rather than pushing the plane of narcosis to the stage of respiratory arrest with the pure gas.

Contrary to previous statements, it has been shown that cyclopropane can cause a rise in blood sugar.[43]

Occasionally a transient erythema similar to an " ether rash " is seen with cyclopropane.[44] It is of no significance.

Indications. The outstanding advantages of cyclopropane are its non-irritative property, the high percentage of oxygen which can be given with it and the slow and shallow respiration which is characteristic. The author has found the gas of great service in major thoracic surgery, in cases of uncompensated heart disease (e.g. total thyroidectomy for congestive heart failure), and in severely shocked and toxic patients such as air raid casualties. It is unfortunate that the increasing use of diathermy so often prevents the gas from being used. Cyclopropane may also be used with advantage in many other cases such as for patients suffering from chronic bronchitis, asthma and respiratory obstruction. In the last two conditions, helium (q.v.) can with advantage be added.[45] Owing to the fact that the gas does not cause liver or kidney damage it is useful for patients suffering from eclampsia.[46] Cyclopropane can be employed as an adjuvant to NO_2—O_2 anæsthesia if more relaxation is required and it is undesirable to add trichlorethylene or ether.

Technique of Administration. Owing to the high cost of the gas the only practical method of administration is by means of a closed circuit apparatus (q.v.) with total rebreathing and CO_2 absorption. A tightly fitting facepiece or an endotracheal tube may be used as desirable. It has been found that, with care, about 2 gallons of cyclopropane are sufficient for an average case.[47] For the induction of anæsthesia the bag is filled with pure oxygen. After applying the facepiece, about 300 c.cm. of cyclopropane per minute and about 250 c.cm. of oxygen per minute are added. After a varying period of one to five minutes anæsthesia is established and the gas is shut off completely, the oxygen rate being adjusted so that the pressure remains constant. This will vary with the type of patient and with his basal metabolic rate. The second stage of anæsthesia is seldom well defined, less then 3 per cent. of patients showing excitement of any kind.[48]   During the course of anæsthesia it may be necessary to add cyclopropane from time to time to compensate for leaks and for diffusion through the rubber bag, etc. It is, however, unnecessary to add the gas continuously, as it is undesirable to eliminate the nitrogen completely. It is, in fact, thought by some that the replacement of nitrogen is responsible for the rare cases of pulmonary collapse reported after cyclopropane anæsthesia.

This theory is based upon the observation that the anæsthetic gases, oxygen and carbon dioxide are absorbed very rapidly from the alveolar epithelium while the " supporting " gases nitrogen and helium are absorbed relatively slowly.   It is therefore desirable to have a " supporting " gas present and if the nitrogen is " washed out " in the course of a long anæsthesia it should either be added by admitting some air or replaced with helium.   This applies especially to cyclopropane since respiration is normally shallow and any bronchial plugging may result in collapse of the lung distal to the plug.[49]   It must be emphasized that cyclopropane is an extremely potent anæsthetic, 10 per cent. in oxygen being a sufficient concentration for light anæsthesia and 14 per cent. to 16 per cent. usually providing fair relaxation.   Sub-anæsthetic concentrations (3 per cent. to 5 per cent.) if inhaled continuously usually produce general analgesia.   Most patients lose consciousness if the gas percentage reaches 6,[50] and it has been estimated that respiratory arrest usually occurs at a concentration of 42·9 per cent. Owing to the depression of respiration it is unwise to employ heavy premedication before cyclopropane, and it may be necessary to cut the CO_2 absorber out of the circuit from time to time.   If extreme bradycardia, tachycardia or arrhythmia occurs, it is usually considered advisable to reduce the gas concentration.[51]   As mentioned before, however, some observers believe that if the plane of narcosis is pushed still deeper, the tendency to cardiac irregularities ceases.[52]

At the conclusion of the operation, more and more air should be admitted to the breathing curcuit so that when the facepiece is finally removed the high oxygen concentration does not become lowered too quickly.

Sequelæ.   A short anæsthesia with cyclopropane-oxygen is usually followed by no more ill-effects than is nitrous oxide-oxygen, but slight nausea and vomiting do occur after prolonged administration.   An endeavour has been made to ascertain remote sequelæ by comparing 2,200 cyclopropane anæsthesias with a control series of 2,200 nitrous oxide-oxygen, ethylene-oxygen and ether anæsthesias. The closed circuit technique was employed in each case and other conditions kept as nearly identical as possible. The figures for respiratory complications and vomiting were definitely in favour of cyclopropane, but those for circulatory complications and post-operative deaths told against the gas.

Derivatives of Cyclopropane

Two chlorine derivatives of cyclopropane, viz. monochlorcyclopropane and dichlorcyclopropane have been tried out as anæsthetics in animals, but both cause so much respiratory irritation that it seems unlikely that they will prove of service.[53]

The cyclopropyl ethers are mentioned in Chapter VI.

CYCLOBUTANE

Cyclobutane, the next higher homologue to cyclopropane, has the structural formula

$$H_2C\text{---}CH_2$$
$$H_2C\text{---}CH_2$$

The gas has similar properties to cyclopropane but its anæsthetic potency appears to be greater.[54]

References

1. HADFIELD, C. F.   *Pro. Roy. Soc. Med.* (An. Sec.), 1926, Feb. 5.
2. LAWRENCE, W.   *Anesth. & Anal.*, 1937, July-Aug., p. 197.
3. HOUSSAY, B. A., and BERCONSKI, I.   *Presse méd.*, 1932, Nov. 23, p. 1759.
4. { PRATT, F. B.   *Brit. Med. Jour.*, 1939, Sept. 9, p. 555.
   { WYNNE, R. L.   *Brit. Med. Jour.*, 1940, June 15, p. 972.
5. HEWER, V. L.   *Brit. Med. Jour.*, 1940, June 15, p. 993.
6. GODFREY, L. *et al.*   *Amer. Jour. Med. Sci.*, 1948, **316,** p. 605.
7. { LOWENBORG, K., *et al.*   *Anesth. & Anal.*, 1938, March-April, p. 101.
   { COURVILLE, C. B.   " Untoward Effects of Nitrous Oxide Anæsthesia,"
   { 1939.
8. ROGERSON, C. H.   *Brit. Med. Jour.*, 1944, Jan. 17, p. 611.
9. WALLIS, R. L. M., and HEWER, C. L.   *Lancet*, 1921, i., p. 1173.
10. HEWER, V. L.   *Lancet*, 1925, Jan. 24, p. 173.
11. PETERSON, R.   *Amer. Jour. Obst. & Gyn.*, 1929, Nov.
12. HERB, I. C.   *Jour. Amer. Med. Ass.*, Nov. 25, p. 1716.
13. ROSEMAN, R.   *Arch. f. exp. Path. u. Pharm.*, 1895, **36,** p. 179.
14. GOLDMAN, A., and J. P.   *Brit. Jour. Anæsth.*, **2,** p. 122.
15. GAUSS, C. J., and WIELAND, H.   *Klin. Woch.*, 1923, **2,** pp. 113, 158.
16. SCHOEN and SLIWKA.   *Z. f. Physiol.*, 1923, p. 131.
17. WIELAND, H.   *Brit. Jour. Anæsth.*, **2,** p. 150.
18. HURLER, K.   *Munch. Med. Woch.*, 1924, **71,** p. 1432.
19. FINCH, G. I.   *Pro. Roy. Soc. Med.* (An. Sec.), 1935, Mar. 1.
20. HENDERSON, V. E.   *J. Pharmacol. exp. Therap.*, 1940, **69,** p. 74.

21. RIGGS, L. K., and GOULDEN, H. D.   *Anesth. & Anal.*, 1925, Oct.
22. SHIPWAY, F., quoted by HADFIELD, C. F.   *Pro. Roy. Soc. Med.* (An. Sec.), 1935, May 3.
23. DAVIDSON, B. M.   *Jour. Pharm. & Exper. Therap. Baltimore*, 1925, Aug.
24. BOURNE, W.   *Lancet*, 1934, July 7, p. 20.
25. FREUND, VON A.   *Monatshefte für Chemie*, 1882, July 13.
26. HAAS, H. B., *et al.*   *Anesth. & Anal.*, 1937, Jan.-Feb., p. 31.
27. ROWBOTHAM, S., *et al.*   *Lancet*, 1935, Nov. 16, p. 1110.
28. ROWBOTHAM, S.   *Pro. Roy. Soc. Med.* (An. Sec.), 1935, Dec. 6.
29. *Research Lab. Ohio, Chem. and Manuf. Co. Pamphlet*, No. 112.
30. TOVELL, R., and EDMONDSON, R. E.   *South Med. Jour.*, 1942, Jan., p. 25.
31. BURGER, O. K.   *Anesth. & Anal.*, 1937, July-Aug., p. 207.
32. SHACKELL, L., and BLUMENTHAL, R.   *Anesth. & Anal.*, 1934, July-Aug., p. 133.
33. ABRAHAMSON, D. I., *et al.*   *Anesthesiology*, 1941, Mar., p. 186.
34. WATERS, R. M.   *Lancet*, 1936, Sept. 12, p. 629.
35. WATERS, R. M., and SCHMIDT, S. R.   *Jour. Amer. Med. Ass.*, 1934, 31, p. 500.
36. THIENES, C. H., *et al.*   *Anesthesiology*, 1941, p. 611.
37. { ROBBINS, B. H.   *Ann. Surg.*, 1939, July, p. 84.
     ROBBINS, B. H., and BAXTER, J. H.   *Anesth. & Anal.*, 1940, July-Aug., p. 201.
38. MILOWSKI, J., and ROVENSTINE, E. A.   *Anesth. & Anal.*, 1942, Nov.-Dec., p. 353.
39. BURNSTEIN, G. L., *et al.*   *Anesthesiology*, 1940, Sept., p. 167.
40. GILLESPIE, N.   Wisconsin, U.S.A.   Personal Communication, 1947, Oct.
41. ROBBINS, B. H.   " Cyclopropane Anæsthesia," Baltimore, 1940.
42. GOULD, R. B.   *Anesth. & Anal.*, 1939, July-Aug., p. 226.
43. PRATT, C. L. G.   *Pro. Roy. Soc. Med.* (An. Sec.), 1938, Apr. 1.
44. { KEATING, V. J.   *Brit. Med. Jour.*, 1938, June 4, p. 1235.
     DALE, H. W. L.   *Brit. Med. Jour.*, 1938, June 11, p. 1286.
45. BONHAM, R. F.   *Anesth. & Anal.*, 1939, Sept.-Oct., p. 288.
46. BOURNE, W.   *Amer. Jour. Surg.*, 1936, Dec., p. 486.
47. GRIFFITHS, H. R.   *Canad. Med. Ass. Jour.*, 1934, Aug., p. 157.
48. BOGAN, J. B.   *Anesth. & Anal.*, 1936, Nov.-Dec., p. 275.
49. JONES, O. R., and BURFORD, G. E.   *Jour. Amer. Med. Ass.*, 1938, April 2, p. 1092.
50. *Rep. Counc. Pharm. & Chem. A.M.A. on Cyclopropane.*
51. WATERS, R. M.   *Brit. Med. Jour.*, 1936, Nov. 21, p. 1015.
52. NOSWORTHY, M. D.   *Pro. Roy. Soc. Med.* (An. Sec.), 1941, April 4.
53. HENDERSON, V. E.   *Jour. Pharmacol. & exp. Therap.*, 1938, Oct., p. 225.
54. KRANTZ, C., *et al.*   *Anesthesiology*, 1948, 9, p. 594.
55. KAYE, G.   *Med. Jour. Austral.*, 1951, April 21, p. 577.
56. *Lancet*, 1952, April-May.   Correspondence.

CHAPTER IV

CARBON DIOXIDE AND HELIUM

Two gases, which are not in themselves narcotics but are used in anæsthesia and medicine generally, must now be discussed. These are carbon dioxide and helium.

CARBON DIOXIDE

Carbon dioxide was distinguished from air by Van Helmont in the seventeenth century, and is a colourless gas with a rather pleasant pungent odour one and a half times heavier than air. It was liquefied by Faraday, and is now stored in cylinders (usually painted green in Great Britain) in the liquid state, a pressure of $52 \cdot 1$ atmospheres being necessary for liquefaction at $15°$ C.[1] Carbon dioxide does not support combustion or life, and until comparatively recently was regarded as a definite poison, although its use in rebreathing from closed inhalers has been practised for more than seventy years. In 1910 it was pointed out in Italy that carbon dioxide was a valuable respiratory stimulant in anæsthesia,[2] but it was not until about fifteen years later that the work of Haldane[3] and Yandell Henderson[4] placed the use of the gas upon a scientific basis.

Effects of Inhalation of Carbon Dioxide.

Man normally breathes air which contains about $0 \cdot 04$ per cent. carbon dioxide and at rest consumes about 7 litres of air per minute.[5] His arterial CO_2 tension is about 40 mm. Hg and the alveolar CO_2 level $5 \cdot 6$ per cent. If, however, 5 per cent. CO_2 is added to the inspired air, an immediate increase in the depth of respiration occurs and in about 20 seconds the volume per minute rises to about 30 litres. By this means the alveolar CO_2 level is kept constant. It is outside the scope of this book to go into all the complicated effects of carbon dioxide on human metabolism, but it may suffice to say that from the anæsthetist's point of view the other main action is an immediate rise in the blood pressure, due to a central action on the vasomotor centre causing constriction of the arterioles. This predominates over a slight local dilating effect which CO_2 shares with other metabolites.[6] The only demonstrable pathological changes following a two-hours' inhalation of 5 per cent. carbon dioxide are stated to be diuresis and increased acidity of the urine.[7] In submarine tests 2 per cent. CO_2 was well tolerated for a period of twenty-four hours. It will thus be seen that carbon dioxide is by far the most potent respiratory stimulant as well as being the natural activator of the respiratory centre.

The above remarks only apply to CO_2 mixtures of less than $5 \cdot 6$ per cent. Directly this concentration is exceeded, the most violent hyperpnœa cannot prevent the alveolar CO_2 level from rising. This in turn leads to a rise in arterial CO_2 tension and when this reaches 100 mm. Hg it causes extreme acidosis,[8] which may be indicated by pallor, low blood pressure, rapid pulse, muscular twitching and rapid irregular breathing. High percentages of carbon dioxide have been shown to produce general anæsthesia in animals,[10] but it is far too dangerous to attempt to utilize the property in man.

There is great variation in patients' reactions to carbon dioxide, but it can be said that acute infections, starvation, dehydration and very hot weather are all factors tending to greater susceptibility.[11]

Technique of Carbon Dioxide Administration

For the reasons stated it is never desirable to administer a mixture containing more than 5 per cent. carbon dioxide for any length of time. The balance is generally composed of air or oxygen. Ready-made mixtures (such as 5 per cent. CO_2 + 95 per cent. O_2) are available in cylinders (painted black, white and green), the name " **dicarbox** " being applied to the gases in Great Britain and " **carbogen** " in America. If such mixtures are available, they can be given conveniently from an intermittent flow apparatus.[22] As a general rule, however, it is preferable to use the pure gas from much smaller cylinders and subsequently to dilute it. For short inhalations, or where little space is available, a " sparklet " bulb B, in a special holder fitted with a needle valve A controlled by the key D, is useful. A rubber tube is attached to the outlet pipe F and can be led to the anæsthetic mask or bag (see Fig. 6). Various patterns of this device are obtainable with different sizes of " sparklet " bulbs, and since 25 g. of liquid carbon dioxide will provide about 12 litres of gas, quite a reasonable supply is available from the smallest sizes.

Two patterns of resuscitation apparatus giving a larger supply of the gas are also available. The first or " Carbetha " type was devised by Professor Haldane and automatically delivers any

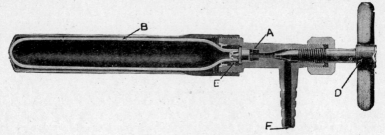

FIG. 6. Briggs' sparklet holder in part section.

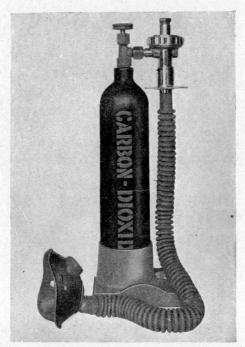

FIG 7. "Carbetha" CO_2—air apparatus.

desired percentage between 3 per cent. CO_2 + 97 per cent. air to 7 per cent. CO_2 + 93 per cent. air to a facepiece. The higher concentrations should not be used for more than brief periods. The mixture in use at the time is indicated on a calibrated dial[11] (Fig. 7).

The second apparatus was designed by Professor Yandell Henderson, and is simply a device for delivering a desired amount of pure carbon dioxide through a water sight-feed of the "depressed level" type (see Chapter V). An automatic "blow-off" prevents more than 2 litres of gas per minute being passed (Fig. 8).

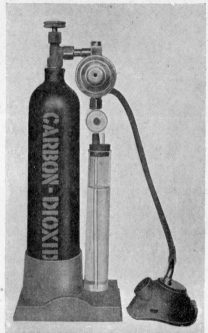

Fig. 8.   Yandell Henderson's CO_2 delivery apparatus.

For anæsthetic purposes, provision is made on most gas-oxygen machines for the administration of carbon dioxide. A common arrangement is to utilize one flow-meter for cyclopropane and CO_2 since the densities of the two gases are practically the same.

If no compressed gas is available, it is possible to use the patient's own carbon dioxide which is present to the extent of about $4 \cdot 1$ per cent. in his expired air. In the conscious patient, mouth breathing through a cardboard tube is possible. A more elaborate arrangement is shown in Fig. 9.[12]

We may now consider the conditions in anæsthetic and general practice in which the administration of carbon dioxide is beneficial.

(i) **During the Induction of Anæsthesia.**   The value of rebreathing in shortening the induction of anæsthesia has been recognized since the introduction of closed ether inhalers in 1863.   If a modern " closed-circuit " technique is being used, it is often advisable to cut out the absorber during the induction period.   In most cases the patient's own breath provides an adequate mixture, but sometimes, particularly in a person with a sensitive larynx, a small

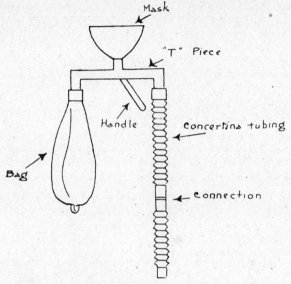

FIG. 9.   Apparatus for " auto-inhalational " CO_2 therapy.
(Harbord, *Brit. Jour. Anæsth.*)

amount of added carbon dioxide conduces to a smoother and quicker induction of ether anæsthesia owing to the increased pulmonary ventilation.   Again, carbon dioxide is useful in inducing anæsthesia in highly nervous patients.   These individuals often breathe deeply and quickly while they remain conscious and thus deplete the carbon dioxide in their blood, so producing acapnia, with consequent shallow breathing or even apnœa.   The judicious administration of carbon dioxide rapidly restores regular breathing. Induction of anæsthesia with intravenous thiopentone often causes a period of respiratory depression which can be shortened by adding CO_2 to the inhaled gases.   Further, if a closed inhaler is not available, the time of an open ether induction can be materially shortened by introducing carbon dioxide through a tube under the mask.

The passage of endotracheal tubes is facilitated by the administration of 5 per cent. CO_2 for a few breaths before intubation, as the lumen of the glottis is greatly increased.

(ii) **During the Maintenance of General Anæsthesia.** The addition of CO_2 to the respired gases is seldom indicated during the progress of general anæsthesia, apart from sudden emergencies. Indeed the percentage of the gas should usually be kept at the lowest possible level so that respiration will continue quietly entailing little exertion from the patient.

Carbon dioxide may possibly be of some service if severe shock should occur during the course of operation (q.v.), although this is stoutly denied by some American workers.

(iii) **After Anæsthesia.** Carbon dioxide is frequently given after long anæsthesia, to expand the bases of the lungs and to increase the rate of elimination of volatile anæsthetics. The subject is discussed under " pulmonary complications " (q.v.).

It has been shown by venous blood analysis that there is a fairly constant fall in the CO_2- content after prolonged anæsthesia, irrespective of the method used. There is thus direct theoretical confirmation of the desirability of CO_2 administration in such circumstances,[13] and it has been proved that a normal acid-base balance is restored more rapidly than if the patient is simply left to recover consciousness by himself.[4]

(iv) **In Persistent Hiccough.** Hiccough is a combined laryngo-diaphragmatic spasm, and it seems reasonable to expect that if the diaphragm could be made to contract regularly and strongly, as in hyperpnœa, its spasm would cease. This supposition is fully borne out in practice.[14] The author has given many patients with most distressing hiccough a CO_2 mixture to inhale, and in every case the spasm has ceased within twenty breaths. The cure may be permanent or a relapse may occur an hour or so later, but as many inhalations as necessary may be given without risk. This method of treatment is of especial value in the intractable type of hiccough sometimes occurring after high abdominal operations, particularly in cases of peritonitis or distension.[9]

(v) **After Tracheotomy.** It has been observed that certain patients, upon whom tracheotomy has been performed for chronic laryngeal obstruction, have stopped breathing and died for no adequate reason. This has usually occurred when the operation has been performed under local analgesia. Negus has pointed out that chronic laryngeal obstruction causes a rise in the CO_2 percentage in the alveolar air (normally $5 \cdot 6$ per cent.). When tracheotomy has been performed, this immediately falls to normal, so that the respiratory centre, which had previously been accustomed to respond to a higher CO_2 concentration in the blood than normal, no longer receives the necessary stimulus, with the result that breathing ceases from acapnia and the patient may die of anoxia.[15] Haldane has described a similar condition in animals when the CO_2 in the tissues and blood is greatly reduced by prolonged and forced artificial respiration. When this is stopped, apnœa occurs, and the animal may die from oxygen deprivation without attempting to draw a single breath. The conception of the condition immediately following tracheotomy suggests that a small percentage of CO_2 added to the air inspired through the tracheotomy tube will prevent apnœa while the respiratory centre is becoming used to the diminished CO_2 concentration in the blood, and it is recommended that this should be a routine proceeding in all cases in which the alveolar CO_2 before operation exceeds 6 per cent.

(vi) **Other Therapeutic Uses.** The use of carbon dioxide in *asphyxia neonatorum* is discussed in Chapter XXIII, whilst the employment of the gas in treating such conditions as *carbon monoxide poisoning*[16] is outside the scope of this book, although there is little doubt that an anæsthetist is really the most suitable person to treat such patients, as he is familiar with the problems involved, and has at hand the most effective apparatus for inhalation therapy.

It has also been shown that the inhalation of carbon dioxide-oxygen mixtures is of value in the treatment of *post-partum hæmorrhage* and *eclampsia*,[17] while it is also employed in *asthma*.[18]

In *psychiatric practice*, the inhalation of a CO_2-O_2 mixture to the stage of producing marked hyperpnœa and restlessness is sometimes used to induce " abreaction ".[23]

There is no doubt that, in the past, extravagant claims have been made for carbon dioxide and the gas has frequently been misused. It appears to the writer, however, that the categorical denial that it is ever beneficial (as has recently been made by some American workers) is equally unsound and should be resisted.

In conclusion it should be reiterated that during a normal inhalation anæsthesia, every effort should be made to **avoid CO_2 accumulation.** This is only too likely to occur when central and peripheral respiratory depressants are used and it is essential to maintain adequate ventilation by assisted or controlled respiration. On the whole it is safer to over-ventilate than to under-ventilate.[24]

HELIUM

Helium is present in air in minute amounts (1 in 185,000) and in natural gas up to 1·84 per cent. in Kansas, Oklahoma and Texas. It was first isolated in 1895 by Ramsey.

Properties. Helium is, with the exception of hydrogen, the lightest gas known, having a density of 0·138 compared with 1 for air. Unlike hydrogen, helium is not inflammable, a property which is beneficial both in aeronautical and anæsthetic practice. Helium will " thin " or lower the density of any gases with which it is mixed, except pure hydrogen, and the resulting mixture can be breathed through a constricted aperture in greater volume and with less effort by the patient. The law governing these conditions states that the velocity of passage of a gas through a small orifice is inversely proportional to the square root of the density of the gas. For example, if the nitrogen in atmospheric air (79 per cent.) be replaced by helium, the artificial atmosphere so created is only one-third as heavy as air, and can be breathed through narrow apertures twice as easily.[19]

Technique of Administration. Helium can be obtained in cylinders and can be added to the anæsthetic mixture by means of a flow-meter. If the nitrous oxide flow-meter is used the reading should be multiplied by 3·3. The closed-circuit method should always be used and even then great care is necessary to avoid leakage.[20]

Indications. Helium is not a panacea for respiratory obstruction, but may be of great temporary value before the cause can be removed. The gas may be used during intrabronchial anæsthesia (q.v.) if breathing is laboured. The addition of helium to cyclo-propane-oxygen mixtures with a view to preventing pulmonary collapse is referred to under cyclopropane. It is possible to use this 3-gas mixture in such proportions that it is non-inflammable. It was thought that this might be useful in thoracic surgery if the diathermy was to be used. Unfortunately the high percentage of helium tends towards light anæsthesia and anoxia. The gas has also been used therapeutically in such conditions as asthma and pneumonia.[21]

References

1.   HEWER, C. L.   *St. Bart's Hosp. Jour.*, 1927, April.
2.   LEVI, E.   *Acad. med. fis.*, 1910, March 16.
3.   HALDANE, J. S.   *Pro. Roy. Soc. Med.* (An. Sec.), 1926, July 13.
4.   HENDERSON, Y.   *Brit. Med. Jour.*, 1925, Dec. 19.
5.   DAVIES, H. W.   *Brit. Jour. Anæsth.*, **4**, p. 148.
6.   BOSTON, F. K.   *Brit. Jour. Anæsth.*, 1939, Dec., p. 13.

7. MEAKINS, J. C., and DAVIES, H. W. " Respiratory Function in Disease," 1925, p. 57.
8. ORTON, R. H. *Pro. Austral. Soc. Anœsth.*, 1951, Oct. 30.
9. HEWER, C. L. *Clin. Jour.*, 1927, July 20, p. 344.
10. LEAKE, C. D., and WATERS, R. M. *Jour. Pharm. & Exp. Ther.*, **33**, 1928, p. 280.
11. WATERS, R. M. *New Orleans Med. and Surg. Jour.*, 1937, Oct. 3, p. 220.
12. HARBORD, R. P. *Brit. Jour. Anœsth.*, 1939, Dec., p. 13.
13. MINNITT, R. J. *Pro. Roy. Soc. Med.* (An. Sec.), 1939, Feb. 2.
14. HEWER, C. L. *China Med. Jour.*, 1927, Oct., p. 854.
15. NEGUS, V. E. *Ann. Otol. Rhinol. and Laryngol.*, 1938, Sept., p. 608.
16. FOG, M., and STÜRUP, G. *Ugeskrift. f. Laeger*, 1934, Dec. 6, p. 1344.
17. MCCORMACK, R. *Anesth. & Anal.*, 1934, Sept.-Oct., p, 213.
18. FARAGO, P. *Zeitschrift f. der gesammte Exper. Med.*, 1933, Oct. 21.
19. SYKES, W. S., and LAWRENCE, R. C. *Brit. Med. Jour.*, 1938, Aug. 27, p. 448.
20. EVERSOLE, H. H. *Jour. Amer. Med. Ass.*, 1938, Mar. 19, p. 878.
21. SISE, L. F. *Amer. Jour. Surg.*, 1936, Dec., p. 423.
22. DEACON, J. N. *Brit. Med. Jour.*, 1936, June 13, p. 1210.
23. MILLIGAN, W. L. *Brit. Med. Jour.*, 1951, June 23, p. 1426.
24. ORTON, R. H. *Anœsthesia*, 1952, Oct., p. 211.

CHAPTER V

MODERN APPARATUS FOR THE ADMINISTRATION OF THE "GAS" ANÆSTHETICS

WHATEVER type of apparatus is employed, a gas-tight **face-piece** is essential. In the past these components left a good deal to be desired, but there are some modern types which are anatomically correct and can be moulded to fit exceptional face contours. Face-pieces should never be sterilized in carbolic or cresol solutions or

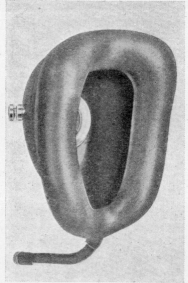

M.I.E LTD.

Fig. 10. Modern facepiece with studs for harness (McKesson).

severe burns may result.[1] A satisfactory method of sterilization is described on p. 352. Alternatively the face-pieces can be washed after use and stored in a 1 in 2,000 solution of biniodide of mercury.

For long operations it is usual to keep the face-piece in position by some retainer such as Clausen's **harness**. This useful device should *not* be interleaved with canvas as has been done by some manufacturers as this destroys the elasticity of the rubber. Furthermore the least possible tension to produce a gas-tight fit should be used and the face-piece must not be allowed to press on the eyelids through maladjustment or incorrect size. Failure to observe these elementary points can give rise to lowered intraocular tension which may last for some time (see Chapter XXV).

Considerable thought has been expended upon the correct shape for pharyngeal **airways.** Two satisfactory patterns, one of metal and one of rubber, are illustrated. If an airway is of correct shape

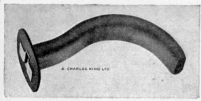
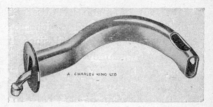

Fig. 11. Rubber airway (Guedel's).   Fig. 12. Metal airway (Waters').

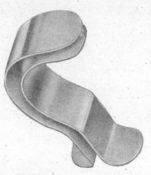

M.I.E LTD.

Fig. 13. Double channel plastic airway.

and size it causes no retching in a conscious patient. This test shows up the deficiencies of many patterns now in use. The main disadvantage of the types shown is the impossibility of cleaning them satisfactorily after use. The modification of removing most of one side of the metal airway enables the inside to be inspected and cleaned with a small brush.[2] This idea has been carried even further in an open-sided double channel airway made of plastic material.

Modern "gas-oxygen" apparatus can be divided into three groups : the continuous flow, the intermittent flow and the closed circuit types, and it will be convenient to consider these separately.

Continuous Flow Machines

The continuous flow machines deliver the mixed gases at a constant rate, and various devices are used to measure the volume of each gas passing in unit time. The flow-meters employed are :

(i) The **Bubble Type,** in which a rough calculation of the rate of flow can be made by observation of the number of holes in a vertical tube through which the gas is bubbling under water. This principle has been used since 1912,[3] and was incorporated in the early "Gwathmey" apparatus. In order to avoid undue disturbance of the water when using large gas flows, "by-pass" taps can be arranged to short-circuit about four-fifths of the gas or the ends of the tubes can be bent back to end above the surface of the water. This type of flow-meter is so inaccurate that it is now obsolete.

(ii) The **Constant Orifice Type.** (a) **Water depression meters.**
If a gas is flowing through a tube AE (Fig. 14) and meets with a

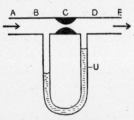

FIG. 14. Principle of water depression flow-meter (after Pask).

constriction at C, the pressure at the point B will be greater than that at D. This difference in pressure can be measured by the manometer U and bears a definite relation to the rate at which the gas is flowing.[4] Actually the flow varies as the square root of the pressure drop (see Torricelli's equation below) and this involves the "square root scale" in which the figures for the small flows are closer together than those for large flows. This type of scale is illustrated in Fig. 16 and the crowding of figures at the lower end is a definite disadvantage.

In practice, the gas is usually led into the top of a vertical tube Z standing in a glass water jar X and escapes through a constricted orifice C situated above the surface of the water (Fig. 15). The level inside the tube will be lowered in proportion to the square of the rate of gas flow. A float inside the tube facilitates the level reading, and if a calibrated scale be placed behind, the gas flow can be read off in litres per minute. One type of " Foregger " apparatus operates on this principle and is extremely accurate.

The foregoing " wet " types of flow-meters are particularly useful when employing the inflammable gases in dry climates, as sufficient

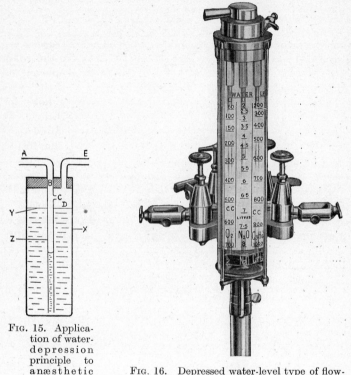

FIG. 15. Application of water-depression principle to anæsthetic practice(after Pask).

FIG. 16. Depressed water-level type of flow-meter for three gases. The "square-root scale " can be seen (Foregger).

moistening occurs to reduce the possibility of explosion from static sparks (see Chapter IX).

(*b*) **Gauge type Flow-meters.** The pressure-drop can also be measured by means of a bourdon type gauge calibrated directly in litres per minute. These are easy to read and have been fitted at times to certain types of Heidbrink, Foregger and Coxeter machines. The gauge actually measures the pressure built up behind a very narrow orifice and under certain conditions may prove misleading.

For example, if the orifice is completely blocked up the gauge will register the reduced pressure of the cylinder connected to it although no gas is actually flowing. The principle of the bourdon gauge is that a length of thin curved metal tubing of oval cross-section and closed at one end tends to straighten out if internal pressure is applied to it. This slight movement is magnified by a ratchet mechanism to a lever moving over a dial. Although the use of such gauges enables a pleasing " dashboard " to be used, the practice cannot be recommended for the reason already given, and they must be regarded as unsuitable for anæsthetic purposes.

The flow of gases through small apertures is determined by Torricelli's equation $Q = A.C.\sqrt{2gh}$ where

    Q is Flow per second.
    A is Area of Orifice.
    C is Coefficient of flow efficiency.
    g is force of gravity.
    h is pressure drop through orifice.

We have seen that in the constant orifice or water-depression flow-meter the *pressure drop* is measured. We can, however, measure the *flow* by varying the size of the orifice, and on referring to the equation above it will be seen that a direct relation exists so that a linear scale is possible.[5]

(iii) The **Bobbin or Variable Orifice Type.** The simplest form of " dry " flow-meter is that which employs a bobbin inside a transparent tube, the height of the bobbin being proportional to the gas flow. Here, direct readings can be taken on a scale. Two principles can be employed to effect this result. Firstly, a tube of uniform bore perforated with holes is placed inside a second transparent tube. Gas entering the inner tube at the bottom pushes up a bobbin and escapes through the holes below it into the outer tube. The greater the gas flow, the larger the number of holes required for its escape, and consequently the higher is the bobbin. Coxeter's dry flow-meter, as used in the standard E.M.S. trolley during the last war is constructed on this principle, as are the units incorporated in one type of McKesson apparatus (see Figs. 17 and 18). In the latter case, however, a sort of opaque inverted test tube " rides " the gas flow instead of an actual bobbin.

Secondly, the same result can be obtained by using a single tapered tube, the small bore end being at the bottom. If gas is led into this tube below a bobbin, the latter will rise proportionally to the flow and the gas will escape *round* the bobbin and can be led away from the top of the tube. By referring to Torricelli's equation (given above) it will be realized that the flow rate varies directly with the annular space between the periphery of the bobbin and the wall of the tapered tube so that a linear scale can be adopted. This is clearly seen in Fig. 19 and is a definite advantage over the

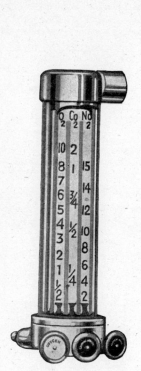

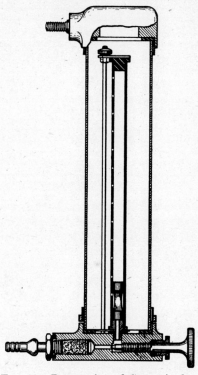

Fig. 17. Coxeter's 3-gas dry flow-meter unit.

FIG. 18. Part-section of Coxeter's dry flow-meter to show principle (A. C. King).

square root scale of constant orifice flow-meters. The bobbins are, in actual practice, fitted into their tubes and the scales are then calibrated individually. At high rates of flow the density of the gas is the predominant factor, but at low rates the viscosity must also be taken into account. The disadvantage of the original bobbins made of vulcanite or similar material was that wear soon occurred with consequent inaccuracy. The modern " Rotameter " bobbins are made of duralumin with diagonal slots so that they rotate in use and do not touch the walls of the tube. The resulting lack of friction eliminates wear and renders great accuracy possible. The indication is said to be correct to within ±2 per cent. The Rotameter principle has been used commercially for measuring gases such as ammonia for many years and was first adopted for anæsthetic gases in Great Britain in 1937 by R. Salt. In some of the latest types of apparatus the oxygen Rotameter tube has a double taper giving fine graduations (100 c.cm. divisions) over the lower half of the scale for use with a closed circuit and a coarse scale (1000 c.cm. divisions) over the upper half when large flows are required. This type of dry flow-meter is deservedly becoming very popular in the United Kingdom and is incorporated into many standard gas-oxygen machines. They must be mounted vertically as any deviation results in inaccuracy. In the "Kinetometer" flow-meter fitted to some Heidbrink models the actual bobbins are hidden, the flow being indicated by attached rods sliding against a scale (Fig. 21). The "Connell" apparatus employs two stainless steel balls instead of a bobbin, the reading being taken from the point of contact between the balls.

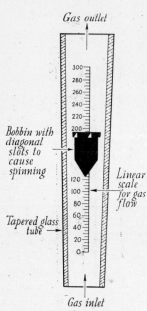

Fig. 19. Diagram showing principle of "Rotameter" (adapted from *Anesthesiology*).

The correct functioning of all types of continuous-flow apparatus depends upon a perfectly steady delivery of the gases. The complete dryness of modern nitrous oxide has eliminated irregular gas flow due to freezing, but it is desirable to incorporate a **reducing valve** between the cylinder and the fine adjustment control for all gases except cyclopropane. A suitable reduction is from cylinder pressure to 10 lb. reduced pressure. This is considerably increased for intermittent-flow apparatus. Reducing valves are a potential source of danger and are discussed more fully in Chapter IX.

If it is intended to use ether or trichlorethylene as the maintenance agent, an **oxygen injector** unit can be interposed between the flow-meters and the trichlorethylene bottle as shown in Fig. 22. Induction of anæsthesia is carried out in the normal way with nitrous oxide, oxygen and ether. The flow-meter controls are then shut and the injector valve A opened until the gauge B indicates

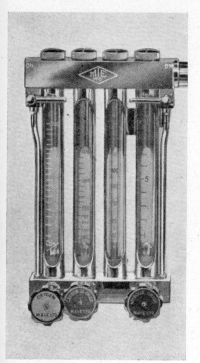

M.I.E LTD.

Fig. 20. " Rotameter " dry flow-meter unit for 4 gases with by- pass taps for O_2 and N_2O.

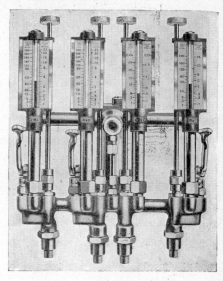

Fig. 21. " Kinetometer " dry flow-meters for four gases (Heidbrink). Fine-adjustment controls at top of apparatus with emer- gency large-volume valves worked by levers below the meters.

an oxygen flow of $1\frac{1}{2}$ to 2 litres per minute. If the disc D is set at 40 per cent. oxygen, atmospheric air is " entrained " so that the resulting mixture will contain 60 per cent. air and 40 per cent. oxygen, and this can be used to vaporize ether or trichlorethylene. Considerable saving in nitrous oxide can thus be effected.[16]

All continuous-flow machines incorporate an arrangement for **partial rebreathing,** the necessary bag usually being situated on the apparatus and connected to the face-piece by unkinkable " concertina " rubber tubing. The size of this bag must be lessened in the case of children or other patients with a diminished respiratory exchange. Partial rebreathing is beneficial in that it conserves respiratory heat and moisture, but the CO_2 concentration is raised so that the depth of breathing is increased. It should be noted that there is a " critical flow " for the mixed gases of about 5 litres per minute. This must always be exceeded so that CO_2 equilibrium may be maintained. If the combined gas flow falls below the critical level, a dangerous accumulation of CO_2 may occur.[8]

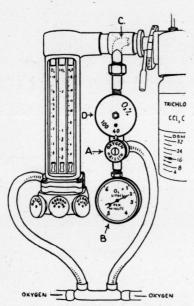

Fig. 22. Oxygen injector interposed between flow-meter and trichlorethylene vaporizer of continuous-flow apparatus. (J. Ives, from *The Lancet.*)

The **expiratory valve** should be situated as close to the face-piece as possible to eliminate dead space. In the past these valves were often flimsy and tended to chatter.

In hospital practice, continuous-flow gas-oxygen apparatus is frequently combined with an anæsthetic trolley, thus saving considerable room.

The Intermittent-Flow Type

This type of apparatus only delivers the gases during the patient's inspirations, the flow ceasing during expiration. The apparatus devised in 1892 by the late Sir F. Hewitt was the forerunner of the highly efficient machines of this type in use at the present time.

The principle on which intermittent-flow machines work is by drawing the gases from two bags at equal pressure through a mixing valve graduated in percentages. The gas supplies are arranged to cut off automatically when the bags reach a certain pressure, which can be varied to suit individual conditions. The principle upon which two common types of cut-off work is shown in the appended diagrams. From the mixing chamber a flexible hose runs to the facepiece with its expiratory valve.

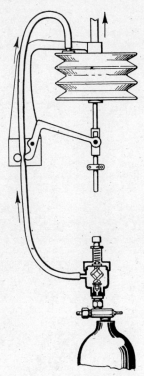

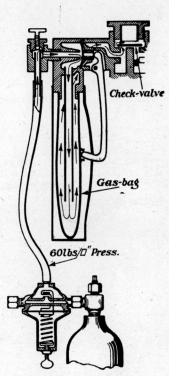

FIG. 23. Diagram illustrating principle of "Walton" cut-off (A. C. King).

FIG. 24. Diagram illustrating principle of "McKesson" cut-off (A. C. King).

The main advantage of this type of apparatus lies in its simplicity of operation. Only one lever is required to control the mixture and one for the pressure. Furthermore, increase of pressure does not upset the mixture, rendering the machine very suitable for continuous nasal gas-oxygen in dentistry. When set to work at a low pressure, the gas flow will cease when the mask is lifted from the face so that this type of apparatus can be used for self-administration as in obstetrics (q.v.). One of the simplest practical intermittent-flow machines is the " Portanaest " illustrated. No rebreathing normally takes place but a rebreathing bag and trichlorethylene vaporizer can be added for long administrations. An " emergency oxygen button " between the gauges enables the lungs to be inflated with oxygen instantly, whatever the setting of the mixture control.

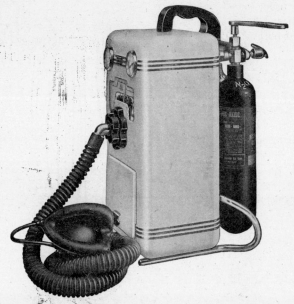

FIG. 25.   Simple intermittent-flow machine for nitrous oxide—oxygen and nitrous oxide—air. (" Portanaest.") The large mixture control and small pressure control surround the exit tube.

The McKesson Model G is of somewhat similar design[9] while the McKesson " Nargraf " has the additional feature of adjustable rebreathing under any desired pressure. This is effected by using a spring-loaded bellows instead of a rebreathing bag.[5] The key adjusting the tension of the spring can be seen in the top right-hand corner of Fig. 31.

Some types of intermittent-flow apparatus with short delivery tubes supply the mixed gases at a temperature lower than that of the atmosphere and it has been shown that a moderate degree of heating enables a slightly higher percentage of oxygen to be used, besides diminishing the heat-loss of the patient.[17] If the usual length of corrugated rubber tubing is used with partial rebreathing, the gases emerge at the facepiece practically at room temperature and no further heating is necessary.

The size of the rebreathing bag is of considerable importance on intermittent-flow machines, as if it is too large and a low pressure is being used, the CO_2 concentration may rise to a dangerous level.[8]

For hospital work intermittent-flow apparatus may be enclosed and incorporated with an anæsthetic trolley.

The Closed Circuit Principle

Since anæsthetic gases are exhaled unchanged from the lungs, it follows that the same gas can be used over and over again. John Snow was probably the first person to use a closed-circuit apparatus for anæsthetizing animals (in 1850). He employed caustic potash to absorb the carbon dioxide.[10] The total rebreathing technique was not adopted until recently owing to a persistent theory that exhaled air contained some poisonous substance. The mythical body was called " anthropotoxin " and it was not until 1923 that the existence of any such toxin was finally disproved.[11] An excellent account of the history of carbon dioxide absorption has been written by R. Waters.[12]

The subjoined diagram illustrates the principle of the method. The rubber bag contains the gas-oxygen mixture and " to and

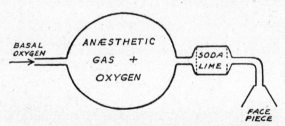

Fig. 26. Diagram showing principle of total rebreathing with carbon dioxide absorption (" to and fro " system).

fro " breathing takes place through a metal chamber containing granulated soda-lime to absorb the carbon dioxide. Theoretically, only just sufficient oxygen for the metabolic rate of the patient (usually called the " basal oxygen flow ") need be added to maintain anæsthesia. In practice, however, small quantities of gas must be added as well in order to compensate for that lost (1) by leakage at joints, (2) by diffusion through the rubber rebreathing bag, (3) by elimination through the skin, and (4) by loss from the surface of the operation wound.[13] It will be remembered that during the induction of narcosis the anæsthetic saturation of the brain is higher than that of the tissues owing to the large carotid circulation, and it may be some little time before equilibrium is established.   During this period of redistribution some fresh anæsthetic gas must be added or the cerebral saturation will fall.

The chief *advantages* of the closed circuit method are :

(*a*) Respiratory heat loss is diminished.

(*b*) Respiratory water-vapour loss is diminished.[14]

These are both of particular importance in endotracheal anæsthesia where the normal air conditioning mechanism of the nose is by-passed.

(*c*) No anæsthetic vapours escape into the atmosphere of the operating theatre, thereby avoiding inhalation by the surgical team and diminishing the risk of explosion.

(*d*) Great economy in gas consumption is possible.[15] For example, it has been estimated that an average consumption with partial rebreathing is about 66 gallons N_2O per hour and 13 gallons O_2. With the absorption technique the rate falls to about $6 \cdot 6$ gallons N_2O and $3 \cdot 3$ gallons O_2 per hour.[16] If expensive gases such as cyclopropane are used total rebreathing is essential.

(*e*) The quiet respiration calls for less exertion on the part of the patient and may facilitate the operative procedure.

(*f*) The nitrogen in the alveolar air is not diminished to any great extent. With a semi-closed circuit and partial rebreathing, it is estimated that all the nitrogen is lost in about an hour.[18] In such a case, if any bronchi or bronchioles are blocked by secretion at the end of operation the gases distal to the block will be absorbed rapidly and an area of atelectasis will develop.

There are two main *techniques* in use at the present time.

The " To and Fro " System

The simplest method of obtaining total rebreathing is to interpose a soda-lime filter between a facepiece and a rebreathing bag and to obtain the necessary gases from a continuous-flow gas-oxygen apparatus equipped with really accurate flow-meters capable of dealing with small flows. The arrangement is, in fact, exactly the same as in the explanatory diagram (Fig. 26), except that the gas inlet should be on the patient's side of the filter in order to effect mixture changes rapidly. This system has the merits of simplicity and efficiency and it will be noticed that no valves are required and that both inspiratory and expiratory gases pass through the filter. It is possible to arrange a cut-out for the " to and fro " type of absorber,[19] but this adds to the complication.

Waters has stressed the importance of correct design and size for the filter.[20] It has been found that the available air space inside the filter (i.e. the inter- and intra-granular space) should equal the patient's tidal air (400 to 500 c.cm.) for maximum efficiency. A metal canister 13 cm. long and 8 cm. in diameter (Fig. 27) accommodates about 500 g. of 4 to 8 mesh soda-lime. Its total volume is

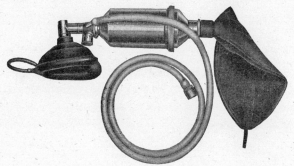

Fig. 27. Waters " to and fro " absorption apparatus.

about 650 c.cm. and its combined inter- and intra-granular air space is just over 400 c.cm. This size is therefore suitable for adult patients.[21] With this technique the average CO_2 concentration in the rebreathing bag is 0 per cent. to 0·02 per cent., at the lips 2·5 per cent. to 4 per cent., and in the pharynx 3·5 per cent. to 6 per cent.[22] The " to and fro " system has four disadvantages. Firstly, it necessitates the presence of a cumbersome and heavy canister adjacent to the facepiece with consequent difficulty in maintaining the essential gas-tight contact. This can be mitigated by interposing a short length of corrugated rubber tubing between the canister and the facepiece although this increases the dead space. About 8 oz. of weight can be saved by substituting a rubber canister for a metal one.[23] In the second place, the inspired gases may become undesirably hot from the chemical action of the CO_2 on the soda-lime. It has been shown that at the point of maximum reaction the temperature may reach 40° C. (104° F.) and, in the case of unsuitable soda-lime, nearly 180° F.[24] As mentioned later, if gases are inhaled at much above body-temperature, excessive sweating and capillary engorgement will ensue. During the late war it was found that the " to and fro " absorption technique should definitely be avoided in tropical conditions.[25] Thirdly, any liquid adjuvant such as chloroform or ether has to be vaporized solely by the basal oxygen feed so that it may be difficult to secure an adequate vapour concentration. Fourthly, it is difficult to avoid the inhalation of irritating dust from the soda-lime, especially in the case of some wartime products.

In order to avoid these drawbacks, the " circle " system was introduced.

The " Circle " System

If the CO_2 absorber is incorporated in the gas-oxygen apparatus it will be clear that a single flexible tube to the facepiece would introduce an inadmissible dead-space. Two tubes are therefore used with suitable valves so that the patient inspires through one

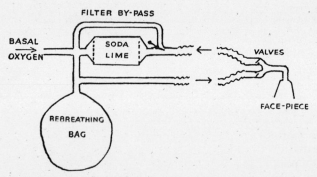

FIG. 28. Diagram to illustrate principle of total rebreathing with filter remote from patient (" circle " system).

tube and expires through the other. The two phases of respiration are therefore kept quite distinct and are separated by the valves. For this reason the term " two-phase " system was used to denote the technique, but to avoid ambiguity the alternative description " circle " system will be used in this book. In the circuit illustrated in the diagram it will be seen that the gases pass through the absorber once only per respiration. A two-way flow can, however,

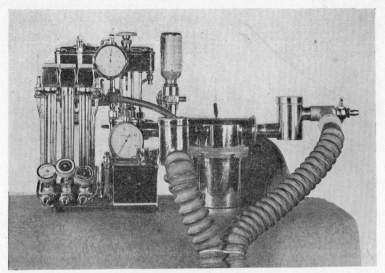

FIG. 29. Author's portable continuous-flow apparatus arranged for circle absorption technique. Di-ethyl and di-vinyl ether can be added by drip-feed vaporizers in the respiratory circuit, the trichlorethylene bottle being out of sight behind the triple rotameters. The upper dial is a pulse timer, the lower one indicating the pressure in the respiratory circuit.

be arranged as in Mushin's absorber,[26] and it is claimed to be more efficient than one-way absorption[27] although this is contrary to previously published work.[28] The "circle" system can be used with a continuous or an intermittent-flow apparatus. In the former case extreme portability and compactness are possible, as illustrated in Fig. 29.

A by-pass can easily be arranged so that the absorber can be cut out of the circuit at will. This facilitates recharging the canister with fresh soda-lime during the course of an operation. There is much less risk of small particles of alkali being inhaled than in the "to and fro" system as deposition in the tubing tends to occur. The only disadvantage of the "circle" system is a slight increased resistance to respiration on account of the tubing and uni-directional valves. This can be minimized by carefully designed apparatus,[28] and need not exceed 2 to 4 mm. H_2O.[26] Although the valves are, for convenience, usually situated on the apparatus, and are of the gravity type, they should really be close to the facepiece so that the expansion of the long corrugated rubber tubing on expiration does not increase the dead space and cause incomplete CO_2 absorption.[29] Such an arrangement is actually used in the " Alfo-Blease " apparatus.

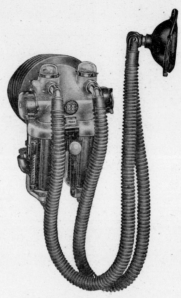

Fig. 30. Mushin's absorber showing luminous knob which moves up and down with the concertina-type breathing bag at the back. The uni-directional valves are situated under the glass domes at the top.

Carbon Dioxide Absorbents

With the exception of the " Primrose " apparatus which makes use of a strong **caustic soda** solution,[30] practically all machines depend upon **soda-lime** for the absorption of CO_2. This substance is important. The ordinary commercial product is unsuitable as it contains dust which may percolate through the gauze mesh of the filter and prove highly irritating. Furthermore, commercial soda-lime is hygroscopic and produces an undesirable drying of the inhaled gases. A special " non-hygroscopic " brand is now obtainable, consisting of firm granules free from dust. These granules should not be larger than 4 to 8 mesh, or " channelling " with inefficient absorption may occur. This means that the

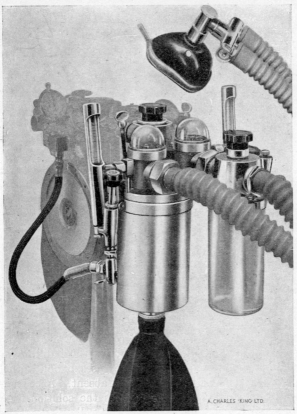

FIG. 31. Intermittent-flow apparatus (McKesson) arranged for circle technique, with Evans's absorber. The uni-directional valves are beneath the glass domes.

smallest granules will not pass a standard screen of 8 apertures to the inch and that the largest will just pass a screen of 4 apertures to the inch. Channelling is particularly likely to occur with horizontal filters, as the soda-lime granules tend to subside by gravity and allow the gases a less resistant channel above them. The canister should therefore be mounted vertically if at all possible.[31] The best soda-lime for anæsthetic purposes is a mixture of from 65 per cent. to 95 per cent. calcium hydroxide and 5 per cent. sodium hydroxide. A small amount of hardening matter (mostly silicates) is added to increase resistance to powdering and the optimum moisture content is from 14 per cent. to 19 per cent.[20] Under average conditions 1 g. of good soda-lime absorbs about 88 c.cm. CO_2. When the patient's respiration becomes progressively

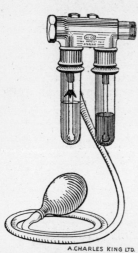

deeper and the pressure rises, the soda-lime has become exhausted and should be changed. Some brands, e.g. " catalytic protosorb " and " sofnolite ", are now coloured green and change to brown when inactive. The American product " dioxorb " changes from pink to yellow as its activity diminishes, while one brand of Wilson soda-lime (" sodasorb " in America) changes from white to violet. If the absorber is constructed of glass or a transparent plastic a visible indication is thus given when the material needs renewing. A more accurate test is to use an indicating solution such as bromcresol purple, buffered with calcium carbonate. A tester, such as that shown in Fig. 32 can be plugged into the circuit on the inspiratory side of the apparatus. One glass tube contains water to trap particles of soda-lime and the other contains the indicator. If the rubber bulb is compressed, some of the gases bubble through the indicator, which remains purple if CO_2 is absent. A concentration of 1·2 per cent. to 1·7 per cent. causes the solution to become colourless, while 2 per cent. is shown by a yellow coloration.[32]

FIG. 32. Carbon-dioxide detector (Heidbrink).

When in use, soda-lime granules gradually acquire a surface coat of sodium carbonate which eventually surrounds completely the remaining alkali within the granules. If " rested ", these change position to some extent, so that a further period of activity can be obtained. Furthermore, actual regeneration of sodium hydroxide occurs as the less active calcium hydroxide which remains, reacts with the sodium carbonate.[21] Thus, even if large absorbers are used, they should always be changed at the end of each case. This practice also allows for cooling off.[33]

A closed-circuit technique is contra-indicated if trichlorethylene is being used as an adjuvant as it is possible for a chemical reaction to take place between this drug and hot soda-lime with the production of toxic substances.[24] (See Chapter VII.) Some

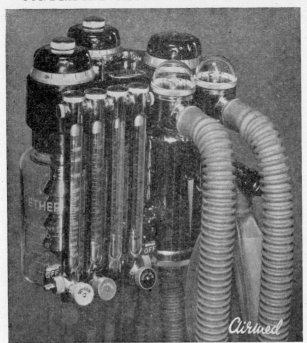

FIG. 33. Head of Marrett's apparatus with automatic device preventing trichlorethylene control (top middle) and absorber control (top right) from being turned on simultaneously.

machines, such as Marrett's, incorporate an automatic device which mechanically prevents this combination.

As a rule the closed-circuit technique should also be avoided if rectal paraldehyde has been used as a basal narcotic. This drug is partly excreted through the lungs and with total rebreathing a concentration can be built up which is so irritating to the respiratory passages that coughing or laryngospasm may occur.

Chloroform vapour can be added to the gases of a closed circuit if indicated as although some carbon monoxide can be formed $(CHCl_3 + 3 NaOH \rightarrow 3 NaCl + CO + 2 H_2O)$ its volume is so small that it can be regarded as innocuous.[34]

A new absorbent is known as " **baralyme** ", and consists of 80 per cent. calcium hydroxide and 20 per cent. barium hydroxide with no inert binder. The advantages claimed for this product over soda-lime are (1) greater efficiency, (2) no periods for recuperation are necessary, (3) it is less caustic, and (4) less heat generation.[35]

Since the soda-lime canister may be used for several cases without change of contents the possibility of cross-infection has been raised. Stringent tests with bacterial cultures have been made with negative results and the opinion has been expressed that " there is certainly no possibility of bacteria being transferred from one patient to another by contamination of the lime in the canister.[36] As a precaution, however, a water-trap can be used on the expiratory side of a closed-circuit apparatus.[37]

Practically every variety of gas-oxygen apparatus embodies means for adding adjustable amounts of ether and chloroform or tri-chlorethylene vapour to the mixed gases, and these features are considered in Chapter VI.

Luminous Indicators

Anæsthetics occasionally must be administered in complete darkness, e.g. for screening fractures, and it is most desirable that the essential indicators should be visible. Already a luminous plaque is often fixed behind the gas flow-meters and the knob on the rebreather control of the Mushin absorber is also visible in the dark. The practicability of using fluorescent colours for the various gas controls has been demonstrated[38] and some interesting developments will probably figure on future types of apparatus.

Gas Cylinders

The large amount of space taken up by the gas and oxygen **cylinders** can be avoided in hospitals by the use of large batteries of cylinders situated in some central room from which pipe lines are laid to each operating theatre. This arrangement also avoids the necessity for changing cylinders between operations and has been adopted in many hospitals in America with considerable economy in operation.[20] In this country an excellent example is provided in the surgical block of St. Bartholomew's Hospital.

Until recently anæsthetic gases have been compressed into heavy carbon-steel cylinders, but considerable research work has been directed towards the production of lighter cylinders to improve portability. For example, Vickers-Armstrong Ltd., under the direction of Dr. C. M. Walter, have produced a nickel-chromium-molybdenum steel of great strength known as " Vibrac ". In spite of an extremely thin wall, a test cylinder did not rupture until the enormous pressure of 10,500 lb. per square inch was attained.   In the case of nitrous oxide, however, the gas is liquefied, and it is impracticable to use pressures exceeding 650 lb. per square inch. Oxygen can be compressed to any reasonable figure, but it is found that after 2,000 lb. per square inch spontaneous fires starting in washers or other fittings are more likely to occur. It is probable, therefore, that the new steels will be used to ensure lightness rather than to employ fantastic pressures for anæsthetic gases.   The Home Office has recently permitted an increased cylinder pressure for oxygen and other permanent gases, the maximum being now 1,980 lb. per square inch.   The advantages of decreasing the weight of oxygen cylinders for such uses as mountaineering or high-altitude aviation can, of course, hardly be over-estimated.[39]

The need for an **international colour code** for anæsthetic gases has been obvious since fatal mistakes occurred during the second World War when British Army anæsthetists used American machines and vice-versa. Since 1943, the Council of the Association of Anæsthetists of Great Britain and Ireland has tried to achieve this end in conjunction with various other organizations, and at last an international code has been agreed and will be implemented in stages.   At the time of writing the actual dates are uncertain, except for nitrous oxide which began to be changed on August 1st, 1952.   The new code together with the existing national colour schemes adopted by the British Standard Specification No. 349— 1932 and the National Bureau of Standards U.S. Dept. of Commerce, 1941, are as follows :

Gas	Existing British Cylinder Colour Code	Existing American Cylinder Colour Code	Agreed International Cylinder Colour Code	Approximate Full Cylinder Pressure (lb. per sq. in.).
Carbon dioxide	Green	Grey	Dark Grey	835
Cyclopropane	Aluminium and red	Orange	Orange	75
Ethylene	Violet and red	Red	Violet	1250
Helium	Brown	Brown	Brown	1500
Nitrous oxide	Black	Blue	Blue	650
Oxygen	Black and white (Commercial cylinder, Black)	Green	White top, Black body	1980

The name of the gas or its chemical symbol must also be painted on the shoulder of the cylinder.

Non-interchangeable couplings usually of the Schrader type, are already standardized on modern British anæsthetic apparatus, but the weak point is the cylinder yoke fitting. A long-term international policy has also been agreed to make these fool proof by means of pins fixed in specified positions on the yokes matching with holes in each cylinder valve. The implementation of this scheme will take time, but when achieved it will be physically impossible to attach cylinders containing a different gas to the corresponding yoke.[41]

As an interim precaution one manufacturing firm has developed an ingenious warning device. If nitrous oxide or carbon dioxide is wrongly piped to an oxygen flow-meter and the gas is turned on, dark liquid is drawn off the indicating chamber and the words " wrong gas " become visible. Similarly if carbon dioxide is connected to the nitrous oxide flow-meter the dark blue liquid in the second indicator changes to a transparent yellow through which the words " wrong gas " appear.

From a perusal of the foregoing chapter, it will be realized that modern anæsthetic apparatus has reached a high standard of mechanical excellence. The most likely danger to arise is the failure of the oxygen supply from emptying of cylinders or other cause. If the anæsthetist does not immediately notice the fact, anoxia will occur. Many reducing valves hum or chatter when the cylinder pressure falls to that of the reduced pressure and audible warning is thus given some minutes before the supply fails. A fitting has been introduced which definitely causes a loud whistle to sound under such circumstances.[40]

In conclusion it should not be forgotten that the skill of the workman is more important than the design of his tools. In other words, a competent anæsthetist should be able to obtain excellent results from any efficient apparatus and should not be dependent upon personal preferences.

References

1. HERWICK, R. P., and TREWEEK, D. N.   *Jour. Amer. Med. Ass.*, 1933, **100**, p. 407.
2. CLUTTON-BROCK, J.   *J. Brit. Jour. Anæsth.*, 1951, July, p. 196.
3. BOOTHBY and COTTON.   *Jour. Surg. & Gyn.*, 1912, Feb.
4. PASK, E. A.   *Lancet*, 1940, Nov. 30, p. 680.
5. FOREGGER, R.   *Anesthesiology*, 1946, Sept., p. 549.
6. IVES, J.   *Lancet*, 1944, April 22, p. 534.
7. ROWBOTHAM, S.   *Lancet*, 1931, Oct. 10, p. 802.
8. WYNNE, R. L.   *Brit. Med. Jour.*, 1941, Feb. 1, p. 155.
9. MCKESSON, E. I.   *Brit. Med. Jour.*, 1926, Dec. 11, p. 1115.

10. SNOW, J. *Lond. Med. Gazette*, 1850, **11**, p. 749, and **12**, p. 622.
11. LEE, F. S. *Rep. New York State Comm. on Ventilation*, 1923.
12. WATERS, R. *Anesthesiology*, 1947, July, p. 339.
13. ORCUTT, F. S., and WATERS, R. M. *Anesth. & Anal.*, 1933, **12**, No. 1, p. 45.
14. WATERS, R. M. *Anesth. & Anal.*, 1932, **11**, No. 3, p. 97.
15. { HEWER, C. L. *Lancet*, 1925, Jan. 21, p. 173.
    { EVANS, F. T. *Brit. Med. Jour.*, 1932, May 21, p. 931.
16. HEWER, C. L. *Brit. Med. Jour.*, 1943, Mar. 13, p. 334.
17. MINNITT, R. J. *Liverpool Med. Chir. Jour.*, 1933, **41**, p. 113.
18. HARRIS, T. A. B. " Mode of Action of Anæsthetics," 1951, p. 530.
19. { MALLINSON, F. B. *Brit. Med. Jour.*, 1940, May 11, p. 774.
    { FRAULD, J. P., and ROBINSON, J. A. W. *Brit. Med. Jour.*, 1940, Nov. 30, p. 746.
    { MALLINSON, F. B. *Brit. Med. Jour.*, 1941, Jan. 4, p. 17.
20. WATERS, R. M. *Pro. Roy. Soc. Med.* (An. Sec.), 1936, Oct. 2.
21. ADRIANI, J. " Chemistry of Anæsthetics," 1946. Oxford.
22. WATERS, R. M. *California & Western Med.*, 1931, Nov., p. 342.
23. KILPATRICK, L. G. *Anæsthesia*, 1951, Oct., p. 236.
24. CARDEN, S. *Brit. Med. Jour.*, 1944, Mar. 4, p. 319.
25. ASHWORTH, H. K. *Pro. Roy. Soc. Med.* (An. Sec.), 1946, Feb. 1.
26. MUSHIN, W. W. *Brit. Med. Jour.*, 1943, Jan. 30, p. 130.
27. MUSHIN, W. W. *Brit. Jour. Anæsth.*, 1943, Jan., p. 97.
28. EVANS, F. T. *Lancet*, 1938, Nov. 5, p. 1050.
29. GOULD, R. B. *Lancet*, 1941, Oct. 18, p. 449.
30. PRIMROSE, W. B. *Brit. Med. Jour.*, 1934, Mar. 17, p. 478 ; Aug. 25, p. 339.
31. WALLS, N. S. *Anæsthesia*, 1950, Oct., p. 171.
32. Designed by DRAPER, W. B., and LONGWELL, B. B.
33. WATERS, R. M. *Anesth. & Anal.*, 1939, Mar.-Apr., p. 75.
34. BASSETT, H. L. *Lancet*, 1949, Sept. 24, p. 561.
35. KILBORN, M. G. *Anesthesiology*, 1941, Nov., p. 621.
36. STOYALL, W. D. Bacteriologist to Wisconsin General Hospital.
37. MAGATH, T. B. *Anesth. & Anal.*, 1938, July-Aug., p. 215.
38. GALLEY, A. H. *Pro. Roy. Soc. Med.* (An. Sec.), 1946, May 3.
39. BLACKER, L. V. S. *Brit. Med. Jour.*, 1933, July, 22, p. 155.
40. DAWKINS, M. *Brit. Med. Jour.*, 1943, Oct. 30, p. 548.
41. *British Standard*, 1319 : 1946.

CHAPTER VI

RECENT WORK ON THE ETHERS

Di-ethyl Ether—Di-methyl Ether—Di-vinyl Ether—N-propyl-ethyl Ether—N-propyl-methyl Ether—Isopropyl-methyl Ether—Isopropyl-vinyl Ether—Cyclopropyl Ether—Other Ethers.

DI-ETHYL ETHER

Despite frequent prophecies to the contrary, di-ethyl ether continues to enjoy great popularity. The reasons for this are its great safety margin and the fact that in moderate dosage it is a stimulator of the sympathetic system with consequent relaxation of the bronchial tree.

It is not proposed to enter into the somewhat prolonged discussion as to whether absolutely pure freshly prepared **di-ethyl ether** does or does not possess anæsthetic properties,[1] although it is not without interest that at least one manufacturing firm has found that purification beyond a certain point calls for complaints on the score of " weakness ". It is, at any rate, agreed by all workers that the common impurities—aldehydes and peroxides—are definitely toxic and should be removed (see also under " Pulmonary Complications ").

Tests for Impurities. The most reliable tests are :

(1) For peroxides. A colourless glass-stoppered bottle is rinsed out with the ether to be examined ; 1 c.cm. of 10 per cent. aqueous solution of potassium iodide is then shaken with 10 c.cm. of the ether. The presence of even $0 \cdot 0005$ per cent. peroxides will be indicated by a yellow coloration within five minutes.

(2) For aldehydes. 3 c.cm. of Nessler's solution are added to 20 c.cm. of the ether in a glass-stoppered bottle and shaken. On allowing the layers to separate, an immediate yellow colour or turbidity shows the presence of aldehydes. On standing for some time a positive result will also be given for alcohol.[3]

Prevention of Decomposition. A considerable amount of research has been undertaken to obtain a pure ether, and manufacturers have been aided in this by the Government decision to allow the use of duty-free ethyl alcohol so that the production of ether from methylated spirit has almost ceased. Even when a purified ether is obtained, however, decomposition tends to occur, but in 1921 it was shown that carbon dioxide has a stabilizing effect[3] and some manufacturers treat their product with this gas before it is bottled. Strong light and heat have also been shown to favour decomposition[4] (see Fig. 34), and most ether is now put up in amber-coloured bottles with instructions for storing in a cool place. In spite of these precautions, however, ether still tends to oxidize when stored for prolonged periods, and efforts have been made to find a suitable anti-catalyst which will inhibit this action. Alcohol and metallic mercury in the form of " grey powder " have both been

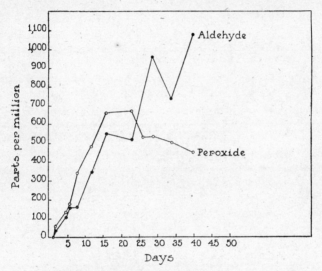

Fig. 34. Chart showing rate of decomposition of ether stored in clear bottle in sunlight. (Hediger, *Jour. Amer. Med. Ass.*)

tried, but it has recently been shown that copper is a most powerful anti-catalyst, and that ether stored in copper cans, or in cans internally copper-plated, shows no tendency to decompose.[5] Not only is this the case, but if anæsthetic gases are bubbled through ether for prolonged periods the rate of decomposition will be greatly diminished if there is an adequate area of metallic copper above and below the ether level.[6] Many makers have applied this observation by using copper tubes in the ether bottles of gas-oxygen apparatus. The addition of 1 part of hydroquinone or diphenylamine to 5,000 parts of ether is also said to arrest oxidation.[7] It has been pointed out that even if an ether is grossly contaminated with peroxide the amount of these impurities actually inhaled by the patient is infinitesimal. This holds good whether an open mask method is used or gases are bubbled through the ether.[8] On the other hand, a series of cases of pulmonary oedema has recently been reported in which the ether used was shown to be grossly contaminated with peroxides.[9]

Various attempts have been made to disguise the taste and smell of ether. Perhaps the most successful has been the addition of about 10 minims of oil of peppermint to the pint of ether.

Effect on Anaphylaxis. For some time it has been held that ether is a desensitizing agent and that anaphylactic shock does not occur if a foreign protein is injected into a sensitive patient under ether anæsthesia. Animal experiments are not conclusive on this point,[10] but observations made by the writer during the late war appear to show that " reactions " after blood transfusions are greatly diminished if the procedure is carried out during an operation performed under general anæsthesia.

"Late ether convulsions", so called to distinguish them from the innocuous " ether tremor " occurring in light anæsthesia, have called for considerable investigation,[11] but their cause remains obscure, because no common factor has been found in all the reported cases. It is possible that in certain persons there exists an inborn tendency to convulsions, and such patients may be " latent epileptics ". A series of twenty-two patients who exhibited ether convulsions were subsequently investigated by electro-encephalo-graphy and three-quarters showed a persisting abnormality of cortical rhythm indistinguishable from that underlying epilepsy.[12] The conditions which may occur during anæsthesia can, on this supposition, be regarded as precipitants of an attack similar in all respects to an epileptic fit. The actual cause, as in all convulsions, is probably interference with cerebral cell respiration, but the means whereby this is brought about is the subject of much discussion.[13] Factors which are thought to have some influence on this phenomenon are :

(a) *Overdosage.* Most of the convulsions have occurred during deep anæsthesia, but simple overdosage of ether results in respiratory arrest without any muscular spasms.

(b) *Impurities in Ether.* Traces of aldehydes and peroxides have been detected in a few cases on subsequent analysis, but usually the drug is found to be reasonably pure. Although di-ethyl ether is much the commonest agent, a similar state has been seen in patients anæsthetized with di-vinyl ether,[14] chloroform,[15] trichlor-ethylene,[16] nitrous oxide-oxygen,[17] cyclopropane,[18] and with local analgesia.[19] It is possible that di-ethyl ether causes convulsions much more commonly than other agents because it produces persistent high-voltage cortical discharges during the induction of anæsthesia.[12] (See Chapter I.)

(c) *Heat Stroke.* Ether convulsions are commonest in hot, damp weather,[20] i.e. when the reading of the wet-bulb thermometer is high or when the ether or its vapour is heated, and in pyrexial and dehydrated patients.[21] It is possible that over-atropinization may be a factor from the diminished heat loss from sweating.[22] On the other hand, anæsthetized patients tend to lose rather than gain heat, and the high temperatures seen after an attack are almost certainly due to the intense muscular activity. In some cases, a neurogenic stimulus has started convulsions in a pyrexial patient.[23] If conditions appear favourable to the occurrence of convulsions, it would seem wise to use an open mask method of anæsthesia in preference to a warmed vaporizer or closed-circuit.[24]

(d) *Carbon Dioxide Imbalance.* It is known that lack of CO_2 and gross overdosage of CO_2 can produce spasms, and both factors have been invoked as the cause of ether convulsions.[25] On the whole, CO_2-lack seems the more probable as the spasms have several times been stopped by the addition of CO_2 to the inspired mixture. Furthermore, ether convulsions have been reported during insufflation endotracheal anæsthesia when the alveolar CO_2 concentration is abnormally low. Lastly, examination of the urine first passed after an attack has shown a high alkalinity so that the patients are presumably suffering from alkalosis.[26]

(e) *Sepsis.* Most of the cases of ether convulsions have occurred in young patients suffering from acute septic conditions. It has been shown that nasal swabs taken from patients during ether convulsions can grow streptococci, which when injected into rabbits cause convulsions when the animals are anæsthetized with ether. Some days later, however, although swabs from the same patients will give a growth of apparently the same organisms, no convulsions can be produced by anæsthetizing injected animals.[27]

(f) *Calcium Deficiency.* There is some evidence to show that if the physiologically active fraction of the serum calcium is diminished, neuro-muscular irritability occurs with a tendency to spasms. Several attacks of ether convulsions have been stopped immediately by the intravenous injection of calcium gluconate.[28]

(g) *Cerebral Congestion.* Several instances have been reported when patients have been placed in a steep Trendelenburg position for some time[29] and the adoption of the opposite slope definitely tends to abort the attack. There is also some evidence to show that a " foot-down tilt " has a prophylactic value against the occurrence of convulsions in young pyrexial patients.[24]

The treatment of ether convulsions consists of (a) raising the head and if necessary sitting the patient bolt upright,[24] (b) sponging the face and limbs with cold water, (c) momentary compression of the common carotid arteries[30] with a view to diminishing the congestion of the Rolandic area.[31] (d) If these simple measures fail, a short-acting barbiturate such as soluble thiopentone should be cautiously injected into a vein.[32] Frequent pauses should be made, and the smallest possible amount of the drug should be used, or serious circulatory and respiratory depression may ensue.[33] It may prove impossible to stop the convulsions without paralysing the respiratory centre in which event prolonged artificial respiration may be necessary, preferably after intubation. A Drinker's respirator may be useful in these circumstances.[21] It is possible that the use of minimal quantities of curare might be safer than thiopentone. The approximate mortality of all reported cases of ether convulsions up to 1936 is stated to be 23 per cent.[34]

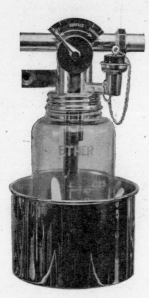

FIG. 35. Standard "through or over" ether bottle with water-bath.

The modern **technique** of administering ether is to add it in the smallest possible amount to nitrous oxide and oxygen in order to obtain the required muscular relaxation. Experience gained in the late war has again emphasized the fact that ether should preferably be avoided altogether in the badly shocked or toxic patient.[35] One school of thought considers that the time has now come to abandon ether completely since less toxic drugs can fill its place.[36] In the author's opinion the time has *not* yet come for this.

There are three ways in which ether can be added to the mixed gases :—

(i) In most types of apparatus operating on the continuous or intermittent flow principles, some or all of the gases can be passed through or over (Figs. 33 and 35) liquid ether or gauze soaked in ether. The internal tubes carrying the gases are usually made of copper in order to retard oxidation of the ether as explained above.

It should be noted that if the ether and trilene bottles of a gas-oxygen machine are connected in " series " it is possible for the ether to become contaminated with trilene (or vice versa, according to the position of the bottles), if the gases are passed over or through both liquids simultaneously. The modification made by Webber avoids this by connecting the bottles in " parallel ".

If certain types of bottles containing chloroform or ether (e.g. early Shipway and Junker inhalers) are connected up wrongly it is possible for liquid to be forced out of the exit tube. The Surgical Instrument Manufacturers' Association has approved certain types of safety devices to avoid this risk, and all apparatus now in use should conform to the standards laid down.[37] It is extremely important that the water jackets of ether bottles operating on this system should not be filled with liquid at a higher temperature than 34° C. (94° F.), which is the boiling point of ether. If the ether should boil, a super-saturated vapour may be obtained with subsequent condensation in the exit tube and in the respiratory passages of the patient. If this occurs an attack of acute pulmonary œdema may follow.[38] It should be noted that during a long narcosis the ether level will fall and its temperature will become lowered. In consequence the vapour concentration will fall and this is a valuable safety-factor which often prevents inexperienced anæsthetists from giving an overdose.

(ii) If the closed-circuit system is used, the basal oxygen flow is so small that it is insufficient to vaporize ether efficiently. This difficulty can be met in the circle system by passing all the patient's respired gases through the vaporizer. In the author's opinion an adjustable drip-feed is the most satisfactory principle to employ. The actual amount of ether being used can be seen, the control is extremely sensitive and the bulk of the ether does not become contaminated by the passage of the gases through it. The subjoined diagram illustrates the principle of an ether vaporizer which has been proved satisfactory. The liquid drips on to a copper gauze tube, through which the respired gases pass. These gases are warm, and heat is also obtained by conduction from the soda-lime canister which is in metallic contact with the gauze tube. If the rate of drip is very high, some ether may drop into a water-jacketed container in which are three copper gauze discs. The basal-oxygen feed impinges upon these discs and assists in vaporizing the remainder of the ether. In this type of vaporizer, the hotter the water in the jacket the better, but in practice the efficiency is such that in most circumstances additional heat is unnecessary. The ether reservoir should have a slightly smaller capacity than the vaporizing chamber so that even if the drip is left on inadvertently between cases, liquid ether cannot enter the breathing tubes.

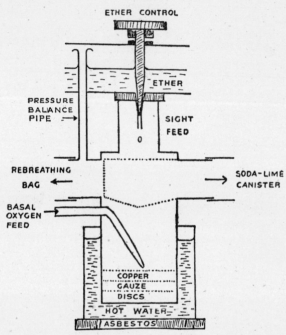

FIG. 36. Diagram illustrating principle of author's ether vaporizer for closed-circuit apparatus (see also Fig. 29).

(iii) Pure ether *vapour* can be added to the gases through a flow-meter. In the " Oxford Vaporizer No. 2 " this is effected in the same way as in Pinson's ether bomb.[39] The liquid ether is maintained at a constant temperature above its boiling point by being enclosed in a double jacket. The outer compartment C holds hot water, and the inner one B crystals of paradichlorbenzene which melt at 52° C. As the water temperature falls, more of this " reservoir substance " passes from the liquid to the solid state giving up its latent heat of fusion so that the temperature remains constant until the whole mass becomes crystalline. At this point more hot water must be added. The undiluted ether vapour is led off through the needle valve H and is measured by the bobbin type flow-meter R[40] (Fig. 37). Since, at the time of writing, this vaporizer is still unobtainable, it need not be considered more fully.

If, owing to circumstances, ether has to be used alone, a " closed " induction is preferable to the open method, owing to the higher

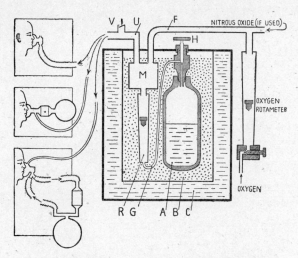

FIG. 37. Diagrammatic vertical section through Oxford Vaporizer No. 2. A contains anæsthetic, B crystals and C hot water, F and G connecting tube, H fine adjustment valve, M mixing chamber, R flow-meter (Rotameter), U connecting tube, V inspiratory valve. (S. L. Cowan, R. D. Scott and S. F. Suffolk, *The Lancet*.)

carbon dioxide percentage maintaining deeper respiration with the consequent more rapid onset of anæsthesia. The well-known " Clover's " apparatus embodied this principle in 1863, although it has been " rediscovered " at intervals ever since.[41]

For the maintenance of anæsthesia with pure ether, it is undesirable to keep up a high CO_2 concentration, but a simple open mask administration falls far short of the ideal both as regards difficulty in maintaining an even concentration and in the low temperature of the inspired vapour. It is not an infrequent occurrence to see frost forming on the outside of the mask. It is true that the specific heat of the gases is low and that the upper air passages are an efficient heating mechanism, but it is clear that the heat necessary for bringing up the temperature of the inspired vapour to 98° F. must come from the patient. The avoidance of using cold gases is particularly important when the endotracheal technique is employed as the normal warming mechanism is largely by-passed. (See Chapter VIII.) During the 1914-18 war, Shipway and Pembrey conducted experiments which led to the construction of the well-known Shipway's warm-ether apparatus in which ether or chloroform vapour or both is passed through a U-tube immersed in a vacuum flask filled with hot water. It was shown that a lower percentage of patients showed a fall in rectal temperature compared with those anæsthetized with open ether.[42] It should be noted that manufacturers tended to fit a longer rubber tube to the mask than was designed. If this is done the temperature of the issuing vapours will approximate to that of the room.

It is also worth noting that the mere application of an " open ether " mask significantly reduces the partial pressure of oxygen in the air under it (153 mm. to 123 mm.) and adding ether causes a further reduction (to 105 mm.). The advantage of adding fresh air or oxygen is thus scientifically shown.[43]

The " Thermanester " inhaler was another attempt to avoid the heat loss associated with open ether.[44]

The " Oxford Vaporizer No. 1 " is designed to deliver a warmed ether vapour of adjustable and known concentration.[45] The patient's inspiration draws air through the inlet valve V and over the surface of ether A (Fig. 38). The vapour concentration depends on the position of the regulator H and can be read off on a dial. The temperature of the ether remains constant because it is jacketed with crystals of hydrated calcium chloride B which are in their turn surrounded by hot water in the chamber C. The " chemical thermostat " acts in the same way as that described under the Vaporizer No. 2, but in this case the ether is kept at a temperature *below* its boiling point as the reservoir substance melts at 29° C. When all this material solidifies, the thermometer T will show a fall and more hot water must be added. With this apparatus there is no appreciable falling off of vapour concentration and this must be gradually reduced as the administration proceeds in order to avoid overdosage. This vaporizer probably affords the most accurate method known of giving an air-ether mixture and has been used successfully under service conditions during the late war. It is particularly useful in maintaining a very light plane of narcosis.

The Connell type rubber bellows enable artificial respiration to be performed if necessary. The chief disadvantages of the apparatus are its weight and bulk, the time taken to attain a working temperature with hot water, and the slow and difficult induction of anæsthesia owing to the absence of rebreathing. The latter

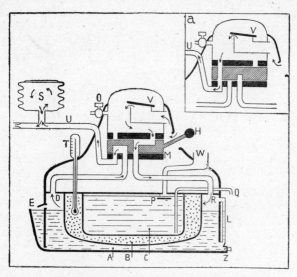

FIG. 38.   Modified vertical section through Oxford Vaporizer No. 1.   A ether chamber, B heat reservoir containing calcium-chloride crystals, C hot-water chamber, D exit for air plus ether vapour, E ether filler, H lever for controlling ether concentration, L ether level indicator, M mixing-tap assembly, O tap for oxygen, P baffle plate, Q water outlet, R inlet for air, S bag, T thermometer, U tube to mask, V inlet valve, W filler for hot water, Z plug for draining ether.   In inset (a) the mixing tap is turned so that air passes direct to the patient (Epstein *et al.*)

difficulty has been overcome to some extent on the later models by the provision of a small rubber bag (i.b.) near the facepiece into which ethyl chloride or di-vinyl ether can be sprayed. (Fig. 39.) In tropical climates it may be necessary to fill the apparatus with *cold* water in order to keep the internal temperature between the prescribed limits. Neglect of this precaution may result in the ether boiling in which case a 100 per cent. vapour will be delivered as in

the Oxford Vaporizer No. 2.[46]   If the apparatus must be used when
a fire risk is present, the exhaled gases can be passed through a
charcoal adsorber (see Chapter IX).

A simpler apparatus working on the same " draw-over " principle
and designed for use with ether, trichlorethylene or both is described
in Chapter VII.   The author's drip-feed apparatus is also con-
vertible to the " draw-over " technique if gases are not available,

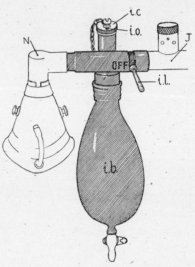

Fig. 39.   " Induction bag " (i.b.) interposed between angle-piece (N) and
expiratory valve (J) of Oxford
Vaporizer No. 1.

by simply substituting an inspiratory valve for the rebreathing bag
(Figs. 29 and 36).

It should be noted that overheating the inhaled vapour causes
profuse sweating.[47]   In general, the patient should breathe an
atmosphere just below body temperature.

The *intravenous* injection of 5 per cent. ether in normal saline[48]
is seldom practised at the present time and the same is true of
rectal oil-ether, both methods having been replaced by endotracheal
administration (q.v.).   It is worth recalling that ether has been
given *by mouth* as in the " Lower sandwich " of the 1914-18 European
war,[49] but frequent enteritis and inadequate narcosis prevented the
method from becoming popular.

Therapeutic Ether Narcosis. The administration of ether to the stage of anæsthesia has been used successfully in the treatment of diphtheritic paralysis[50] and of asthma (see Chapter XXIV). Daily ether enemata have also been employed in whooping cough.[51]

DI-METHYL ETHER

Investigations have been carried out for many years upon the anæsthetic properties of the other ethers[52] (see later). **Di-methyl ether** (CH_3—O—CH_3) showed some promise, but was soon abandoned[53] as many patients became congested and cyanosed.

DI-VINYL ETHER

Di-vinyl ether (di-vinyl oxide) has the formula

$$CH_2 = CH$$
$$|$$
$$O$$
$$|$$
$$CH_2 = CH$$

History. The anæsthetic properties of di-vinyl ether were first demonstrated by Leake and Chen in 1930.[54] The first trial on the human subject was carried out three years later by Gelfan and Bell, who used the anæsthetic on themselves.[55]

Properties. Di-vinyl ether is a clear colourless liquid with a smell reminiscent of ethylene. The specific gravity is 0·77 and the boiling point 28° C., i.e. lower than that of di-ethyl ether. There is little difference between the two ethers as regards inflammability when pure and explosibility when mixed with air, oxygen or nitrous oxide. The limits of inflammability are said to be from 1·7 per cent. to 27 per cent. di-vinyl ether in air and from 1·85 per cent. to 85 per cent. in oxygen (Guedel). Pure di-vinyl ether is unstable and should be used from a freshly opened bottle. The slightest trace of acid accelerates decomposition with polymerization and the appearance of formaldehyde and formic acid.[56] The proprietary preparation known as " **vinesthene** " (syn. " **vinethene** ") is di-vinyl ether with the addition of 3·5 per cent. absolute alcohol and 0·01 per cent. phenyl-anaphthylamine put up in an atmosphere of nitrogen. This is much more stable than the pure drug and the bottle when opened can be resealed by screwing up the cap tightly. It is stated that the fluid remaining can be used within ten days without fear of deterioration.[57] For further details of the physical properties and methods of preparation of di-vinyl ether the reader is referred to the papers indicated by the reference.[58]

Action. From determinations of the concentration in the blood necessary to produce anæsthesia, it has been estimated that the anæsthetic potency of di-vinyl ether is about four times that of di-ethyl ether and slightly greater than that of chloroform.[59] The actual *anæsthetic* blood concentration is said to be about 28 mg. per 100 c.cm. in dogs and 11 to 18 mg. in man.[60] The *lethal* blood concentration in dogs is about 68 mg. per cent. There is no appreciable change in the blood coagulation time.[61] The induction of anæsthesia is quicker and more pleasant than with di-ethyl ether as the odour is not pungent. If given by the open method (an undesirable technique), an average of 2 c.cm. per minute of di-vinyl ether is required. In order to avoid waste from rapid volatilization, Bourne recommends a mixture of 75 per cent. di-ethyl ether and 25 per cent. di-vinyl ether. This is now available in Great Britain under the title, **" vinesthene anæsthetic mixture "** or " V.A.M. ". It contains 0·83 per cent. absolute ethyl alcohol as a stabilizer. Such a mixture will vaporize in approximately proportional percentages, and somewhat resembles a C.E. mixture without the risk of primary cardiac failure. Salivation and irritation of the respiratory passages are on the average less with pure di-vinyl ether than with the di-ethyl variety.[62] Muscular relaxation varies but is usually good. On the other hand, muscular movements may persist during apparently deep narcosis and in animals " running movements " may be present until respiratory paralysis occurs from overdosage.[53] There is no inhibition of intestinal peristalsis nor of uterine contractions.[64]

Sequelæ. The absence of nausea and vomiting constitute one of the chief advantages of di-vinyl ether. With a " single-dose " technique the patient usually wakes up feeling quite well, while in 200 consecutive administrations of varying times only three patients vomited at all.[65]

Toxic Effects. The blood sugar rises at the beginning of anæsthesia but falls more rapidly than is the case with di-ethyl ether or chloroform (see Chapter I). In over-dosage, respiration always appears to cease before the circulation fails.[66] In animals, no gross pathological changes have been observed in the liver, heart, lungs and kidneys, and in man very slight impairment of the liver function was detected by the bromsulphalein dye test.[67] On the other hand, two deaths from liver necrosis have been reported in America,[68] and some anæsthetists consider that the drug is more toxic than di-ethyl ether in this respect,[69] especially in the presence of anoxia. Cases of convulsions[70] indistinguishable from those seen with di-ethyl ether have been recorded[69] while others have occurred during the recovery stage in children anæsthetized with only 3 c.cm. of the drug for dental extractions.[72]

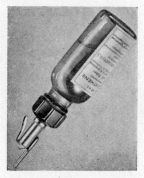

Fig. 40. Bottle of di-vinyl ether fitted with spray attachment.

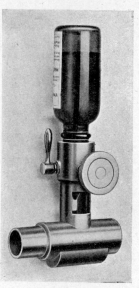

Fig. 41. Drip-feed vaporizer for di-vinyl ether (Goldman's), showing wheel control and tap for pressure balance.

Marked tachycardia has been noted when using the vinesthene mixture.[72]

Indications. Di-vinyl ether is useful in reinforcing nitrous oxide-oxygen anæsthesia when it is undesirable to add the toxic effects of chloroform or the irritative effects of di-ethyl ether. For example, in a few cases it is difficult to " settle " a partial thyroidectomy case with pure gas-oxygen, and a trace of di-vinyl ether produces a much smoother anæsthesia. The drug is of some value in thoracic surgery if cyclopropane is unobtainable. The rapid action of di-vinyl ether and its negative effect on uterine contractions render it of great service in obstetrics, although it is usually impossible to produce analgesia alone.[73] The single-dose technique is useful in dentistry and in guillotine tonsillectomy in children (q.v.).

Technique of Administration. As mentioned above, di-vinyl ether can be given by the open method, in which case it is convenient to screw a spray attachment into the bottle as illustrated. The warmth of the hand is enough to generate sufficient pressure for the drug to be forced out of the nozzle as in an ethyl chloride tube. It is preferable, however, to add the vapour of di-vinyl ether to nitrous oxide and oxygen. In view of its great potency and high volatility, a finer adjustment is necessary than that provided by the usual ether vaporizer. A small adjustable drip-feed outfit is usually interposed in the circuit of a gas-oxygen apparatus.[74] The volatility of the drug is so high that it vanishes in the most annoying manner, but in Goldman's vaporizer (Fig. 41) this difficulty is surmounted by screwing the original bottle into a leak-proof mount. Very prolonged administration is undesirable, as is any trace of anoxia, since this undoubtedly increases the toxic effect of the drug on the liver. A simple type of closed inhaler for a single-dose administration is described in Chapter XIX.

N-PROPYL-ETHYL ETHER

This has the structural formula C_2H_5—O—C_3H_7 and is a colourless liquid with an odour less pungent than that of di-ethyl ether. The potency is somewhat greater, its B.P. is $63\cdot6°$ C. and S.G. $0\cdot75$. Preliminary experiments on animals suggest that there is little respiratory irritation, that the safety margin is wide and that after-effects are slight.[75] A series of fifty administrations of the drug as an adjuvant to N_2O—O_2 in human subjects has shown encouraging results[76] and a relative lack of bleeding at operation has been observed.

N-PROPYL-METHYL ETHER

This ether, also known as **metopryl** and **neothyl,** is an isomer of di-ethyl ether with the formula CH_3—O—$CH_2\cdot CH_2\cdot CH_3$. It was first described by Chancel in 1869. It is a volatile colourless inflammable liquid with a B.P. of $39°$ C. and a S.G. of $0\cdot73$. It is supplied with the addition of $0\cdot002$ per cent. diphenylamine as a stabilizer against oxidation. It has a slightly pungent odour and tends to cause headaches in the operating team unless given in a closed circuit. It is about 25 per cent. more potent than di-ethyl ether, and causes less irritation to the respiratory tract and less post-operative vomiting.[77]

ISOPROPYL-METHYL ETHER

This ether, known as **isopryl** is also an isomer of di-ethyl ether

$$CH_3{-}O{-}\overset{\displaystyle CH_3}{\underset{\displaystyle CH_3}{\overset{|}{\underset{|}{CH}}}}$$

with the formula :

The potencies of the two drugs are said to be about the same.[71]

ISOPROPYL-VINYL ETHER

This compound, also known as **propethylene,** has the structure

$$\overset{\displaystyle H}{\overset{|}{C}} = \overset{}{\underset{\displaystyle CH_3}{\overset{|}{C}}}{-}O{-}\overset{}{\underset{\displaystyle H}{\overset{|}{C}}} = \overset{\displaystyle H}{\underset{\displaystyle H}{\overset{|}{C}}}$$

and is an isomer of cyprethylene ether (q.v.). Its B.P. is 55° C. and S.G. 0·786, and it has a characteristic smell resembling that of cyclopropane. It is less volatile than di-ethyl ether but is a much more potent anæsthetic in animals and man. Preliminary trials have been promising[79] and the drug appears to be definitely less toxic to the liver and kidneys (in animals) than di-ethyl and di-vinyl ethers and chloroform.[80]

THE CYCLOPROPYL ETHERS

Various compounds can be made by substituting an ether radicle for one of the hydrogen atoms in cyclopropane. Three such ethers have been prepared and have been shown to have anæsthetic properties.

(1) **Cyclopropyl-methyl ether (cyprome ether)**

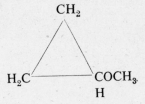

It has a B.P. of 44° C. and S.G. of 0·786.   It smells like cyclo-propane.

(2) **Cyclopropyl-ethyl ether (cypreth ether).**   Its B.P. is 68° C. and S.G. 0·780.

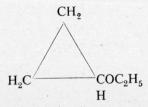

In animals, its potency is greater and its toxicity is less than that of di-ethyl ether, but in man it is a respiratory irritant.[81]

(3) **Cyprethylene ether.**

$$H_2C \overset{CH_2}{\diagup \diagdown} COC = C \begin{smallmatrix} H \\ H \end{smallmatrix}$$

It is possible that (1) and (3) may prove useful in human anæsthesia,[82] but work on them has not yet passed the experimental stage.

OTHER ETHERS

The properties of the commonly available ethers of from 2 to 10 total carbon atoms have been determined and tabulated.[83]   The figures are based on experiments on white mice and must not be taken as applying exactly in man.   The percentage figures given for anæsthetic and lethal concentrations mean the number of animals per hundred anæsthetized or killed respectively by the given vapour concentration inhaled.

Ether	Molecular Weight	Boiling Point °C at 760 mm. Hg.	Vapor pressure at 25 C. in mm. Hg.	Specific Gravity at 20 C.	Solubility in Water Weight Per Cent at 25 C.	Anesthetic Concentration 50%	Anesthetic Concentration 95-99%	Lethal Concentration 1-5%	Lethal Concentration 50%	Therapeutic Index	Certain Safety Factor
1. Dimethyl	46.05	−23.5	>760	—		14	20	35	37	2.6	1.7
2. Methyl ethyl	60.06	7.9	>760	0.73		6	9	14	18	3.0	1.8
3. Divinyl	70.05	28.3	684	0.77	0.78	1.5	1.75	3.7	4.7	3.1	2.1
4. Ethyl vinyl	72.06	35.5	500	0.76	0.6	1.5	1.75	3.5	4.5	3.0	2.0
5. Methyl cyclopropyl	72.06	44	410	0.78	5.1	1.4	1.75	1.4	1.75	1.25	—
6. Methyl isopropyl	74.08	32.5	550	0.74	6.7	2.0	2.5	4.0	5.5	2.75	1.6
7. Diethyl	74.08	34.5	537	0.71	6.3	1.75	2.0	4.0	6	3.4	2.0
8. Methyl propyl	74.08	37	500	0.78	3.25	1.25	1.5	3.0	3.5	2.8	2.0
9. Ethyl cyclopropyl	86.08	68	150	0.78	2.0	0.8	1.0	0.8	1.0	1.25	—
10. Ethyl isopropyl	88.09	53.5	250	0.72	2.4	1.0	1.3	2.0	2.5	2.5	1.5
11. Methyl ter-butyl	88.09	55.2	244	0.74	5.16	0.8	1.2	1.5	1.6	1.6	1.25
12. Methyl sec-butyl	88.09	58	230	0.74	1.10	0.9	1.1	1.5	1.6	1.8	1.4
13. Methyl isobutyl	88.09	60	210	0.74	1.60	1.0	1.1	1.5	1.6	1.6	1.4
14. Ethyl propyl	88.09	61.4	185	0.73	1.87	0.8	1.0	2.0	2.5	3.1	2.0
15. Methyl butyl	88.09	70.3	160	0.74	0.89	0.7	0.8	1.5	2.0	2.9	1.9
16. Di isopropyl	102.11	67.5	170	0.73	0.93	0.7	0.8	1.2	1.5	2.1	1.5
17. Ethyl ter-butyl	102.11	72.8	155	0.74		0.7	0.8	1.0	1.2	1.7	1.25
18. Ethyl sec-butyl	102.11	81.2	98	0.74		0.6	0.7	1.2	1.4	2.3	1.7
19. Ethyl isobutyl	102.11	81.1	98	0.75		0.6	0.7	1.2	1.5	2.5	1.7
20. Propyl isopropyl	102.11	83	85	0.75	0.67	0.55	0.65	1.25	1.5	3.0	1.9
21. Methyl amyl	102.11	88.5	55	0.75		0.4	0.5	1.0	1.3	3.2	2.0
22. Dipropyl	102.11	90.1	60	0.74		0.4	0.5	1.2	1.6	4.0	2.4
23. Ethyl butyl	102.11	91.4	52	0.75		0.5	0.6	1.2	1.5	3.0	2.0
24. Ethyl ter-amyl	116.12	101.0	43	0.77		0.4	0.5	0.5	0.7	1.75	2.0
25. Ethyl isoamyl	116.12	112	30	0.76		0.35	0.45	0.8	1.0	2.8	1.0
26. Ethyl amyl	116.12	119.5	18	0.76		0.35	0.45	0.9*	1.0*	2.8	1.8
27. Di sec-butyl	130.14	121	17	0.76		0.5	0.6	0.8*	1.0*	2.4	2.0
28. Di isobutyl	130.14	122.5	15	0.76	<0.01	0.4*	0.5*	1.0*	1.2*	3.2	1.8
29. Dibutyl	130.14	142.4	—	0.77				1.0*	1.3*		1.7
30. Di isoamyl	158.17	172.5	—	0.78		Not anesthetic					
31. Diamyl	158.17	187.5	—	0.77		Not anesthetic					

* Chamber and contents must be heated to 35 C. for this concentration to be volatilized.

Properties of various ethers (MARSH & LEAKE, "Anesthesiology", July, 1950)

References

1. {
   COTTON, Y. *McGill University Lecture*, 1917, June 13.
   WEBSTER, W. *Amer. Jour. Surg.*, 1922, July.
   WALLIS, R. L. M. *Pro. Roy. Soc. Med.* (An. Sec.), 1921, April.
   LEEUWEN, S. VON. *Pro. Roy. Soc. Med.* (An. Sec.), 1924, March.
   CASSIDY, P. *Amer. Jour. Surg.*, 36, No. 7.
   }
2. NEFF, W. B. *Canad. Med. Ass. Jour.*, 1933, June.
3. WALLIS, R. L. M. *Lancet*, 1921, *i.*, p. 1173.
4. {
   HADFIELD, C. F. *Pro. Roy. Soc. Med.* (An. Sec.), 1928, **21,** p. 1699.
   HEDIGER, E. L., *et al.* *Jour. Amer. Med. Ass.*, 1940, Apr. 13, p. 1424.
   }
5. NITARDY, F. W., and TAPLEY, N. W. *Brit. Jour. Anœsth.*, 1928, p. 53.
6. HEWER, C. L. *Lancet*, 1929, April 13, p. 770.
7. {
   NOLAN, H. O. *Lancet*, 1933, July 15, p. 129.
   LINGREN, C. "Autoxidation of di-ethyl ether." 1946, Stockholm.
   }
8. COSTE, J. H., and GARRATT, D. C. *Pro. Soc. Pub. Anal.*, 1936, May.
9. STOUT, R. J. *Anœsthesia*, 1950, Jan., p. 41.
10. {
    QUILL, L. M. *Jour. Amer. Med. Ass.*, 1937, Sept. 11, p. 854.
    KOONTZ, A. R., and SHACKLEFORD, R. T. *Bull. Johns Hopkins Hosp.*, 1939, Feb., p. 125.
    }
11. {
    WILSON, S. R. *Lancet*, 1927, *i.*, p. 1117.
    HADFIELD, C. F. *Pro. Roy. Soc. Med.* (An. Sec.), 1928, p. 33.
    SYKES, W. S. *Brit. Med. Jour.*, 1930, *i.*, p. 147.
    CLEMENTS, F. V. *Anesth. & Anal.*, 1928, March, p. 72.
    }
12. WILLIAMS, D., and SWEET, W. H. *Lancet*, 1944, Sept. 20, pp. 430 and 444.
13. KEMP, W. N. *Brit. Med. Jour.*, 1944, Apr. 1, p. 447.
14. DAWKINS, C. J. M. *Brit. Med. Jour.*, 1938, June 4, p. 1236.
15. MATHEWS, W. *Brit. Med. Jour.*, 1941, May 3, p. 697.
16. {
    GARLAND, Y. *Brit. Med. Jour.*, 1942, Nov. 21, p. 607.
    CULBERT, T. P. *Brit. Med. Jour.*, 1942, Dec. 5, p. 679.
    }
17. OSBORNE, S. E. *Brit. Med. Jour.*, 1941, May 3, p. 689.
18. GEBAUOR, P. W., and COLEMAN, F. P. *Ann. Surg.*, 1938, Apr., p. 481.
19. {
    HUDSON, R. V. *Brit. Jour. Anœsth.*, 1936, July, p. 151.
    Rep. Australian Soc. of Anœsth., 1937, May 3.
    }
20. WRIGHT, A. D. *Brit. Med. Jour.*, 1933, Dec. 30, p. 1210.
21. WOOLMER, R. F., and TAYLOR, S. *Lancet*, 1936, May 2, p. 1005.
22. DODD, H. G. *Brit. Jour. Anœsth.*, 1939, April, p. 90.
23. BRENNAN, H. J. *Brit. Med. Jour.*, 1941, Nov. 29, p. 765.
24. SMITH, A. *Lancet*, 1944, Jan. 8, p. 52.
25. HEWER, C. L. *Brit. Med. Jour.*, 1938, Oct. 29, p. 921.
26. KEMP, W. *Brit. Jour. Anœsth.*, 1932, July, p. 169.
27. {
    ROSENOW, E. C., and TOVELL, R. M. *Amer. Jour. Surg.*, 1936, Dec., p. 474.
    ROSENOW, E. C., *et al.* *Anesthesiology*, 1945, Jan., p. 12.
    }
28. HOSEASON, A. S. *Brit. Jour. Anœsth.*, 1936, July, p. 142.
29. PASK, E. A. *Brit. Med. Jour.*, 1940, Sept. 7, p. 337.
30. DALY, A. *Brit. Jour. Anœsth.*, 1932, Jan., p. 67.
31. CLARK, L. T. *Brit. Med. Jour.*, 1931, Aug. 22, p. 358.
32. {
    CHADWICK, T. H. *Brit. Med. Jour.*, 1936, June 20, p. 1253.
    PINKERTON, H. H. *Brit. Med. Jour.*, 1938, April 9, p. 780.
    }
33. TAYLOR, S., and GOLDMAN, V. *Brit. Med. Jour.*, 1938, Oct. 8, p. 744.
34. PAYNE, R. Y. *Guy's Hosp. Rep.*, 1936, Oct., p. 461.
35. MALLINSON, F. B. *Brit. Jour. Anœsth.*, 1941, Jan., p. 98.
36. MALLINSON, F. B. *Lancet*, 1943, Dec. 11, p. 729.
37. *Brit. Jour. Anœsth.*, 1935, Apr., p. 142.
38. NEGUS, V. E. *Pro. Roy. Soc. Med.* (An. Sec.), 1933, May 5.
39. WILSON, S. R., and PINSON, K. B. *Lancet*, 1921, Feb. 12.

40. Cowan, S. L., *et al.* *Lancet*, 1941, July, p. 64.
41. { Henkel. *Ztschrft. f. Geb. v. Gyn.*, 1927, p. 91.
{ Ombrédanne. *Deut. Zeits. f. Chir.*, 1928, Mar., p. 179.
42. Shipway, F., and Pembrey. *Lancet*, 1916, *i.*, pp. 70 and 1001.
43. Faulconer, A., and Latterell, K. E. *Anesthesiology*, 1949, **10**, p. 247.
44. King, G. *Journal-Lancet Minneapolis*, 1936, Oct., p. 536.
45. { Macintosh, R. R., and Mendelssohn, K. *Lancet*, 1941, July 19, p. 61.
{ Bannister, F. B. *Pro. Roy. Soc. Med.* (An. Sec.), 1942, Sec. 4.
46. Blackiston, P. M. *Brit. Med. Jour.*, 1944, Apr. 29, p. 601.
47. Hewer, C. L. *Pro. Roy. Soc. Med.* (An. Sec.), 1928, **21**, p. 352.
48. Rood, F. *Brit. Med. Jour.*, 1911, Oct. 11.
49. Gwathmey, J. T., and Karsner, H. T. *Brit. Med: Jour.*, 1918, *i.*, p. 254.
50. Hennerbert and Schuermans. *Scalpel, Liége*, 1937, Jan. 9, p. 336.
51. Bloise, N. L., and Perez. *Arch. de Pediat. del. Uruguay*, 1937, Mar., p. 137.
52. Pinson, K. B. *Pro. Roy. Soc. Med.* (An. Sec.), 1923, Dec. 3.
53. { Richardson. *Med. Times and Gazette*, 1868, May 30, p. 581.
{ Hewitt, F. *Lancet*, 1904, Nov. 19, p. 1408.
54. Leake, C. D., and Chen, M. Y. *Pro. Soc. Exper. Biol., N.Y.*, **28**, p. 151.
55. Gelfan, S., and Bell, I. R. *Jour. Pharmacol.*, **47**, p. 1.
56. Leake, C. D., *et al.* *Jour. Pharm. & Exp. Therap.*, 1933, Jan.
57. Adriani, J. *Anesthesiology*, 1941, Mar., p. 191.
58. { Ruich and Major. *Jour. Amer. Chem. Soc.*, 1931, **53**, p. 2662.
{ Miles and Menzies. *Jour. Phys. Chem.*, 1933, **37**, p. 425.
59. Goldschmidt, S., *et al.* *Jour. Amer. Med. Ass.*, 1934, Jan. 6, p. 21.
60. Ravdin, I. S., *et al.* *Jour. Amer. Med. Ass.*, 1937, Apr. 3, p. 1163.
61. Bourne, W., *et al.* *Anœsth. & Anal.*, 1937, Jan.-Feb., p. 46.
62. Roberts, K., and Johnson, W. *Amer. Jour. Surg.*, 1933, Dec. p. 461.
63. Orth, O. S., *et al.* *Anesthesiology*, 1940, *i.*, p. 246.
64. Bourne, W. *Canad. Med. Ass. Jour.*, 1935, **33**, p. 629.
65. { Dorffel, G. W. *Deut. Med. Woch.*, 1935, June 14, 955.
{ Goldman, V. *Brit. Med. Jour.*, 1936, July 18, p. 122.
66. Bourne, W., *et al.* *Brit. Jour. Anœsth.*, 1935, Jan., p. 69.
67. Rosenthal, S. M., and Bourne, W. *Jour. Amer. Med. Ass.*, 1928, **90**, p. 377.
68. Shipway, F. *Brit. Med. Jour.*, 1933, Jan. 12, p. 71.
69. { Dawkins, C. J. M. *Brit. Med. Jour.*, 1938, Jan. 4, p. 1236.
{ Guerrier, S. M., and Dafoe, C. S. *Brit. Med. Jour.*, 1940, March 2, p. 366.
70. Smith, A. *Lancet*, 1944, Jan. 8, p. 52.
71. { Dawkins, C. J. M. *Brit. Med. Jour.*, 1940, Feb. 3, p. 163.
{ Boston, F. K. *Brit. Med. Jour.*, 1940, June 8, p. 929.
72. Cartwright, F. F. *Brit. Med. Jour.*, 1939, May 27, p. 1081.
73. Caine, A. M. *Amer. Jour. Surg.*, 1936, Dec., p. 463.
74. Harris, T. A. B. *Brit. Med. Jour.*, 1938, May 14, p. 1054.
75. Brown, W. E. *Anesth. & Anal.*, 1941, March-April, p. 38.
76. Brown, W. E., and Lucas, G. H. W. *Canad. Med. Ass. Jour.*, 1940, Dec., p. 526.
77. Fisher, A. J., and Whitacre, R. J. *Anesthesiology*, 1947, Mar., p. 156.
78. Carr, C. J., *et al.* *Anesth. & Anal.*, 1947, July-Aug., p. 173.
79. Davis, E. H., and Krantz, J. C. *Anesthesiology*, 1944, Mar., p. 159.
80. Evans, W. E., *et al.* *Anesthesiology*, 1945, Jan., p. 39.
81. Krantz, J. C., *et al.* *Jour. Pharmacol. Exp. Therap.*, 1941, **72**, p. 233.
82. Krantz, C. K., *et al.* *Anesth. & Anal.*, 1942, July-Aug., p. 234.
83. Marsh, D. F., and Leake, G. P. *Anesthesiology*, 1950, July, p. 455.

CHAPTER VII

THE HALOGEN-CONTAINING ANÆSTHETICS

Ethyl Chloride—Methyl Chloride—Methylene Dichloride—Isopropyl Chloride —Chloroform—Trichlorethylene.

MANY compounds whose molecules contain one or more halogen atoms are used in anæsthesia. The basal narcotics, bromethol, trichlorethanol, pernocton and eunarcon have already been mentioned.

ETHYL CHLORIDE
(chlorethyl, monochlorethane, narcotile, kelene, chloryl anæsthetic)

Ethyl chloride continues to be used extensively for the induction of anæsthesia and for short operations in children. In many patients it is possible to produce analgesia without anæsthesia[1] (see Chapter XVIII). Portability, safety and rapidity of action constitute the main advantages of ethyl chloride.[2] Ethyl chloride is explosive in mixtures between 5 per cent. and 15 per cent. by volume in air, the resulting vapour containing hydrochloric acid being extremely irritant.[3] ($C_2H_5Cl + 3O_2 \rightarrow 2CO_2 + 2H_2O + HCl$.) An innovation has been made in scenting the drug with chemicals, giving an odour resembling that of eau de Cologne. One preparation in particular is so successful that the rather unpleasant smell of ethyl chloride is completely disguised and children can often be anæsthetized before they realize that the " scent " is of an unusual nature. A combined mask and tube holder has been introduced and facilitates the administration of ethyl chloride, using one hand only. From time to time attempts are made to adapt ethyl chloride for anæsthesia in prolonged operations, and Caillaud has devised an ingenious apparatus for maintaining the temperature and vapour percentage constant,[4] *vide* also Chapter XVIII. The method has, however, made little progress in Great Britain. Ethyl chloride can also be used as an adjuvant to nitrous oxide and oxygen by the simple expedient of spraying it into the trichlorethylene bottle of the apparatus and adding the vapour to the mixed gases as required.[5] Mixtures containing the drug are " **anesthol** " (ethyl chloride 17 per cent., chloroform 36 per cent. and ether 47 per cent.), " **Schleich's mixture** " (containing the same three drugs) and " **somnoform** " (ethyl chloride 35 per cent., methyl chloride 60 per cent. and ethyl bromide 5 per cent.). These have some vogue on the Continent.[6] " **Novanest** ", which is popular in Italy, contains ethyl chloride, methyl chloride, chloromethylene and di-ethyl ether. These constituents, however, cannot be separated by such methods as fractional distillation. Novanest is prepared by dropping concentrated sulphuric acid on to a mixture of alcohol and chloroform containing aluminium chloride and granulated zinc. The resulting product is fractionated to 40°. It is said that recovery from novanest anæsthesia is rapid and that vomiting is uncommon.[7]

Ethyl chloride is still used to a limited extent in rendering tissues insensitive by freezing. Mixtures of ethyl chloride and methyl chloride (e.g. " **anestile** ") are also used for the same purpose and produce a lower temperature.

METHYL CHLORIDE

Methyl chloride is, at the present time, not used alone, although its action as a general anæsthetic was investigated as long ago as 1879 by a Committee of the British Medical Association.[8] Since the employment of this compound in refrigerators several cases of poisoning have been reported[10] and in one fatal case cirrhosis of the liver had occurred.[9]

METHYLENE DICHLORIDE

Methylene dichloride was used as a general anæsthetic by Richardson in 1867 but was soon abandoned. At the present time the compound is extensively employed as a paint remover and cases of poisoning have been described.[11]

ISOPROPYL CHLORIDE (proponesin)

Isopropyl chloride (proponesin) has the structural formula $CH_3CHClCH_3$ and is an inflammable colourless liquid with S.G. 0·859 and B.P. 36·6° C. It is prepared commercially by the action of hydrochloric acid on isopropyl alcohol in the presence of zinc chloride and is then distilled and purified. When used as an inhalation anæsthetic isopropyl chloride gives a rapid induction and recovery and has a marked analgesic effect which it was thought might prove useful in obstetric practice.[12] Unfortunately cardiac arrhythmias are common[13] and since a case of primary cardiac failure occurred early in a series of administrations in man[14] the present view is that its use is unjustifiable.

CHLOROFORM (Trichlormethane.   CHCl₃)

Chloroform is now rarely given alone but is occasionally added in the smallest possible amounts to nitrous oxide and oxygen. Until recently, chloroform was infrequently used in **closed circuits** owing to the impression that phosgene could be produced by the action of soda-lime.   Although this is theoretically possible, it has been shown that under normal working conditions, the chemical reaction is as follows. $CHCl_3 + 3NaOH \rightarrow 3NaCl + CO + 2H_2O$. The amount of carbon monoxide generated is so small (less than 16 c.cm.) that in practice no harm will result.[15]

The **indications** for chloroform are now few since cyclopropane also causes no irritation to the respiratory passages.   The fact that chloroform does not burn or explode in mixtures of air, oxygen or nitrous oxide constitutes its only real asset, and it seems probable that trichlorethylene may oust it even when a source of ignition may be present.   If used by itself, the concentration of chloroform in air necessary to produce anæsthesia is from 2 per cent. to 3 per cent. and narcosis can usually be maintained by 1 per cent. or 2 per cent.

Various dosimetric **inhalers** have been designed to provide a definite percentage of vapour, such as Vernon Harcourt's, Levy's and Rowling's,[16] but they are now little used, although an apparatus for dropping with paratroops was designed during the late war and known as the " E.S.O."

It seems established that chloroform can exert **toxic effects** in at least four different ways.   (i) Primary cardiac failure by (*a*) vagal stimulation.[17]   This effect has been rather discounted in recent years but there is little doubt that it does exist.   In animals under the influence of atropine this effect is not obtained, and it is possible that in man full doses of atropine may give some protection from vagal stimulation.   (*b*) Ventricular fibrillation due to an intermittent administration or to stimulation before the patient is fully anæsthetized, or to the administration of adrenaline.[18] Recent work with the electrocardiograph seems to show that the site of origin of systole may change from the sinoauricular node to the atrioventricular node in the early stages of chloroform anæsthesia,[19] and a definite " prefibrillation phase " has been demonstrated.[20]   This probably occurs at the end of the second stage and just before full surgical anæsthesia is reached.[21]   It is possible that preliminary basal narcosis with one of the barbiturates may afford some protection against ventricular fibrillation.[22] (ii) Gradual paralysis of the respiratory centre from overdose.

The " secondary cardiac failure " which ensues if this condition is not promptly treated may be due in part to a decrease of glycogen and an increase of lactic acid in the heart muscle, chloroform being said to have a similar effect to the cyanides in this respect.[23] (iii) Delayed chloroform poisoning. A fatal dose has been recorded in which only 4 drachms of the drug were used.[24] It used to be thought that the liver was damaged by derivatives of chloroform such as carbonyl chloride and hydrochloric acid, but it has recently been proved that chloroform as such is toxic to parenchymatous organs in direct ratio to the lipoid content of their cells.[25] There is some evidence (in animals) to show that preliminary medication with sulphanilamide affords some protection against liver damage by chloroform.[26] It is clear that it would be most unwise to administer chloroform to patients in a poor nutritional state particularly if they have recently vomited or are suffering from any toxæmia. The latest work on the toxic effects of chloroform is embodied in an admirable monograph written by the anæsthetic staff of Madison.[27]

Occasional fatalities still occur from mistaking chloroform for ether. The difference in weight and smell should make the distinction obvious, but there is a good deal to be said for the practice of one manufacturer who colours chloroform with a red dye.

TRICHLORETHYLENE

Trichlorethylene has the chemical formula $CCl_2 . CHCl$, and was first described in 1864.

Properties. It is a colourless liquid with a smell resembling chloroform without its pungency. The specific gravity is 1·47, the vapour density 4·53 and the boiling point 87° C. It is not inflammable nor will its vapour explode when mixed in any proportion of air. If, however,[28] the air is enriched with oxygen, or if trichlorethylene vapour is mixed with pure oxygen, at temperatures higher than 25·5° C. (78° F.), inflammable mixtures may be formed which ignite at 419° C. In Great Britain, it is unlikely that the gases issuing from unheated vaporizers should exceed 78° F., but it would seem wise to use air in preference to oxygen if an ignition risk is present. If the diathermy cautery is used in the presence of strong trichlorethylene (or chloroform) vapour, a minute quantity of phosgene may be formed, but in practice this can be ignored.[29] On the other hand, it is dangerous to smoke in the presence of trichlorethylene vapour, as all the decomposition products are inhaled by the smoker. The drug has a high solvent power for fats but is practically insoluble in water. It will mix with di-ethyl ether in any proportion without chemical reaction. Pure trichlorethylene tends to decompose in strong sunlight and air and should therefore be stored in stoppered amber bottles. The main action of decomposition is one of oxidation to dichloracetyl chloride, carbon monoxide, hydrochloric acid and phosgene. The addition of $0 \cdot 01$ per cent. thymol retards decomposition and the resultant product is known under the trade name **Trilene** (**Inalene** in Italy). A similar preparation is known as **Trimar** in America. At the author's suggestion this is now coloured with 1 in 200,000 " waxoline blue" to distinguish it from chloroform. Trichlorethylene is used commercially for such purposes as the dry-cleaning of clothes, the de-waxing of lubricating oils and the de-greasing of metals. For these uses the substance is known under a variety of trade names such as triklone, gemalgene, chlorylene, trethylene and westrosol. These preparations are too impure for inhalational use and industrial poisoning is not very infrequent, the symptoms including giddiness, vomiting, optic neuritis and various palsies.[30]

Preparation. Trichlorethylene is prepared by the controlled chlorination of acetylene to give tetrachlorethane. $C_2H_2 + 2Cl_2 \rightarrow C_2H_2Cl_4$. This is followed by treatment with lime slurry $2C_2H_2Cl_4 + CaO \rightarrow CaCl_2 + H_2O + 2C_2HCl_3$ and subsequent distillation.

Tests for Impurities. If decomposition is suspected, the following three tests will show whether trichlorethylene is sufficiently pure to be used for anæsthetic purposes.

10 c.cm. of the sample are shaken for three minutes with 20 c.cm. of freshly boiled and cooled distilled water. The aqueous layer is separated into three lots, two of 5 c.cm. and one of 10 c.cm.

(1) To 5 c.cm. a few drops of bromcresol purple are added. The colour should be the same as that produced by the addition of the same quantity of the indicator to 5 c.cm. of freshly boiled and cooled distilled water. If it is not, an excess of acid is present.

(2) To 5 c.cm. are added an equal volume of distilled water, 1 drop of concentrated nitric acid and $0 \cdot 2$ c.cm. of 5 per cent. silver nitrate solution. The liquid should remain clear. Any opalescence indicates an excess of chlorides.

(3) To 10 c.cm. are added 1 c.cm. of 5 per cent. cadmium iodide solution and 2 drops of freshly prepared starch solution. Any blue coloration shows the presence of free chlorine.[31]

Therapeutic Uses. Trichlorethylene has been used externally to clean up dirty wounds and burns and also as an inhalant to

TRICHLORETHYLENE 115

mitigate the pain of trigeminal neuralgia. The origin of this procedure is curious. It was reported by two separate observers that patients suffering from chronic trichlorethylene poisoning showed complete bilateral paralysis of all divisions of the trigeminal nerve.[30] It was then assumed that the drug had some specific action on this nerve and its administration for trigeminal neuralgia was suggested[32] and found to be effective.[33] It is much more probable that the pain is relieved because a state of general analgesia is induced. The question of nerve palsies is considered below.

Anæsthesia in Animals. A great deal of experimental work has been done by repeatedly anæsthetizing various animals with trichlorethylene. Microscopical examination of the viscera suggests that the drug has much less toxic effects than chloroform.[34]

Analgesia and Anæsthesia in the Human Subject. Trichlorethylene was first used rather tentatively to anæsthetize patients in America[35] but after a full investigation in Great Britain[36] its use spread very rapidly and after its definite limitations were realized it has found a recognized place in anæsthesia.[37]

Effects on Cardio-vascular System. Cardiac arrhythmias are not uncommon under trichlorethylene narcosis particularly in the induction stage.[38] They are usually auricular extra systoles but the ventricular type have also been noted (see also Chapter I). Very occasionally cardiac arrhythmias may persist during the post-anæsthetic period.[39] Primary cardiac failure, probably from ventricular fibrillation, is an exceedingly rare event[40] and is probably due to employing an excessive concentration of the drug in a patient already showing the signs of ventricular extra systoles. It is a sound practice to avoid the use of trichlorethylene with patients known to be suffering from cardiac irregularities. Blood pressure usually remains within normal limits during trichlorethylene narcosis but bleeding from cut surfaces is noticeably less than with ether.

Effects on Respiratory System. Trichlorethylene has practically no irritating effects on the respiratory passages so that the induction of anæsthesia is usually smooth and free from coughing. If " pushed " the drug causes tachypnœa (see Chapter I) and this sign should be regarded as signifying overdosage. If muscular relaxation is essential it should be obtained by a peripheral relaxant such as curare. Occasionally the respiratory rate is undesirably high under quite light narcosis and under these circumstances a *small* intravenous dose of pethidine will often bring about a significant reduction. If not, a change to some other anæsthetic should be made. The reason for the often dramatic reduction in the respiration rate with pethidine is obscure, one suggestion being that bronchiolar dilatation occurs which ensures the efficient elimination of carbon dioxide.[54]

Effects on Nervous System.   Analgesia is usually marked in the first stage and occurs so rapidly that the drug is tending to replace nitrous oxide in midwifery[41], dentistry (q.v.), minor surgery, burn dressings and for the many painful or frightening procedures in medical paediatric practice.[42] Amnesia is often present after trichlorethylene has been used in this way. It has been estimated that if consciousness is to be completely lost, the concentration of the drug in the blood is from 6 to 12·5 mg. per 100 c.cm. (Powell, 1945).

Toxic Effects and Complications.   Post-anæsthetic nausea and vomiting would seem to be definitely less than with ether.   Some cases of cranial nerve palsies have been recorded[43] but either impure trichlorethylene had been used,[44] or the drug had been given in a closed-circuit with soda-lime[45] (see below).   Up to date only one case of liver necrosis has been recorded and here the influence of the drug was extremely doubtful.[46]   The toxic action on the liver is almost certainly less than that of chloroform or of di-ethyl ether.[47] Changes in blood-sugar and blood-urea values appear to be negligible.

Technique of Administration.   Owing to its low volatility, trichlorethylene is unsuitable for administration by an open mask method, and the apparatus illustrated has been devised.[48]   On

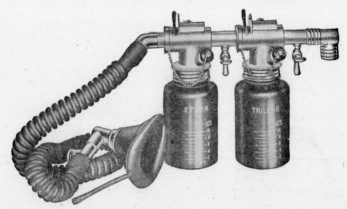

Fig. 42.   " Draw-over " type of apparatus for producing analgesia or anæsthesia with trichlorethylene or ether or with both (Marrett).

inspiration the patient draws air through a valve. This passes through the vaporizing bottle, which contains a circular wick and the strength of trichlorethylene vapour can be regulated with some precision by a lever fixed on a rotating drum. Expiration takes place through a standard valve close to the facepiece, but partial rebreathing into a small bag can be used if desired. The addition of a second and similar bottle enables practically any type of operation to be performed under anæsthesia with trichlorethylene, ether or both. Either a facepiece or an endotracheal tube can be used provided that air leaks are avoided. The provision of a side tap permits ethyl chloride to be admitted or, if oxygen is available, the " blow-through " principle can be used for such purposes as pharyngeal insufflation with a Davis gag for dissection tonsillectomy (q.v.). The construction of this vaporizer is such that resistance to respiration is very small and no water jacket is necessary for either bottle. It is also light in weight and relatively inexpensive.

A pocket inhaler weighing only 10 oz. for insertion into a nostril is a useful device where portability is of paramount importance.[49] A spring-loaded plunger is used to snap a 6 c.cm. ampoule of trilene and one charge will suffice for self-administered analgesia for about an hour (Fig. 43).

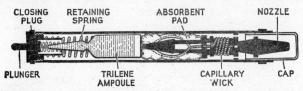

FIG. 43. Section of " Trilite " inhaler for auto-analgesia. (Hayward-Butt, *The Lancet.*)

Special types of inhaler have been evolved for producing analgesia in dentistry and midwifery (q.v.).

If desired, trichlorethylene can be used as an adjuvant to nitrous oxide and oxygen by placing it in the " chloroform bottle " of any standard apparatus. It should be noted that the bottle should be made of tinted glass and the trichlorethylene changed every few days. Neglect of these precautions may lead to the formation of small quantities of hydrochloric acid and phosgene.[55] It should be remembered that the drug has a relatively low volatility and is consequently excreted slowly. It will be found that, once anæsthesia is attained, an extremely small maintenance dose is sufficient, and the drug should be cut off altogether some time before the end of the operation. If these precautions are not taken, anæsthesia may become unnecessarily profound and recovery will be unduly prolonged.

Trichlorethylene should *not* be used in a closed circuit as it is possible for a chemical reaction to take place between it and soda-lime with the production of dichloracetylene.[45]

$$\begin{matrix} CHCl \\ \| \\ C.Cl_2 \end{matrix} + NaOH \rightarrow \begin{matrix} C.Cl \\ \||| \\ C.Cl \end{matrix} + NaCl + H_2O$$

This decomposition product is certainly toxic and is probably the cause of cranial nerve palsies. The effect is much more likely to occur with unsuitable soda-lime, which becomes unduly hot, while the presence of moisture and of ether minimizes the reaction.[50] It is wise, however, to eschew closed circuits altogether when using trichlorethylene. Various mechanical devices to prevent this occurrence have been described such as a by-pass tap for fitting to existing apparatus[51] and an ingenious lock which is an integral part of Marrett's gas-oxygen apparatus.[52] (See Chapter V).

Trichlorethylene has also been used with success as a " single-dose " anæsthetic in Goldman's vinesthene inhaler for such operations as dental extractions and guillotine tonsillectomies in children[53] (see Chapter XIX).

References

1. AMOILS, M. *Brit. Med. Jour.*, 1934, June 23, p. 1143.
2. HEWER, C. L. *Brit. Med. Jour.*, 1930, Feb. 8, p. 262.
3. COSTE, J. H., and CHAPLIN, C. A. *Brit. Jour. Anæsth.*, 1937, April, p. 115.
4. CAILLAUD, E. *Presse Méd.*, 1928, Dec. 1, p. 1531.
5. WESTELL, V. M. *Lancet*, 1941, Nov. 29, p. 666.
6. FLEXER-LAWTON. *Brit. Jour. Anæsth.*, 1933, Jan., p. 51.
7. GIORDANENGO, G. *Anesth. & Anal.*, 1939, Sept.-Oct., p. 251.
8. GORHAM, A. P. *Brit. Med. Jour.*, 1934, March 24, p. 529.
9. BIRCH, C. A. *Lancet*, 1935, Feb. 2, p. 259.
10. WOOD, M. W. *Lancet*, 1951, Mar. 3, p. 508.
11. COLLIER, H. *Lancet*, 1936, Mar. 14, p. 594.
12. MACDONALD, T. J. C. *Brit. Jour. Anæsth.*, 1950, Apr., p. 92.
13. ELAM, J. E., and NEWHOUSE, M. L. *Brit. Med. Jour.*, 1951, Jan. 6, p. 13.
14. ROUALLE, H. L. M. *Brit. Med. Jour.*, 1950, Sept. 23, p. 712.
15. BASSETT, H. L. *Lancet*, 1949, Sept. 24, p. 561.
16. ROWLING, S. T. *Brit. Jour. Anæsth.*, 1932, Jan., p. 59.
17. { *B.M.A. Chloroform Commission*, 1910, July.
    { EMBLEY. *Lancet*, 1915, *ii*, p. 283.
18. LEVY, A. GOODMAN. *Chloroform Anæsthesia*.
19. OSBORNE, W. A. *Brit. Jour. Anæsth.*, 1932, Jan., p. 87.
20. HILL, I. G. W. *Lancet*, 1932, May 28, p. 1139.
21. MILLS, A. *Brit. Med. Jour.*, 1935, Oct. 26, p. 821.

22. GUEDEL, A. E., and KNOEFEL, P. K.   *Amer. Jour. Surg.*, 1936, Dec., p. 497.
23. MAXWELL, I.   *Med. Jour. Australia*, 1933, p. 626.
24. TODD, T. F.   *Lancet*, 1934, Sept. 6, p. 597.
25. MACNIDER, W. de B.   *Anest. & Anal.*, 1935, **14,** p. 97.
26. FORBES, J. C., and EVANS, E. I.   *War Medicine*, 1943.   Chicago, Oct., p. 418.
27. WATERS, R. M.   " Chloroform," 1950.   University of Wisconsin Press.
28. JONES, C. W., and SCOTT, G. S.   *Bureau of Mines. Rep.* 3666.   Pittsburg, Pa., U.S.A.
29. HEWER, C. L.   *Brit. Med. Jour.*, 1943, Apr. 10, p. 453.
30. { PLESSNER, W.   *Berlin klin. Wchr.*, 9116, **53,** p. 25.
     { GERBIS, H.   *Zbl. Gewerbehyg*, 1928.
31. Information kindly supplied by Imperial Chemical Industries, Ltd.
32. OLJENICK, I.   *Jour. Amer. Med. Ass.*, 1928, **91,** p. 1085.
33. GLASER, M. A.   *Jour. Amer. Med. Ass.*, 1931, **96,** p. 916.
34. { JOACHIMOGLU, G.   *Berlin klin. Wschr.*, 1921, **58,** p. 47.
     { KRANTZ, J. C., et al.   *Pro. Amer. Pharmaceut., Ass.*, 1935.
     { LANDE, P., et al.   1939.
35. { STRIKER, C., et al.   *Anesth. & Anal.*, 1935, March-April, p. 68.
     { JACKSON, D. E.   *Anesth. & Anal.*, 1934, Sept.-Oct., p. 198.
36. HEWER.   C. L.   *Brit. Med. Jour.*, 1941, June 21, p. 924.
37. HEWER, C. L.   *Pro. Roy. Soc. Med.* (An. Sec.), 1942. Mar. 6.
38. BARNES, C. G., and IVES, J.   *Pro. Roy. Soc. Med.* (An. Sec.), 1944, May 5.
39. CONDON, H. A.   *Brit. Med. Jour.*, 1948, ii, p. 340.
40. { HAWORTH, J., and DUFF, A.   *Brit. Med. Jour.*, 1943, Mar. 27, p. 381.
     { LLOYD-WILLIAMS, K. C., and HEWSPEARE, P.   *Brit. Med. Jour.*, 1942, ii, p. 170.
41. ELAM, J.   *Lancet*, 1942, Sept. 12, p. 309.
42. THOMSON, J.   *Brit. Med. Jour.*, 1949, Dec. 24, p. 1449.
43. MCAULEY, J.   *Brit. Med. Jour.*, 1943, Dec. 4, p. 713.
44. HEWER, C. L.   *Pro. Roy. Soc. Med.* (An. Sec.), 1943, May 7.
45. { HUMPHREY, J. H., and MCCLELLAND, M.   *Brit. Med. Jour.*, 1944, Mar. 4, p. 316.
     { CARDEN, S.   *Brit. Med. Jour.*, 1944, Mar. 4, p. 319.
46. DODDS, G. H.   *Brit. Med. Jour.*, 1945, June 2, p. 769.
47. ARMSTRONG, D. M.   *Anœsthesia*, 1947, April, p. 45.
48. MARRETT, H. R.   *Brit. Med. Jour.*, 1942, May 23, p. 643.
49. HAYWARD-BUTT, J. T.   *Lancet*, 1947, Dec. 13, p. 865.
50. FIRTH, J. B., and STUCKEY, R. E.   *Lancet*, 1945, June 30, p. 814.
51. GALLEY, A. H.   *Brit. Med. Jour.*, 1948, May 22, p. 996.
52. MARRETT, H. R.   *Brit. Med. Jour.*, 1948, Feb. 28, p. 403.
53. GALLEY, A. H.   *Pro. Roy. Soc. Med.* (An. Sec.), 1943, May 7.
54. JOHNSTONE, M.   *Brit. Med. Jour.*, 1951, Oct. 20, p. 943.
55. OSTLERE, G.   *Brit. Med. Jour.*, 1952, June 28, p. 1405.

CHAPTER VIII

RECENT DEVELOPMENTS IN ENDOTRACHEAL ANÆSTHESIA

Historical. Intubation of the trachea in animals was, so far as is known, first performed and recorded by Vesalius[1] in 1542. Snow gave chloroform vapour through a tracheotomy tube to animals in 1858. It is interesting to observe that he used a closed-circuit with caustic potash to absorb the carbon dioxide[2]. Trendelenburg applied Snow's method to man in 1871,[3] while MacEwen in 1880 was the first to administer an anæsthetic (chloroform) through a metal tracheal tube introduced through the mouth.[4] Kuhn and Elsberg[5] both used endotracheal anæsthesia in suitable cases between 1900 and 1910 while Magill and Rowbotham developed the technique to deal with plastic facial surgery occasioned by the 1914-18 European war.[6]

Two main **principles** can be utilized :

(*a*) The *insufflation* method in which anæsthetic gases are forced through a tube whose distal extremity lies in the trachea, the return flow either taking a natural course or an artificial one through a second tube also lying in the trachea. The true insufflation technique is now obsolete, the chief disadvantage being loss of heat and water vapour and prolonged acapnia from the low alveolar CO_2 concentration. If allowed to continue, alkalosis accompanied by a fall in blood pressure occurs, a similar condition to that produced by prolonged hyperventilation. A modified form of insufflation anæsthesia with some rebreathing is referred to in Chapter XXIII.

(*b*) The *inhalation* method in which to and fro respiration takes place through one wide-bore tube which may be regarded as a continuation of the trachea. This tube may be passed through the nose, mouth or through laryngotomy or tracheotomy wounds as required. Any type of open-, semi-closed-, or closed-circuit technique may be employed.

The chief **indications** for endotracheal anæsthesia are :

(i) Operations in which obstruction to the airway may be expected either from the nature of the disease, the surgical technique, the position of the patient or the presence of fluids in the air passages.

(ii) Most major operations on the head and neck.

(iii) Most prolonged upper abdominal operations where shallow respiration is desirable and in which spinal, splanchnic or other local blocks are not employed.[7] It is specially useful in gastro-enterostomy or partial gastrectomy where the passage of a stomach tube is desirable. This can be effected with no interruption of the anæsthesia.

The routine use of endotracheal anæsthesia for every type of operation and patient cannot be too strongly deprecated.

Apparatus Required. Practically any type of continuous-flow, intermittent-flow or closed-circuit gas-oxygen apparatus can be used for inhalation endotracheal anæsthesia (see Chapter V). An adapter connects the breathing tube to the tracheal tube instead of to the normal facepiece, and, since the resulting circuit is gas-tight, it is desirable that some form of automatic blow-off be incorporated, so that excessive intra-pulmonary pressure is impossible. It is, for example, extremely dangerous to employ the emergency oxygen valve fitted to many machines when using endotracheal anæsthesia, as a high pressure is rapidly built up. Some divergence of opinion exists on the maximum pressure permissible. It has been stated that, even with the chest laid open, a dog's lungs can withstand a pressure of over 120 mm. Hg without injury.[8] Later work has suggested that much lower pressures can cause pulmonary emphysema[9] and in practice it is rarely necessary to go above 8 mm. Hg (*vide* also Thoracic Surgery).

Massive surgical emphysema has occasionally occurred during endotracheal anæsthesia, the first case having been reported in 1912.[10] The condition is probably due to a minute perforation of the pharyngeal mucosa during intubation through which gases under pressure are forced into the fascial planes of the neck and mediastinum. The onset may occur with alarming rapidity and continuous aspiration through a wide-bore needle passed through the deep fascia of the neck may be necessary.[11]

It should be remembered that all methods of endotracheal anæsthesia by-pass the nose with its natural mechanism for warming and moistening the inspired air. Experiments have shown that the temperature at the tracheal bifurcation is 5° to 7° lower than the rectal temperature if $N_2O—O_2$ and ether are given by the semi-closed endotracheal method. This heat-loss is greatly diminished by using a closed-circuit and whenever possible this should be done.[12]

If no gas-oxygen apparatus is available, " open " ether or chloroform can be given by means of a Hahn's cone or gauze vaporizer connected to the intubation tube, or chloroform or ether vapour can be pumped from a Junker's bottle or a Shipway's apparatus into the inlet of an Ayre's T-piece (see Chapter XXVII). A certain amount of rebreathing can be arranged through a wide-bore rubber tube open to the air. Although Cobb's adapter (Fig. 44) was primarily designed for tracheal suction, it can equally well be used as a T-piece for open endotracheal work.[13]

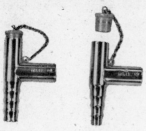

FIG. 44. Endotracheal adapter (oral or nasal) which can either be used for tracheal suction or as a T-piece (W. A. Cobb).

The usual "push on" metal adapter has been known to come adrift from old or perished tubes, a mishap which can be obviated by a modified adapter with a locking device. After insertion, the proximal end of the endotracheal tube is slipped on to the inner tube of the adapter. The ring is then pushed home which causes the claws of the outer part to grip the tube securely.[14]

A great many modifications of Magill's original endotracheal tube adapter have been made, the one most generally useful, in the author's opinion, being the Nosworthy type illustrated. This is made in two parts, the straight one being pushed well home into the mouth of the tracheal tube and the other curved portion being ground to an airtight push fit. The breathing tube can be moved to any convenient position without having to disconnect or twist the rubber, and kinking is rendered unlikely.

If no apparatus of any description is available, the end of the intubation tube can be used in the same way as an ordinary airway

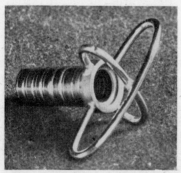

FIG. 45. Bell's endotracheal adapter. (*Lancet.*)

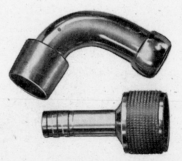

FIG. 46. Nosworthy's endotracheal connector. (M.I.E.)

and chloroform or ether administered from a lint or mask held over the face as in the usual inhalation anæsthesia. The adapter illustrated is useful for this purpose as it can be used under the facepiece of a gas-oxygen apparatus, the wire frame ensuring that no obstruction to the orifice can occur.[15]

Technique of Passing Endotracheal Catheters and Tubes

Preliminary Medication. Whatever other drugs are given before operation, an adequate dose of atropine or scopolamine is desirable in order to diminish secretions.

Cocainization of the Larynx. Rosenberg[16] used cocaine to diminish the laryngeal and pharyngeal reflexes in anæsthesia as long ago as 1895, and some anæsthetists cocainize the larynx as a routine before intubation.[17] In spite of theoretical objections the method has much to commend it, as a much lighter initial

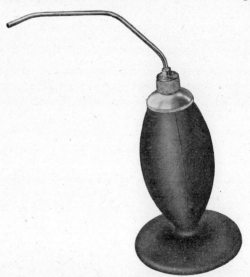

Fig. 47. Spray suitable for cocainization of nose or larynx which can be operated by one hand. (A. C. King, Ltd.)

anæsthesia is required. In nasal intubation, at any rate, both sides of the nose should be sprayed with 20 per cent. cocaine in a fine nebulizer. If this is done during inspiration, some of the solution will be carried down to the larynx so that the glottis will become less sensitive and there will be more room in the nose from shrinkage of the turbinates. It is possible that less absorption occurs from strong cocaine solutions than weak ones, but great caution must be exercised in children. It should be noted that some sprays deliver a jet of liquid if used on the recumbent patient. If this is swallowed toxic symptoms may occur. Most authorities consider it inadvisable to cocainize the glottis before nasal and oral operations owing to the danger of inefficient closure when the patient is returned to bed.[18] On the other hand, it is undeniable that the passage of tracheal tubes under light general anæsthesia only can give rise to reflex disturbances of the respiratory and circulatory mechanisms and even death.[19] (This is not surprising since each year many instantaneous deaths occur in persons who have had food lodged on the glottis. These fatalities are not due to asphyxia, as was once supposed, but are reflex in origin.[20]) Investigations have shown that electrocardiographic charges are very common at the moment of tracheal intubation.[21] For example, in one series 68 per cent. of all patients showed E.C.G. disturbances during intubation but if intravenous procaine was given previously this figure was reduced to 24 per cent.[22] Cardiac arrhythmias are particularly likely to follow intubation under light cyclopropane and the barbiturates[23] and are apparently caused by irritation of vagal fibres in the larynx and trachea.

If no analgesic effect is required, a few drops of one of the many paraffin-ephedrine preparations instilled into each nostril will give a clearer passage and act as a lubricant. For long operations in which a very light narcosis is adequate (e.g. craniotomy) lubrication of the tracheal tube with nupercaine ointment will lessen the incidence of coughing if the head is moved. Both nupercaine (1 per cent.) and xylocaine (5 per cent.) are now obtainable as lubricants in a water-miscible base which has no deleterious effect on rubber. The routine use of strong laryngeal analgesics, on the other hand, cannot be too strongly condemned. For example the cough reflex can be inhibited for several hours after tonsillectomy and the possibility of inhaling blood is correspondingly increased.

Use of Carbon Dioxide. The administration of 5 per cent. carbon dioxide for a few moments before intubation increases the size of the glottic opening and facilitates the passage of tubes.[24]

Oral Intubation

The passage of catheters and tubes into the trachea by direct laryngoscopy has often been described and rarely presents any difficulty.

Magill's laryngoscope is a convenient instrument incorporating a battery in the handle. A wide slot for manipulation is provided and the lens-fronted bulb directs the light downwards, thus giving good illumination without undue reflection. In the latest pattern the lamp is more proximal and is set at an angle in a recess so that there is no projection to impede manipulation. Most American instruments have the handle (sometimes folding and incorporating an automatic lamp switch) mounted at an acute angle to the spatula, so that it does not touch the chest when the head is flexed[25] (Fig. 48). In difficult cases a piece of sheet lead can be used to

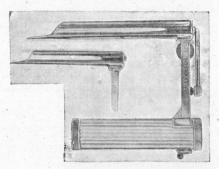

Fig. 48. Magill's laryngoscope with semi-proximal illumination, showing interchangeable spatulæ for adults and children. Some later models have hinged handles and three alternative sized blades.

protect the upper incisor teeth, but this is usually unnecessary. A strip of strapping placed over the front teeth is, however, a wise precaution to avoid the possibility of chipping the enamel. As a general rule, a curved soft rubber tube is well lubricated and passed through the glottis. The proximal end is then connected by a curved metal angle-piece to the breathing tube of the gas-oxygen apparatus. If it is desired to employ tracheal suction, one of the T-shaped adapters shown in Figs. 44 and 128 is substituted for the angle-piece, and a suction catheter can then be passed down the lumen of the tracheal tube. The largest tube which will enter the glottis easily with the cords abducted should be employed. Magill's tubes are made of mineralized rubber in the sizes shown. The stiffer tubes are intended for oral intubation and the thin-walled

Dimensions and Catheter Gauge Equivalents of Magill Oral and Nasal Tubes.

Oral	Nasal	Approx. External Diameter	Approx. Internal Diameter		Length	Nearest French Catheter Gauge
			Oral	Nasal		
00	—	$\frac{11}{64}''$	$\frac{1}{8}''$	—	$8''$	13
0	—	$\frac{7}{32}''$	$\frac{11}{64}''$	—	$8\frac{1}{2}''$	16
1	—	$\frac{1}{4}''$	$\frac{3}{16}''$	—	$8\frac{3}{4}''$	19
2	2	$\frac{9}{32}''$	$\frac{13}{64}''$	$\frac{7}{32}''$	$9\frac{1}{4}''$	21
3	3	$\frac{5}{16}''$	$\frac{7}{32}''$	$\frac{1}{4}''$	$9\frac{3}{4}''$	24
4	4	$\frac{21}{64}''$	$\frac{15}{64}''$	$\frac{17}{64}''$	$10\frac{3}{8}''$	25
5	5	$\frac{23}{64}''$	$\frac{17}{64}''$	$\frac{9}{32}''$	$10\frac{7}{8}''$	27
6	6	$\frac{3}{8}''$	$\frac{9}{32}''$	$\frac{19}{64}''$	$11\frac{3}{8}''$	29
7	7	$\frac{13}{32}''$	$\frac{19}{64}''$	$\frac{5}{16}''$	$12\frac{3}{8}''$	31
8	8	$\frac{27}{64}''$	$\frac{5}{16}''$	$\frac{21}{64}''$	$13''$	33
9	—	$\frac{15}{32}''$	$\frac{11}{32}''$	—	$13\frac{3}{8}''$	36
10	—	$\frac{1}{2}''$	$\frac{3}{8}''$	—	$14\frac{1}{4}''$	38

ones for passage through the nose.[26] The distal end of the tube must lie between the glottis and the tracheal bifurcation, a rough

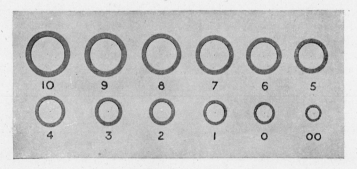

FIG. 49. Actual size of Magill's tubes.

guide to the correct length being twice the distance between the lobe of the ear to the ala of the nose.

If the widest possible lumen is desirable (as in thoracic surgery), a soft, specially shaped rubber tube can be slipped through a

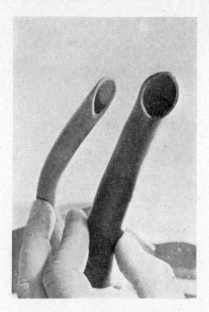

Fig. 50. Wide-bore tapered endotracheal tube (Macintosh) contrasted with No. 10 Magill tube above. (*Anœsthesia.*)

completely paralysed glottis by threading it over a gum-elastic catheter. This tube is tapered and the tracheal end has a cross-section twice that of a No. 10 Magill tube.[27]

Owing to the shortage of natural rubber during the late war, various substitutes have been tried for tracheal tubes. Synthetic rubber lacks elasticity but vinyl acrylic resin has been found satisfactory.[28] " Portex " white tubes made from this material will stand repeated boiling well provided that they are cooled off in the required curve. The tendency to kinking seems to be about the same as that of a similar tube made from natural rubber.

Various positions of the head have been recommended for direct laryngoscopy but it would seem clear that the correct posture should ensure that the three axes of the mouth, pharynx and larynx should coincide.[29] With a normal patient lying flat, these axes are not in the same plane (Fig. 51A). Flexion of the head on a firm pillow straightens out the cervical spine and makes the axes of the pharynx and larynx coincide (Fig. 51B). Nasal intubation with a well curved tube is often successful in this position (see below). The chin is now pulled upwards causing extension of the head at the atlanto-occipital and upper cervical joints (Fig. 51c). The axes should now be coincident and the blade of the laryngoscope is made to lift up the tongue and epiglottis thus exposing the vocal cords.

It is said that direct-vision laryngoscopy can be performed under a lighter plane of narcosis if the tip of the laryngoscope blade is only passed as far as the angle made by the epiglottis with the base of the tongue (this area is innervated by the glossopharyngeal nerve which plays no part in the laryngeal reflex, whereas the posterior surface of the epiglottis is supplied by the superior laryngeal nerve, stimulation of which results in adduction of the vocal cords). If the laryngoscope be now lifted the tongue with the attached epiglottis will be forced upwards, bringing the glottis into view. A short curved laryngoscope blade has been designed to facilitate this proceeding.[30] It should be noted that the skill of the anæsthetist is of much greater importance than the exact design of his laryngoscope.

Occasionally there is real difficulty in exposing the glottis adequately, and in this case a small guide such as a bent gum-elastic catheter can be passed through the cords and the tracheal tube threaded over it as suggested before for passing very wide-bore orotracheal tubes.[27]

It is quite often possible to intubate " blindly " through the mouth by some modification of Kuhn's original method or by means of a divided metal airway.[31]

For the beginner, really deep narcosis induced by N_2O—O_2—E is undoubtedly the safest preliminary to the passage of tracheal tubes. The " crash induction " technique using curare and thiopentone saves time, and is more spectacular, but it is essential to be sure that the stomach is empty or regurgitation may occur before intubation can be effected.

Packing. If there is any possibility of fluids entering the air passages, or if the closed-circuit technique is to be used, some form of airtight seal must be used. A *gauze roll* soaked in weak antiseptic or in liquid paraffin can be packed round the tube, but

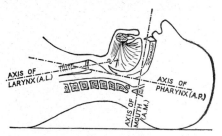

(A) Relative positions of the axes of mouth, pharynx, and larynx with patient lying flat.

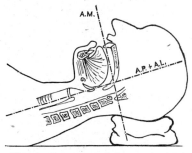

(B) Showing how axes of pharynx and larynx may be made to coincide when the head is raised. The cervical spine is also straightened out.

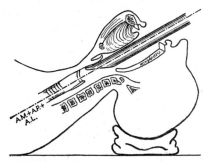

(C) Axis of mouth is now made to coincide with the other axes by extension of the head around the atlanto-occipital and *upper* cervical joints.
(Bannister & Macbeth, *The Lancet.*)

Fig. 51.

however carefully this is done, post-operative pharyngitis is common and displacement of the pack may be followed by leakage of fluid into the trachea round the outside of the tube.   If a pack is used, one end should be left visible or an attached thread should be secured outside the mouth.   Furthermore the person who inserts the pack *must* be responsible for seeing that it is removed later.   Deaths have occurred from respiratory obstruction due to retained packs.   On the whole inflatable *tracheal cuffs* fitting on the tubes are more satisfactory than packs (Figs. 52 and 53).   These are passed in the deflated condition through the glottis until their upper edge lies just beneath the vocal cords.   Air is then injected from a syringe until the trachea is just filled,[32] a state which can be verified by compressing the rebreathing bag with the expiratory valve shut and ascertaining that no leakage occurs.   The author has added a small pilot balloon to the inflating tube as a guide to the degree of cuff distension and to give warning in case of accidental puncture. The importance of some such indication is shown by a recorded case of rupture of a tracheal cuff with fatal results.[33]   Ballooned tubes if new and properly made are so smooth that they can be passed through the nose in the deflated condition,[34] especially if the inflating channel is in the wall instead of a separate rubber tube.

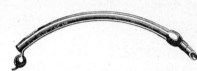

Fig. 52.   Tracheal tube fitted with distal inflatable cuff and proximal pilot balloon (Hewer's modification of Magill's).

Such tubes should not be lubricated with vaseline or oil preparations as these have a deleterious effect on the rubber which tends to thin out in one place so that inflation causes an aneurysmal swelling instead of an even distension.

In America, large cuffs made from extremely thin rubber have been tried. In this case the cuff lies both above and below the

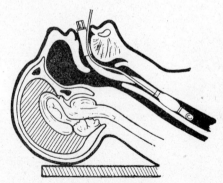

Fig. 53.   Diagram showing inflated tracheal cuff in position (after G. J. Thomas).

cords and is inflated by an air bulb connected to a water manometer, the usual pressure being 15 to 18 cm. H$_2$O. A suction catheter can be built into the tube.[35]

Some anæsthetists prefer a *pharyngeal cuff* on the tracheal tube, but this is not so efficient as a tracheal cuff, and its bulk renders oral intubation more difficult and nasal intubation impossible. On the other hand, secretions collecting proximal to the cuff are more easily removed than with the orthodox tracheal balloon.[36]

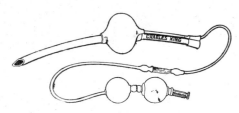

Sterilization of Tubes. Tracheal tubes lose their elasticity after

FIG. 54. Tracheal tube fitted with pharyngeal cuff and double inflating bellows (Rowbotham's).

frequent boiling, and in view of the rubber shortage some other means of sterilization is advisable. In hospital practice, the author has found the following method satisfactory. After use, the tubes are thoroughly cleaned internally with the brush of appropriate size. They are then washed and kept in a large enamelled bowl of 1 in 2,000 biniodide of mercury. Immediately before use they are rinsed in water and their distal 3 inches lubricated with a non-oily preparation such as K.Y. jelly.

Nasal Intubation

The nasal endotracheal technique is extremely useful for operations in the mouth or for other cases where an oral tube is inconvenient. The obvious theoretical objection is that the tube must be passed through a septic cavity and might introduce infection into the trachea. In practice this risk, although slight, is not negligible, cases of pneumonia following this technique having occurred in which the same organisms were cultivated from the nasal mucosa and from the pneumonic lesions in the lungs.[37] The method is, of course, definitely contra-indicated if there is a history of recent sinusitis. Several cases of laryngeal granulomata have been reported following nasal intubation,[38] whilst intranasal adhesions are not unknown. These probably follow infection caused during *extubation*, the septic material being then drawn over previously damaged tissues.[39] An exhaustive survey of over 2,700 endotracheal anæsthesia in America revealed that nasal intubation showed a higher incidence of minor respiratory sequelæ than oral, while in patients with pre-existing pulmonary disease, the incidence of both major and minor complications was higher if the nasal route was adopted.[40] In thoracic surgery (q.v.) naso-tracheal intubation is usually contra-indicated as the largest possible tube should be used. For these reasons, the author and others[41] prefer to use the mouth rather than the nose for intubation, unless the latter is specially indicated.

Technique. The patient's nose and larynx are cocainized, his head slightly extended, and the lubricated curved rubber tube is introduced into the nostril which has the freest passage. Magill's tubes are cut with the bevel to the left and are meant for passing through the right nostril. In actual practice, however, there is little difference between the two sides.[42] When the end of the tube is lying in the pharynx an attempt at "blind" intubation should first be made.[43] If the patient has a reasonably straight nasal septum the bevelled end of the tube will frequently enter the glottis if pushed gently onwards during expiration. Success is notified by the free passage of air through the mouth of the tube. An initial failure may sometimes be rectified by partial rotation of the tube in either direction followed by another attempt. If this also fails, it is the author's practice to withdraw the tube until its end lies in the naso-pharynx and then connect up to the anæsthetic apparatus giving a mixture of N_2O—O_2 and ether with about 5 per cent. CO_2. When the respiration has become deep a further trial is made, the tube being advanced and twisted so that a maximum excursion of the rebreathing bag is maintained. This technique usually succeeds but occasionally, as in the case of a large posterior septal spur, it may be impossible to induce the tube

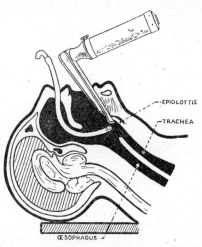

EPIGLOTTIS

TRACHEA

ŒSOPHAGUS

Fig. 55. Diagram illustrating nasal intubation under vision (after G. J. Thomas).

to enter the glottis. If this occurs, a laryngoscope should be passed through the mouth, the epiglottis lifted forwards (Fig. 55) and another attempt made under vision. This may be helped by actually picking up the end of the tube with long forceps (Fig. 56)

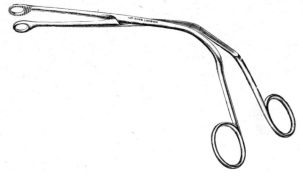

FIG. 56. Magill's forceps.

and guiding it into the desired orifice. If nasal obstruction is evident, either from a deflected septum or from turbinal hypertrophy, no force whatever is permissible and the naso-tracheal route should be abandoned.

Endotracheal Anæsthesia Conducted through Laryngotomy and Tracheotomy Tubes. This proceeding may be advisable for the removal of extensive pharyngeal and laryngeal growths in which septic material might be carried down the trachea during intubation or where the presence of the tube might impede the surgeon.[44] Such operations as lateral pharyngotomy, laryngofissure and laryngectomy may be cited as examples. (It is often possible to avoid tracheotomy or laryngotomy in laryngofissure for the excision of small growths. A modified endotracheal technique for this purpose is described in Chapter XX.) Laryngotomy is preferable to tracheotomy if the site of operation permits and this procedure will now be described briefly. The patient is anæsthetized in the usual way and his head is extended into the thyroid position. The interval between the cricoid and thyroid cartilages is next determined, and a small fold of skin over the mid-line is pinched up and transfixed with a scalpel so that a transverse incision about $\frac{1}{2}$ inch long results. A closed pointed laryngotome is then pushed through the crico-thyroid membrane and the handles are approximated. Air should be heard entering and leaving the aperture, and the laryngotomy tube is then inserted by means of its pilot. The latter being withdrawn, an adapter is inserted and anæsthesia maintained by any desired method. The changes in respiration which occur after laryngotomy and tracheotomy are discussed in Chapter IV.

Extubation. At the end of a long operation, the throat reflexes are often absent and a nasotracheal tube can often be left *in situ* with advantage. It is usual to transfix the end of the tube with a large safety pin to avoid any possibility of its disappearance down the trachea. The pin should be exactly in the middle of the tube and as near its proximal end as possible. This will discourage nurses from inserting a glass connection and blowing oxygen down the tube direct from a cylinder. This practice has caused fatalities[45] from ruptured lungs. If the patient begins to " buck " on the tube, it should be gently withdrawn. It is rarely safe to send a patient back to bed with an orotracheal tube in position. If this is essential, the end must be secured and a prop or gag inserted so that the patient cannot bite the tube while recovering consciousness. A cuffed tube must not be withdrawn until the clip has been loosened and it is *certain* that the cuff is actually deflated.

Intrabronchial anæsthesia is dealt with under thoracic surgery (q.v.), and endopharyngeal anæsthesia under dental surgery (q.v.). For further details, the reader is recommended to peruse the exhaustive book by N. A. Gillespie entitled " Endotracheal Anæsthesia ", 2nd edit., 1948 (University of Wisconsin Press).

References

1. VESALIUS, A. " De Humanis Corporis Fabrica," 1542, p. 653.
2. SNOW, J. " On Chloroform and Other Anæsthetics," 1858. London, p. 117.
3. TRENDELENBURG, F. *Arch. f. Klin. Chir.*, 1871, **12,** p. 121.
4. MacEWEN, W. *Brit. Med. Jour.*, 1880, ii, p. 122.
5. ELSBERG. *New York Medical Record*, 1910, Mar.
6. ROWBOTHAM, E. S., and MAGILL, I. W. *Pro. Roy. Soc. Med.* (An. Sec.), 1921.
7. { HEWER, C. L. *Brit. Med. Jour.*, 1926, Aug. 14.
   { TANNER, W. E. *Post-Grad. Med. Jour.*, 1932, Jan., p. 25.
8. McKESSON, E. I. *Brit. Med. Jour.*, 1926, Dec. 12, p. 1117.
9. { MACKLIN, C. C. *Canad. Med. Ass. Jour.*, 1937, xxxvi, p. 414.
   { MARCOTTE, R. J., et al. *Jour. Thorac. Surg.*, 1940, ix, p. 346.
10. WOOLSEY, W. C. *New York State Jour. Med.*, 1912, **15,** p. 93.
11. BARRETT, N. R., and THOMAS, D. *Brit. Med. Jour.*, 1944, Nov. 25, p. 692.
12. GILLIES, J. *Pro. Roy. Soc. Med.* (An. Sec.), 1943, Mar. 5.
13. COBB, W. A. *Brit. Med. Jour.*, 1943, May 29, p. 667.
14. OWEN-FLOOD, A. *Brit. Med. Jour.*, 1945, Mar. 17, p. 371.
15. BELL, H. E. *Lancet*, 1951, Mar. 17, p. 619.
16. ROSENBERG. *Berlin klin. Wschr.*, 1895, 1 and 2.
17. MAGILL, I. W. *Pro. Roy. Soc. Med.* (An. Sec.), 1928, Nov.

18. NEGUŠ, V. E.   *Brit. Jour. Anœsth.*, 1933, July, p. 177.
19. HARRISON, G.   *Anœsthesia*, 1949, Oct., p. 181.
20. SIMPSON, K.   *Lancet*, 1949, Apr. 2, p. 558.
21. REID, L. C., and BRACE, D. E.   *Surg. Gyn. & Obst.*, 1940, **70**, p. 157.
22. BURSTEIN, C. L., *et al*.   *Anesthesiology*, 1950, May, p. 299.
23. BURSTEIN, C., and ROVENSTINE, E. A.   *Jour. Pharmacol. & Exp. Thor.*, 1938, May, p. 42.
24. GALE, J. W., and WATERS, R. M.   *Jour. Thor. Surg.*, 1932, Apr., p. 432.
25. GOLDMAN, V.   *Brit. Med. Jour.*, 1936, Aug. 22, p. 394.
26. MAGILL, I. W.   *Ann. Jour. Surg.*, 1936, Dec., p. 450.
27. MACINTOSH, R. R.   *Anœsthesia*, 1950, Apr., p. 97.
28. THORNTON, H. L.   *Brit. Med. Jour.*, 1944, July 1, p. 14.
29. BANNISTER, F. B., and MACBETH, R. C.   *Lancet*, 1944, Nov. 18, p. 651.
30. MACINTOSH, R. R.   *Lancet*, 1943, Feb. 13, p. 205.
31. SYKES, W. S.   *Anesth. & Anal.*, 1937, May-June, p. 133.
32. GUEDEL, A. E., and WATERS, R. M.   *Ann. Otol., Rhinol. & Laryngol.*, 1931, Dec.
33. LENNON, E. B., and ROVENSTINE, E. A.   *Anesth. & Anal.*, 1939, July-Aug., p. 217.
34. TOVELL, R. M.   *Anesth. & Anal.*, 1937, Sept.-Oct., p. 105.
35. GRIMM, J. E., and KNIGHT, R. T.   *Anesthesiology*, 1943, Jan., p. 9.
36. ROWBOTHAM, E. S.   *Lancet*, 1944, July 1, p. 15.
37. DAWKINS, C. J. M.   *Brit. Jour. Anœsth.*, 1937, Jan., p. 45.
38. { GOULD, R. B.   *Brit. Med. Jour.*, 1935, Sept. 14, p. 499.
     COHEN, M.   *Brit. Med. Jour.*, 1938, Feb. 5, p. 283.
     ROBIN, I. G.   *Pro. Roy. Soc. Med.* (Lar. Sec.), 1946, Mar. 1.
39. DINGLEY, A. R.   *Brit. Med. Jour.*, 1943, June 5, p. 693.
40. GILLESPIE, N. A., and CONROY, W. A.   *Anesthesiology*, 1941, Jan., p. 28.
41. MILNE, R. M. P., and MACKENZIE, J. R.   *Brit. Med. Jour.*, 1939, Dec. 9, p. 1136.
42. GILLESPIE, N. A.   *"Endotracheal Anœsthesia,"* 1948, p. 103.
43. MAGILL, I. W.   *Anesth. & Anal.*, **10**, No. 9, p. 166.
44. MORRIS, C. W.   *Pro. Roy. Soc. Med.* (An. Sec.), 1932, Mar. 4.
45. *Lancet*.   (Annotation), 1952, July 26, p. 195.

CHAPTER IX

THE EXPLOSION RISK IN ANÆSTHESIA

IN the last few years the use by surgeons of electrical and other apparatus producing heat and sparks has greatly increased, and it behoves the anæsthetist to bear in mind the possible risk of fire and explosion. If such an accident should occur, it is quite possible that he will become involved in medico-legal proceedings.

Incidence

One of the first reports of an anæsthetic explosion in Great Britain was in 1892.[30]

It has been estimated that at least 100 cases of burns of the eyebrows, lips, pharynx, etc., occur in Great Britain every year from ether explosions.[1]

In a recent American series of statistics compiled from the records of eighty-seven anæsthetists, the explosion rates for ether ethylene and cyclopropane were all in the neighbourhood of 2 to 4 per 100,000 anæsthesias, and the explosion mortality was 1 in 1,150,000 cases.[2]

It will be convenient to discuss the matter under (a) the explosive mixture, (b) the source of ignition, and (c) means of separating (a) from (b).

The Explosive Mixture

The anæsthetic agents capable of igniting or exploding in suitable conditions are ethylene, acetylene, cyclopropane, ethyl chloride, and the anæsthetic ethers. The mixture of oxygen, nitrous oxide or both with any of these agents will usually increase the violence of the explosion, and in certain cases a catastrophic detonation can occur.[3] It should be particularly noted that nitrous oxide and ether without any air or oxygen are explosive, the necessary oxygen being derived from the breaking down of nitrous oxide. The liberation of the " energy of dissociation " of nitrous oxide into nitrogen and oxygen adds to the violence of the explosion. Since ether vapour will ignite at 190° C.[4] and liquid ether contaminated with peroxides at 100° C., it will be realized that excessive heat is by no means necessary. Thus a cautery at a temperature of 300° to 350° C. *below* visible red heat may ignite an oxygen-ether vapour.[5] The limits of inflammability and explosibility of ether are from 3 per cent. to 80 per cent. in oxygen[6] and 3 per cent. to 9 per cent. and 19 per cent. to 34 per cent. in air. The higher percentages of ether can ignite by means of a slowly travelling " cool flame " which is a particularly insidious type of ignition, since it cannot be seen in daylight. This " cool flame " is initiated by hot wires but not by sparks.[7] Since the vapour density of ether is more than double that of air, any escaping vapour tends to run downwards in a concentrated stream so that ignition at floor level at some remote point is not impossible.[8] The limits of inflammability of the other volatile anæsthetics are given under the individual agents.

It is possible for explosions and fires to take place apart from the anæsthetic agent employed. For example, fatal accidents have occurred from use of a diathermic needle on skin which had just previously been sterilized with ether or spirit.

The detection of an inflammable or explosive gas mixture can be effected by an instrument known in America as a " Vapotester ".[9] This consists essentially of a Wheatstone bridge with a balanced electrical circuit (Fig. 57). The circuit includes two incandescent platinum wires, one of which (A) is enclosed while the other one (B) is situated in a test chamber through which a sample of the gas can be drawn. If this is combustible, the temperature of the wire (B) rises and its electrical resistance is increased, thus unbalancing the circuit and showing a current on the ammeter (C).[10] (See Fig. 57.)

A simpler apparatus for determining if a sample of a gas mixture is inflammable or explosive consists of a 2 inch length of 1 inch steel rod drilled through and tapped at one end to take a sparking plug and turned at the other end to hold a toy rubber balloon. This

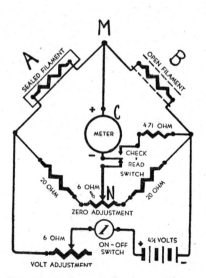

FIG. 57. Diagram to show principle of " Vapotester " to ascertain if a gas mixture is inflammable. (J. W. Uhl, *et al.*, *Anesthesiology*.)

fitting is fixed to a stand by a side tube through which the balloon can be filled with a sample of the gas mixture. A 6-volt battery, car induction coil, flex and switch complete the outfit.[11] This will convince the most obtuse surgeon of the inadvisability of using

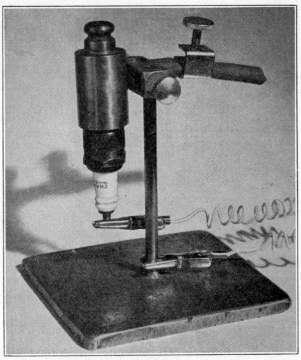

Fig. 58.   Morton's apparatus for testing explosive properties of anæsthetic gases.   (*Brit. Med. Jour.*)

the diathermy on the air passages of a patient anæsthetized with cyclopropane.

The Source of Ignition

The probable sources of ignition in an operating theatre are (*a*) static electricity, (*b*) non-static electricity, (*c*) other sources of heat, and (*d*) spontaneous ignition.

Static Electricity.   In extremely dry climates, such as those of certain parts of America, sparks from static electricity constitute a serious risk, and elaborate systems of earthing all metal apparatus have been adopted,[12] while the humidification of the atmosphere inside operating theatres has also been suggested,[13] as no danger is to be apprehended if the relative humidity exceeds 54 per cent.[14] Static sparks are unlikely to occur unless the difference in potential exceeds 350 volts and even then they are less than 1/1000 inch long and incapable of igniting an inflammable vapour. Voltages of from 5,000 to 15,000, however, have been recorded and the resulting sparks are extremely dangerous.[15] In general, the duration of static sparks is very short : of the order of one millionth of a second and the discharge is oscillatory in character.[16] In some countries the danger from static sparks is regarded so seriously that recommended precautions include the earthing of patient and anæsthetist by spring clips encircling their wrists![17] Until recently, no explosions from static sparks had been reported in Great Britain, but there are now several " incidents " which appear to have been due to this cause.[18] It seems likely that the drier and hotter atmospheres becoming fashionable in modern operating theatres from the use of conditioned air will increase the risk. There is no doubt that gases passing through pipes, the motion of rebreathing bags, the drawing of blankets over rubber-topped trolleys, etc., can all produce charges of sufficiently high potential to cause long sparks.

In the case of anæsthetic apparatus, if no provision is made for equalizing the electrical potentials of the component parts, a high local charge can be built up which eventually sparks across to another component at a lower potential and if the spark happens to traverse an inflammable mixture, a " spontaneous " fire or explosion results.[29]

An instrument known as a " statometer " or " staticater " has been developed in America to record dangerous static charges. One model of this apparatus emits a buzzing sound when a charged object is within a certain distance of it.[10]

A conducting type of rubber has been prepared by the Dunlop Rubber Co., and is a development from earlier work on anti-static tyres for aircraft. Conductivity is achieved by adding finely divided carbon to the rubber mix.[19] The use of this material in anæsthetic apparatus should greatly diminish the risk of generating local charges of high potential. It should also be used for all rubber theatre furniture such as the mattresses on operating tables, footwear, trolley wheel tyres, etc.[20] Conducting rubber is black and usually carries a distinctive red marking. As a temporary measure, the painting of rubber articles with a high-grade aluminium paint gives a surface of fairly high conductivity. A further factor of safety when using the CO_2 absorption technique is the saturation of the respired gases with water vapour so that the corrugated tubing is covered internally with a layer of moisture which acts as a conductor. If an apparatus has been unused for some time, it is wise to rinse out the tubing and rebreathing bag with water before the induction of anæsthesia. If it becomes necessary to make or unmake metallic connections during anæsthesia, it is always wise to change over to a non-inflammable agent *some time before* the event.

It has been shown that intercoupling connections should not be made of low resistance wire, but should have a resistance of about 1 megohm. A patient included in such an intercoupled group of objects runs less risk of being injured by the accidental contact of a lethal current. Furthermore, the intercoupled group does not have a greater electrostatic capacity than any one of its component parts as occurs with ordinary wire couplings. The resistance does not appreciably affect the time required for the equalization of potential, this being of the order of 1/1000 sec.[21]

Most modern operating theatres have floors of the " granolithic " or " terrazzo " type in which a matrix of marble chips is made solid with magnesium oxychloride and then ground smooth. Such floors have sufficient conductivity to prevent the accumulation of dangerous static charges if all the equipment is fitted with chains which trail for a few inches. Non-conducting rubber flooring, cork carpet and wood blocks, on the other hand, have a high resistance, and unless metal strips are sunk every few inches it is impossible for trailing chains to disperse charges effectively.[8] A committee was recently set up in America to make recommendations for theatre floors in Government hospitals.[28] It recommended *inter alia* that floors should have a resistance of less than 500,000 ohms as measured between two electrodes 3 ft. apart. The resistance should also be more than 25,000 ohms as measured between two electrodes placed 3 ft. apart at any location on the floor and more than 3 ft. from any earthed object. It is worth noting that if the theatre staff are not provided with conducting rubber shoes, ordinary leather soles are considerably safer than standard rubber ones.[31]

Non-static Electricity. Certain operative procedures such as use of the diathermic cautery unavoidably provide a source of ignition, and in such cases it is the anæsthetist's duty to avoid any possibility of inflammable vapours coming into contact with it. The use of endoscopes fitted with electric lamps calls for care. In order to provide maximum illumination such lamps are often grossly over-loaded with consequent rise of their outside temperature. It is recommended that such lamps should always be lit from batteries whose maximum voltage does not exceed the rated voltage of the lamps by more than 25 per cent.[7] This is very much safer than obtaining the current from A.C. mains with a transformer. It is most important that all electrical wiring of endoscopes should be regularly inspected for short circuits and poor connections.

Electrical apparatus some way from the site of operation must be spark proof, as in certain circumstances inflammable vapours can travel for a considerable distance. The armatures of electric motors driving suction pumps or bone saws are not always above suspicion, nor are the spark-gap interrupters of some diathermy apparatus. Although modern X-ray apparatus is said to be spark-proof, it is unwise to use an inflammable vapour while the plant is working. Many explosions have occurred with obsolete plant.[22]

In modern operating theatres the electrical switchgear should be laid out with a view to rendering sparks impossible. Not only should the switches themselves be spark-proof, but they should be fitted with interlocking adapters so that the flexible leads cannot be removed with the current on. The switches should be at least 3 feet from floor level to avoid contact with heavy layers of inflammable vapour.

Other Sources of Heat. When operations are to be performed in private houses it is necessary to make sure that the heating of the rooms is not effected by means of open fires, gas stoves or electric radiators with exposed elements. Some old-fashioned sterilizers are still operated by naked flames from spirit stoves or gas rings. In dental practice the operator sometimes dries a cavity by blowing hot air into it, and this has resulted in an explosion of ether vapour in the mouth. Surgeons have been known to smoke in anæsthetic rooms and operating theatres !

Spontaneous Ignition. If oil or grease comes into contact with highly compressed oxygen a spontaneous fire may start which may prove impossible to extinguish. For this reason the greatest care must be taken to ensure that the screw threads and washers of oxygen cylinders are dry. Leather washers should never be used as it is difficult to free them entirely from grease. Fibre washers are safe, but so hard that gas-tight joints are sometimes difficult to secure. The most satisfactory washer to date is constructed of lead in a brass casing which prevents spreading of the soft metal.

Reducing Valves are a potential source of danger, the writer having had a narrow escape when a valve blew to pieces. On reference to Figs. 59 and 152, which show the working principles of two typical reducing valves, it will be appreciated that if the main cylinder pressure be turned on suddenly and the outlet (low pressure) tap is shut, the sudden strain may rupture the diaphragm or otherwise cause a leak from the high to the low pressure side with disastrous consequences. It is therefore recommended that (1) reducing valves should be arranged to point at the floor or a blank wall, (2) that they should be fitted with some type of safety blow-off, (3) that a tap should not be rigidly connected to the outlet but at the distal end of rubber pressure tubing, (4) that cylinders should be turned on gently with the outlet taps open (if fitted), and (5) that separate reducing valves should be kept for different gases, e.g. a valve used on a nitrous oxide cylinder should never subsequently be used for oxygen.

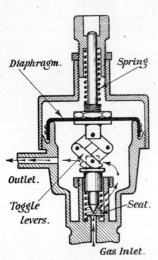

Diaphragm.   Spring.
Outlet.
Toggle
levers.   Seat.

Gas Inlet.

Fig. 59.   Section of reducing valve (Adams) to show working principle (A. C. King).

Separation of the Explosive Mixture from the Source of Ignition

As a general principle it would seem sound practice to avoid explosive anæsthetic mixtures if there is any source of ignition present.

The various methods of anæsthesia at our disposal in this event are : basal narcotics (all), intravenous anæsthesia with the barbiturates, local analgesia, nitrous oxide (with such adjuvants as curare and pethidine), chloroform, trichlorethylene in air (see Chapter VII) and their various possible combinations. Unfortunately other considerations may make it most desirable for a patient to have an inflammable anæsthetic and, as a rule, this is possible provided that a rigid closed-circuit technique is used. The mixture will then be confined within the patient's respiratory passages and the apparatus, and consequently the source of ignition cannot come into contact with it. It has been estimated that a slight leak in a closed system will not result in an explosive risk at a distance exceeding 1 foot from the leak.[23] It need hardly be said that diathermy of lung tissue or indeed anywhere inside the pleural cavity is not permissible. The possibility of a bronchial fistula must also be borne in mind. If a closed system is not available, ether vapour can be " adsorbed ", by passing the expired gases through activated charcoal. In an emergency the container of a service respirator is efficient for a short time, but for prolonged periods a larger container such as a Waters' canister is necessary.[24]

Explosions have occurred when the anæsthetist has imagined that he was administering a non-inflammable vapour, e.g. nitrous oxide-oxygen-chloroform. Such accidents are invariably due to faulty apparatus, as it is possible in some cases for an explosive mixture containing ether to be delivered although the indicator is set at " chloroform ".[25] This may be due to positive pressure in the ether bottle from a hot water jacket or to a partial vacuum occurring from the gases passing over it.[26] If there is any doubt of the correct functioning of such apparatus, the ether bottle should be removed entirely when an ignition risk is present.

All sorts of unlikely circumstances have actually caused fires and explosions in operating theatres, some of which are described in an excellent paper which appeared recently.[32]

An exhaustive survey initiated by the American Society of Anæsthetists concludes with the assertion, " Our present-day knowledge of the ætiology and prophylaxis of all anæsthetic fires and explosions is sufficient to prevent all further anæsthetic combustions."[27] Unfortunately it has not done so up to the present time.

References

1. PINSON, K. B.   *Brit. Med. Jour.*, 1930, *ii.*, p. 312.
2. WOODBRIDGE, P. D.   *Jour. Amer. Med. Ass.*, 1939, Dec. 23, p. 2308.
3. *New Eng. Med. Jour.*, 1933, May 4, p. 949.
4. MORGAN, J. P.   *Pro. Roy. Soc. Med.* (An. Sec.), 1931, Nov. 6.
5. *H.M. Stationery Office, Memo.*, **191**, *Med.* and **191** *Med.* (Revised).
6. THORNTON, W. M.   *Pro. Inst. Elect. Engin.*, 1939, Feb.
7. SWANN, H. W.   *Brit. Med. Jour.*, 1938, July 30, p. 234.
8. RAYNER, E. H.   *Pro. Inst. Elect. Engin.*, 1938, Feb.
9. JARMAN, R.   *Pro. Roy. Soc. Med.* (An. Sec.), 1948, Mar. 5.
10. UHL, J. W., *et al.*   *Anesthesiology*, 1949, July, p. 479.
11. MORTON, H. J. Y.   *Brit. Med. Jour.*, 1951, Feb. 10, p. 298.
12. HERB, I. C.   *Jour. Amer. Med. Ass.*, 1925, Dec. 5.
13. BUCHMAN, M. A.   *Anesth. & Anal.*, 1932, **11**, No. 3, p. 42.
14. ROVENSTINE, E. A.   *Amer. Jour. Surg.*, 1936, Dec., p. 460.
15. THOMAS, G. J.   *Amer. Soc. Anesth. Newsletter*, 1950, No. 8.
16. LOW, W. A.   *Pro. Roy. Soc. Med.* (An. Sec.), 1950, Dec. 1.

17. GAUSS, C. J., and MARGRAF, C.   *Deut. Med. Woch.*, 1933, April 21, p. 598.
18. { IRONSIDE, R.   *Pro. Roy. Soc. Med.* (An. Sec.), 1935, March 1.
     { CHIVERS, E. H.   *Lancet*, 1943, April 24, p. 527.
19. *Lancet* (annotation), 1947, Apr. 5, p. 469.
20. BULGIN, D., *et al.*   *Lancet*, 1949, May 7, p. 789.
21. WOODBRIDGE, P. D.   *Jour. Amer. Med. Ass.*, 1939, Aug. 26, p. 740.
22. { HEWER, C. L.   *Pro. Roy. Soc. Med.* (An. Sec.), 1930, Apr.
     { GREENE, B. A.   *Amer. Jour. Roent.*, 1941, **45,** p. 737.
23. HORTON, J. W.   *Anesthesiology*, 1941, March, p. 122.
24. EPSTEIN, H G.   *Lancet*, 1944, Jan. 22, p. 114.
25. FEATHERSTONE, H. W.   *Pro. Roy. Soc. Med.* (An. Sec.), 1931, Nov. 6.
26. PRIMROSE, W. B.   *Brit. Med. Jour.*, 1939, Feb. 4, p. 215.
27. GREENE, B. A.   *Anesthesiology*, 1941, March, p. 160.
28. *Rep. Cte. on Explosions in Hospital Operating Suites*, 1950, Jan. 1.
     Washington, D.C., and *Bureau of Mines Report of Investigation,* **4833,**
     1952, Jan.
29. *Anæsthesia* (editorial), 1952, June.
30. *Brit. Med. Jour.*, 1892, *ii*, p. 1457.
31. GREENE, B. A.   *Anesthesiology*, 1952, March, p. 203.
32. LOW, W. A.   *Pro. Roy. Soc. Med.* (An. Sec.), 1950, Dec. 1.

CHAPTER X

INTRAVENOUS ANÆSTHESIA AND ANALGESIA INTRAMEDULLARY ANÆSTHESIA

Chloral Hydrate—Di-ethyl Ether—Hedonal—Ethyl Alcohol—Sterols—Soluble hexobarbitone—Soluble thiopentone—Kemithal sodium—Venesetic—Eunarcon—Narconumal—Surital sodium—Techniques—Intravenous Analgesia with Procaine and Pethidine—Intramedullary Anæsthesia—Rectal Analgesia.

Drugs

A VARIETY of drugs has been used for producing complete anæsthesia by intravenous injection, but in man a very limited number are satisfactory. The first successful human intravenous anæsthesia was accomplished in 1872 by Ore, of Lyons, who administered **chloral hydrate** by this route.

Di-ethyl ether at one time had a considerable vogue as an intravenous anæsthetic, given as a 5 per cent. solution in normal saline.[1] Since the introduction of the endotracheal technique the method has fallen into disuse.

Hedonal (methyl propyl urethane, $CO(NH_2)(OC_5H_{11})$) was introduced as an intravenous anæsthetic in 1909, but largely abandoned owing to its prolonged effect and marked fall of blood pressure (about 27 per cent.).[2] Farkin, however, has obtained good results with minimal doses used in conjunction with ether,[3] while a solution containing hedonal, sodium chloride and gum acacia has been used successfully in animals,[4] as also has a mixture of hedonal and isopral (trichlorisopropyl alcohol).[5] It has been demonstrated that there is a remarkable antagonism between nikethamide and hedonal, and the former drug can be used as a stimulant in hedonal narcosis.[6]

Ethyl alcohol has been used intravenously to produce anæsthesia, and is stated to be useful in patients suffering severely from shock, loss of blood or other debilitating conditions.[7] A light anæsthesia is secured but muscular relaxation may not be complete. The alcohol is usually combined with a glucose solution and the average dose required is 2 to 3 c.cm. of 90 per cent. alcohol per kilogramme body weight.

Therapeutic Use. Considerable success has been obtained by the treatment of suppurative pulmonary diseases with intravenous alcohol : 20 parts of absolute alcohol with 80 parts normal sterile saline are given in doses of 20 to 50 c.cm. on successive days up to 20. Insulin in daily doses of 6 to 10 units is also given.[8]   Intravenous glucose and alcohol has also been used in the treatment of puerperal pyæmia.[9]

Bromethol.   The method of giving bromethol intravenously has been referred to in Chapter II.

Sterols.   It has recently been shown in animals that some of the sterols which are active as hormones have anæsthetic properties when given in large doses by the oral, intravenous or intraperitoneal route.   They also potentiate the effects of the volatile anæsthetics so could possibly be used for basal narcosis, but no work on man has yet been carried out.   The two most promising sterols appear to be progesterone and desoxycorticosterone.[10]   12 mg. of progesterone will suffice as the sole anæsthetic in rats, half this dose being sufficient if partial hepatectomy has been carried out beforehand.   In monkeys, however, very large doses are required and this is also probably true in man.[11]

The Rapidly-acting Barbiturates

As previously mentioned under basal narcosis, the very quick-acting barbiturates can be given intravenously in sufficient dosage to produce true anæsthesia, and one or other of this group has practically ousted all other drugs for intravenous anæsthesia.   It is essential that the compounds used should have a high safety factor (ratio of minimum lethal dose to minimum anæsthetic dose).

Pharmacological   Effects.   Intravenous   barbiturates   produce unconsciousness very rapidly and pleasantly.   The patient feels extremely sleepy, usually yawns and relapses into anæsthesia with little evidence of the second or excitement stage.   Muscular twitching is common, particularly with hexobarbitone, and actual convulsions have been reported.[12]   It is stated that there is less tendency to twitching if the solution is warmed and allowed to stand for some minutes before use.[13]   Occasionally a sudden muscular contraction occurs when narcosis appears to be deep. This may be induced by operative stimuli.   Muscular relaxation is, however, usually good and the tongue may drop back necessitating the introduction of an artificial airway.   There is some evidence to show that the barbiturates act mainly on the hypothalamic area in contrast to the volatile anæsthetics whose chief action appears to be on the cells of the cerebral cortex (see Chapter I).   The oil/water coefficient of the barbiturates rises in approximately the same proportion as the rapidity of action.   For example it is 4·7 in the case of the rapidly-acting thiopentone and 0·214 for the slow-acting barbitone.[116] The initial high uptake of thiopentone in the brain accounts for the rapid onset of unconsciousness. Redistribution occurs largely in fat in which levels of from 5 to 10 times those of plasma can be found.[117] This acts as a buffering mechanism as the thiopentone is stored in fat and slowly released and detoxicated by oxidation, probably in the liver. Only traces of the short-acting barbiturates appears in the urine.[118] (Observations on the elimination of the medium and long-acting barbiturates will be found in Chapter II.) The intracranial and blood pressures fall and respiration is depressed. The drugs have only a slight effect on the blood-urea and blood-sugar values. It was stated that the oxygen capacity of the blood could be seriously reduced for some time,[14] but later investigations have suggested that this effect is not quite so great as had been previously thought.[15] The skin temperature of the extremities rises but lymph flow is reduced (compared with ether anæsthesia). This suggests that the tissue oxygen supply is diminished—a factor to bear in mind when dealing with cases of gangrene.[16] Laryngeal spasm may be an annoying and occasionally a dangerous, complication. The condition is often initiated by a plug of mucus dropping from the naso-pharynx on to the glottis, when the soft palate muscles have relaxed. The usual explanation is that the barbiturates first stimulate the parasympathetic nervous system causing brick reflexes with a tendency towards laryngeal spasm. In the author's opinion, it is more likely that the sympathetic system is first paralysed leaving a temporarily unopposed parasympathetic. An analogous effect probably occurs during high spinal block where the sympathetic supply to the intestines is paralysed leaving an unopposed vagus which causes contraction and increased peristalsis. Masseteric spasm is relatively common and is combated by the insertion of a dental prop before the administration of a barbiturate is started.

The characteristics of the individual drugs must now be considered briefly.

Soluble hexobarbitone (evipan sodium, evipal soluble, methexenyl sodium, cyclural sodium, cyclonal sodium, endorm, and hexanostab) is sodium

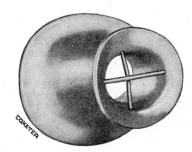

Fig. 60. Oral prop (Hewer's).

N-methyl-c-c-cyclo hexenyl methyl barbiturate and was introduced by H. Weese in 1932.

Soluble hexobarbitone is a white powder supplied in $0·5$ g. and 1 g. ampoules. As a freshly prepared 10 per cent. solution is used, the contents of each ampoule must be dissolved in either 5 c.cm. or 10 c.cm. of distilled water respectively. The resulting fluid should be clear and colourless and has a pH of $11·5$. Muscular twitching is rather common during injection. The safety-factor is given as $2·7$.

Soluble thiopentone (pentothal sodium, thiobarbiturate 8064, intraval sodium, sodium thio-pentobarbital) is sodium ethyl

$$CH_3CH_2CH_2CH\underset{\underset{CH_3}{|}}{\overset{\overset{\displaystyle CH_3CH_2}{\diagdown}}{C}}\underset{\underset{CO-\!\!-\!\!-N}{|}}{\overset{\overset{\displaystyle CO-\!\!-\!\!-NH}{|}}{C}}-SNa$$

(1-methyl-butyl) thiobarbiturate and is put up in $0·5$ g. and 1 g. ampoules as a pale yellow powder mixed with 6 per cent. anhydrous sodium carbonate. Since the 10 per cent. solution causes more respiratory depression than hexobarbitone and produces more irritation if inadvertently injected outside the vein,[18] a 5 per cent. solution is now commonly employed. For example, the contents of a 1 g. ampoule are dissolved in 20 c.cm. of distilled water. A gas smelling of sulphuretted hydrogen is evolved and the fluid should be straw-coloured and clear. Thiopentone solution is more stable than was at first supposed, and can be used after some days' storage.[19] If kept for a very long time, however, decomposition into insoluble thiopentone acid may occur. This change can be detected by the solution looking cloudy from the fine precipitate.[20] In one clinic in America it is stated that phlebitis occurs in about 1 in 1,000 cases with 5 per cent. soluble thiopentone and a concentration of $2·5$ per cent. is recommended.[21] Muscular twitching is not common during injection but the patient may notice a sulphurous taste. Since the drug contains a sulphur atom in its molecule it was thought to be contra-indicated during sulphonamide therapy in case sulphæ-moglobinæmia might occur.[22] This danger was undoubtedly exaggerated[23] but the fact remains that in some animals such as in rats receiving sulphanilamide in therapeutic doses, there is a markedly decreased tolerance to all barbiturates, especially to those containing sulphur.[24] Thiopentone, unlike hexobarbitone, is extremely toxic to the liver in small animals such as mice,[25] and it is worth noting that toxic jaundice has occurred in man.[26] The safety factor is stated to be 2·3.[27] Thiopentone has largely displaced hexobarbitone in Great Britain.

Venesetic (sodium thioethamyl) is sodium iso-amyl ethyl thiobarbiturate and is thus the sulphur homologue of sodium amytal. It is supplied as a yellow powder in 1 g. capsules. The usual strength of the intravenous solution is 7·5 per cent. so that the contents of each capsule are dissolved in 13 c.cm. of distilled water. The safety factor is 3·75.[28] The drug acts in a very similar way to thiopentone.

Kemithal sodium (thialbarbitone) is sodium 5 cyclohexamyl-5-allyl-2-thiobarbiturate and is a pale yellow powder usually dissolved as a 10 per cent. solution which has a pH of 11·2 and is stable for 4-5 hours.[29] Kemithal is about half as potent as thiopentone per unit weight and generally resembles its effects.[30] Kemithal probably produces rather less respiratory depression than thiopentone for an equal degree of muscular relaxation and possibly has rather less tendency to cause laryngeal spasm and postanæsthetic restlessness and excitement.[31]

Eunarcon (R. 1238). Eunarcon is a 10 per cent. solution of sodium c-c-isopropyl-β-bromallyl-N-methyl barbiturate. Like pernocton, the drug is stable in solution and can thus be used direct from ampoules (containing 5 or 10 c.cm.).

The rate of injection is slower than with most other drugs. Some authorities recommend that the first cubic centimetre should take from one and a half to two minutes, the subsequent amount being given at a somewhat faster rate.[32] In any event, at least thirty seconds should be taken for each c.cm. of fluid, as a fast rate may induce severe muscular twitchings. In an average adult patient, about ten minutes' anæsthesia results from 5 c.cm. intravenous eunarcon and the maximum single dose is regarded as 9 c.cm. Eunarcon is very similar to hexobarbitone in its effects with possibly less tendency to post-operative headache and more to restlessness.[33] The safety factor is said to be 2·5. A case of fatal respiratory failure has been reported two minutes after the injection of 10 c.cm. of eunarcon in an elderly patient (a definite overdose),[34] and another occurred in an asthmatic woman after 4·4 c.cm.[35]

Narconumal is 1-methyl-5-5-allyl isopropyl barbituric acid. It must on no account be confused with the long-acting barbiturate numal. The drug is put up in 1 g. ampoules, which are freshly dissolved in 10 c.cm. of distilled water. The rate of intravenous injection should not exceed 1 c.cm. in thirty seconds and should preferably be as slow as 1 c.cm. per minute. Narconumal resembles hexobarbitone in its effects,[36] but has the exceptionally high safety factor of 4.

Surital sodium (thioquinal barbitone) is sodium 5-allyl-5 (1 methyl ethyl)-2-thiobarbiturate. The drug acts in a very similar way to

$$CH_2{=}CHCH_2 \quad CO{-}{-}NH$$
$$CH_3CH_2CH_2CH{-}C \qquad C{-}SNa$$
$$\qquad\qquad\quad CH_3 \quad CO{-}{-}N$$

thiobarbitone but in a series of 1,200 cases it was thought that on the average, recovery was more rapid and that there was less tendency to laryngeal spasm. Four asthmatics were included in this series and in two of them acute attacks were precipitated.[37] Some observers consider that surital sodium causes less respiratory and circulatory depression for a given depth of narcosis than does thiopentone.[38]

Technique of Venepuncture

It should be noted that any accessible vein can be used except a varicosed one, in which the drug may stagnate and produce slow anæsthesia and possibly thrombosis.[39]

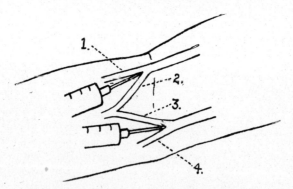

Fig. 61.   Diagram of veins of right antecubital fossa (after Muldavin).   1. Superficial radial vein.   2. Median cephalic vein.   3. Median basilic vein.   4. Superficial ulnar vein.

The commonest difficulties encountered during venepuncture are (*a*) complete transfixion of the vein by the needle, and (*b*) excessive mobility of the vein. Both these troubles can be minimized if the needle is aimed at the angle formed by the junction of two veins, as shown in the accompanying diagrams (Figs. 61, 62).[40]

For continuous intravenous anæsthesia, a narrow adjustable garter can be made to encircle the arm and to cover that part of the needle which lies beneath the skin. The point of the needle, however, should be left free.

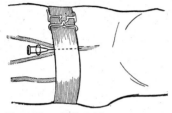

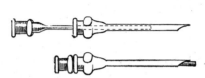

Fig. 62. Adjustable arm garter for retaining needle in vein (Macintosh and Pask).

Fig. 63. Needle and cannula for large veins (Macintosh and Pask).

If a large vein is available, a 1·5 mm. needle can be used through which passes a blunt-ended cannula. The latter is pushed home after introduction and projects into the vein beyond the end of the needle. This renders accidental displacement unlikely.[41]

An ingenious needle to avoid clotting during repeated injections was devised by Gordh.[42] The proximal end contains a rubber diaphragm and injections are made by a second fine needle through it. The elasticity of the rubber maintains a very slight positive pressure which prevents any blood from entering the intravenous needle after injection. The original needle was rather large and needed frequent resharpening but Robertshaw's modification avoids both these disadvantages by making the diaphragm holder separate from the intravenous needle as shown. Any suitable Record type

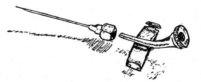

Fig. 64. Non-clotting intravenous needle (Robertshaw's, modification of Gordh's).

needle can be inserted into the vein and a size 15 hypodermic needle is used to pierce the rubber diaphragm.[43]

Technique of Administration

The preparation of the various solutions has already been considered under the individual drugs. Three distinct techniques of administration can be employed.

(*a*) **The Single-dose Method.** When hexobarbitone was first introduced it was recommended that the solution should be injected intravenously at a rate not exceeding 1 c.cm. in fifteen seconds until consciousness was lost. The volume injected is noted and an equal volume added (in elderly or feeble patients half the volume). This relatively slow injection gives about fifteen minutes' anæsthesia since the concentration of the drug is approximately the same in all tissues and little " redistribution " occurs as in very rapid injection (see Chapter II). There is, however, a period of extremely deep narcosis at the beginning accompanied by a low blood pressure and depressed respiration. These disadvantages can be overcome to a certain extent by making a " safety pause " of at least thirty seconds after the injection of the first 3 c.cm. of solution. The method is, of course, applicable to any other of the short-acting barbiturates such as thiopentone. This technique renders it possible for one practitioner to give the anæsthetic and do a minor operation, but it is absolutely essential that a nurse or other helper should keep the jaw forward or insert an artificial airway if any respiratory obstruction should occur. Owing to the fall in blood pressure, care must be taken if the patient is in the sitting[44] or reversed Trendelenburg position.[45] For example, fatalities have occurred from injudicious intravenous anæsthesia in the dental chair. It need hardly be said that preparation is necessary as for any other general anæsthetic but ignorance of this elementary fact has been responsible for deaths from regurgitation.[46]

(*b*) **The Repeated-dose or Fractional Method.** If an anæsthetist is available, it is preferable for him to inject just sufficient solution to abolish reflex movements. The needle is kept in the vein and very small quantities of the drug are injected from time to time as requisite. In this way respiratory depression and the fall in blood pressure are minimized.

With these two techniques an ordinary Record syringe with an eccentric needle mount is quite adequate, but for the fractional method the " third hand " illustrated is most convenient.[47]

A self-locking syringe has been devised to avoid regurgitation of blood with the consequent risk of clotting in the needle. After each of the fractional doses has been given, the knurled end of the piston rod is turned clockwise with a slight forward thrust (Fig. 66).

This locks the piston in position until the next dose is required when
an anti-clockwise turn is made.[48] Alternatively, Gordh's non-

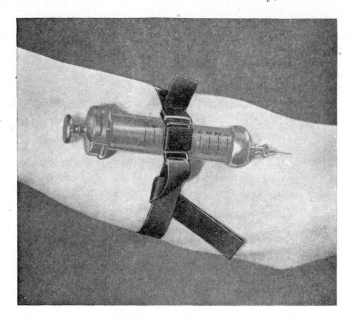

Fig. 65. A " third hand " for fractional intravenous
anæsthesia (I. W. Magill).

clotting needle, already described, can be used. The sterilization
of syringes is discussed later.

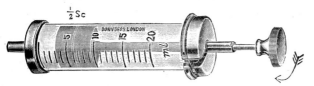

Fig. 66.   Self-locking syringe for giving fractional thiopentone
(Freedman).
A quarter-turn locks the piston in position.

If a long operation is contemplated it is preferable to add the
barbiturate solution from time to time to an intravenous drip of
normal saline or glucose-saline. The simplest method is merely
to puncture the drip tubing with the needle and inject the solution

from a 20 c.cm. syringe.[49] It has been said that saline only should be used if thiopentone is the selected barbiturate as a precipitate may be formed with glucose which may block the needle.[50] The writer has not encountered this difficulty.

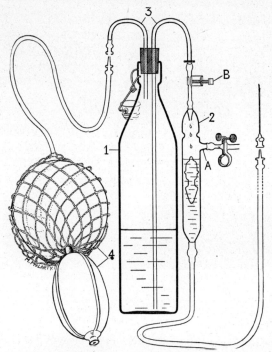

Fig. 67. Single bottle apparatus for continuous intravenous or intramedullary anæsthesia (Macintosh
and Pask).
1. Standard bottle.
2. Drip chamber with float.
3. Stainless steel tubing.
4. Hand bellows.
A. Side tube to regulate level.
B. Screw clip to regulate flow.

The number of modifications of this method is legion and during the late war many Service anæsthetists made up ingenious pieces of apparatus from local materials which proved very effective.

A gravity drip-feed is not always satisfactory even with a wide-bore needle and a two-bottle apparatus using air pressure from a hand-bellows can be used.[51]

(c) **The Continuous Method.** If a quick-acting barbiturate is added to sterile saline in a standard bottle (e.g. thiopentone 0·5 per cent. to 1 per cent.) the second bottle can be dispensed with as shown in Fig. 67. A float inside the drip chamber acts as a safety device by bedding down on to its seating if the bottle becomes empty, thus avoiding the risk of air embolism.[52] Alternative methods of obtaining pressure are from the gases generated from the electrolysis of water[53] or from an oxygen cylinder fitted with a reducing valve and control tap.[54]

The continuous administration of a dilute barbiturate solution does not give the same quickness of control as the previously discussed technique of adding a strong solution at intervals to a saline-drip, nor is it so economical.

In the event of collapse, nikethamide or other analeptics can be given through the same needle or blood transfusion can be carried out.

Oxygen inhalation through a nasal tube is said to be beneficial during continuous intravenous anæsthesia,[55] and in any event it is desirable to have at hand an apparatus capable of inflating the lungs instantly with oxygen.[56] The emergency oxygen valve of a gas-oxygen machine is ideal for such a purpose, but a simple fitting on an oxygen cylinder such as that shown in Fig. 151 is quite adequate.

During prolonged operations under intravenous anæsthesia it is convenient to have some indicator of respiration. A " butterfly " of cotton wool strapped below the nostrils is commonly used, while an even more sensitive indicator is a sheet of cellophane placed over the nose and mouth. The slightest expiration causes a clouding of the transparent sheet.

It is probable that prolonged administration of barbiturates compares unfavourably as regards safety with inhalation anæsthesia. Animal experiments suggest that after a time a cumulative effect occurs and that the margin of safety becomes progressively less.[57] The possibility of liver damage must also be borne in mind and cases of this have been recorded.[58] The very prolonged period of unconsciousness with depressed respiration which may follow fractional and continuous intravenous anæsthesia can be shortened by the injection of an analeptic such as leptazol (q.v.).[59]

Intravenous anæsthesia can be combined with various other methods, e.g. to render a patient unconscious during spinal block or when curare is being used (q.v.). The intravenous barbiturates can also be used as an adjuvant to procure relaxation when the patient is having pure nitrous oxide and oxygen inhalation.[57]

Although a preliminary injection of morphine and scopolamine is used by some anæsthetists, and is stated to minimize post-operative restlessness, it seems inadvisable as a general rule to depress respiration further, and dosage should be minimal.[60] On the other hand a full dose of atropine as a prophylactic against vagal stimulation has been recommended.[61] Picrotoxin can be used to antagonize respiratory failure, 2 c.cm. of a 0·3 per cent. solution being injected into the deltoid muscle immediately before starting the barbiturate administration.[62] Alternately, 1 c.cm. of nikethamide can be mixed with the injected solution. This may be of great service in shocked patients (q.v.).

The technique of producing *basal narcosis* with the short-acting barbiturates is described in Chapter II, as is the treatment of inadvertent overdosage.

Sequelæ. As a rule patients awake from the narcosis with no after-effects, but some degree of excitement is not uncommon,[63] and the author has seen one case of actual mania lasting three hours. A fatality has been recorded from a similar case following hexobarbitone anæsthesia in an alcoholic.[64] In some continental clinics the patients are actually strapped in bed until fully conscious in order to prevent injury.[65] Amnesia is common and may persist up to twelve hours after recovery seems to be complete. This fact shows that outpatients should never be allowed to go home unaccompanied after intravenous anæsthesia,[12] and should not be allowed to drive a car until the next day.[66] Occasionally patients relapse into a second period of unconsciousness after apparent recovery.[67] Nausea and vomiting are not usual but may prove troublesome.[68] Prolonged drowsiness, photophobia, headache, nystagmus and bradycardia have all been described as sequelæ,[69] as has extensive muscular paralysis.[46]

It is worth noting that, in dogs recovering from barbiturate narcosis, intravenous glucose sends them back to sleep again as if they had received a further barbiturate injection.[70] Although this phenomenon has not yet been confirmed in man, caution should be employed if this treatment is necessary.

Remote Effects. Severe cases of mental changes following hexobarbitone anæsthesia in children have been reported.[71] Agranulocytosis and toxic jaundice are occasionally seen in susceptible patients.[72] Although, strictly speaking, it is not a complication of intravenous anæsthesia, the possibility of transmitting the virus of infective hepatitis must be borne in mind. As the incubation period of this disease may be three months, it is probable that many cases have been missed. The most certain method of preventing infection is to sterilize syringes, needles, etc., by dry heat in an electric oven. Unfortunately this is, at the time of writing, a counsel of perfection as the cement used in the composite glass and metal " Record " type syringes disintegrates in the oven. All-glass syringes can be sterilized by dry heat, but the small " Record " type needle mounts are fragile and tend to crack. A satisfactory syringe is an all-glass pattern fitted with a wide-bore ("Luer") eccentric needle mount. A small metal adapter enables " Record " needles to be used if necessary. Such syringes can be sterilized by wrapping in " Kraft " paper and kept for one hour at 160° F. in an electric oven. Special glass-metal syringes with high melting point cement are becoming available for similar sterilization. There is no doubt that in large hospitals a " syringe service " is the most efficient and economical method of dealing with intravenous syringes.

Local Toxic Effects are usually due to some of the fluid having been injected outside the vein, in which case tissue necrosis may occur.[73] In this connection it is interesting to note that an anæsthetist developed dermatitis after cutting his finger on an evipan ampoule.[74] The author has seen a very severe generalized rash with œdema which persisted for three weeks after a hexo-barbitone narcosis. With thiopentone, at any rate, a true cutaneous allergy can occur and to disregard a history of previous trouble may lead to a patient becoming gravely ill with pyrexia and an erythematous vesication which may end in a pustular eruption.[75] It has been shown that tissue sloughing in animals following the extravenous injection of thiopentone can be avoided by the immediate infiltration of the affected area with 1 per cent. procaine in normal saline.[76] The probable mechanism is vaso-dilatation counteracting the vaso-spasm and this prophylactic treatment is well worth trying in man if some of the thiopentone solution has been inadvertently injected into the tissues. Alternatively hyaluronidase can be injected into the affected area to aid the rapid dispersal of thiopentone. Venous thrombosis can occur even if all the solution is injected into the vein and cannot be regarded necessarily as a sign of faulty technique. Cases of extensive thrombosis following the intravenous injection of 5 per cent. pentothal sodium have been recorded.[77]

It might be supposed that **intra-arterial injection** was virtually impossible but this accident has occurred on many occasions. The incidence in Great Britain has been estimated at 1 in 55,000 injections of thiopentone.[78] In a small proportion of patients, the brachial or ulnar artery takes an abnormally superficial course through the ante-cubital fossa, and might be mistaken for a vein if the pulsation was ignored or masked by a tourniquet (see Fig. 68). Intra-arterial

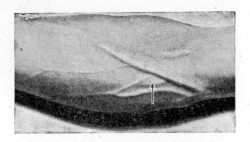

FIG. 68. Veins distended with rubber band. Arrow indicates superficial ulnar artery. Gliding of needle to enter median basilic vein may lead to puncture of artery. (Cohen, *Lancet*, 1948.)

injections are usually accompanied by severe burning pain radiating down to the fingers and if any complaint of pain is made, the injection must be stopped at once. The mishap is a serious one and may be followed by intense vaso-spasm and arterial thrombosis resulting in gangrene of the fingers.[79] These untoward effects are probably due to the high pH of the solution making it intensely irritating. In a series of eight cases, five of the patients subsequently underwent arm or forearm amputation.[78] The pulse in the affected limb may immediately become weak or imperceptible, but even if it remains full, this does not preclude impending disaster as it has been known to fail as late as the tenth day after injection. Loss of consciousness after an average dose of thiopentone occurs but it is slightly delayed compared with an intravenous injection. If the anæsthetist is certain that a considerable volume of the barbiturate has been injected into an artery, the operation should, if possible, be abandoned and a brachial plexus block (q.v.) performed with a long-acting analgesic such as amethocaine. Heparinization should be carried out at once, a suggested dose of 15,000 units (in the adult) being injected into the artery. The anti-coagulant treatment is later continued with dicoumarin. The limb is carefully watched and a decision as to exploration must be reached within six hours. If this is decided upon, the artery should be opened proximal to the site of injection and the clot removed. A distal intra-arterial injection of heparin should be given before closing the wound. Arterectomy is contra-indicated. The limb should be wrapped up in a sterile towel and well covered with wool, but it should *not* be heated. If the operation must continue, cyclopropane is the anæsthetic of choice as it relaxes peripheral blood vessels.

Mortality. Statistics are notoriously misleading, but some indications may be gathered from the following published mortality rates. An early series of 6,500 administrations was reported with eight deaths presumably due to the drug.[80] This gives a mortality of 0·123 per cent. Menegaux and Sechehaye worked out the figures for 20,000 hexobarbitone anæsthesia and found that there were twenty-two immediate deaths, 90 per cent. of which took place within five minutes of the injection. This series gives practically the same mortality rate of 0·11 per cent.[81] In the deaths directly attributable to the anæsthetics employed in the principal hospitals of the Union of South Africa during the period 1931-35, hexobarbitone ranks next to chloroform in danger with a mortality rate of 0·14 per cent.[82] An identical figure is given for thiopentone in a small series recently published in Australia.[83] The Council of Pharmacy and Chemistry (U.S.) has published a critical survey of forty-three deaths which were considered to be partly or entirely due to the administration of hexobarbitone.[84] Niederland in an analysis of fifteen deaths and fifty non-fatal complications considers that the risks attendant on intravenous anæsthesia have been greatly under-estimated.[85]

There is, however, little doubt that many deaths have been due to faulty technique, to a disregard of known contra-indications and to the missing of severe laryngeal spasm until too late. It has been said with grim truth that " the danger with intravenous anæsthetics is that they are so fatally easy to give ". It cannot be stressed too often that it is impossible to calculate dosage beforehand and the anæsthetist must observe the reaction of the individual patient to the drug given. It is unfortunate that the dangerous practice of inducing anæsthesia in the patient's bedroom with intravenous thiopentone has become popular. The anæsthetist is usually without the means of inflating the lungs with oxygen under pressure and may be separated from the operating theatre by passages and lifts. Emergencies are thus difficult to deal with and the risks generally are increased.

Indications. The vast majority of patients prefer a needle prick to a facepiece and the induction of anæsthesia is now usually effected by the intravenous route. Intravenous barbiturates are also useful for producing a short anæsthesia where inhalation methods such as nitrous oxide-oxygen are inconvenient or inapplicable, e.g. under Service conditions (see Chapter XVII). They are particularly useful for short operations on the mouth or face, for procedures involving the use of the diathermic cautery, and for examinations such as sigmoidoscopy and cystoscopy.[86] The method is also serviceable in patients suffering from chronic respiratory diseases and where good muscular relaxation is required for a short time, e.g. for manipulation of joints or setting of fractures. It has been found, however, that the musculature of the pregnant uterus is not fully relaxed so that the technique should not be employed for version. Some gynæcologists dislike intravenous anæsthesia for the injection of lipiodol for salpingo-hysterography and for tubal insufflation with carbon dioxide on the grounds that the Fallopian tubes may contract spasmodically. The author's observation does not bear out this objection. The barbiturates decrease the intraocular tension in both normal and glaucomatous eyes, and this effect is frequently of advantage in ophthalmic surgery.[87] On the other hand, occasional reflexes such as sneezing, coughing or twitching may occur and prove disastrous during an ophthalmic operation.[68] The cause of these reflexes has already been discussed. It is also possible that instilled solutions may pass down the naso-lachrymal duct and irritate the nasal mucosa so causing a reflex sneeze. It has been suggested that preliminary cocainization of the eye reduces this risk.[88]

Therapeutic Uses. The short-acting barbiturates have been used with success as anti-convulsants in such conditions as chorea,[89] delirum tremens,[90] and late ether convulsions (q.v.). They are also used extensively for " narco-analysis " in such conditions as sudden loss of memory[91] and in psychiatry generally.[92]

Contra-indications. It is generally held that the barbiturates should not be used for patients who suffer from severe cardiac or respiratory embarrassments or who show signs of grossly impaired hepatic or renal function. Whatever may be the exact mechanism of elimination (see Chapter II) it is a fact that patients with very poor renal and hepatic function (e.g. after extensive burns) recover very slowly, if at all, after the normal intravenous dose of a barbiturate.[93] It has also been observed during the late war that patients suffering from malaria are extremely susceptible to even small doses of these drugs.[94] Intravenous anæsthesia is extremely dangerous in quinsy, two fatalities having been reported from one clinic within a few weeks of each other.[95] The same remarks apply to cervical suppuration generally, e.g. parotid[96] and submaxillary[97] abscesses and Ludwig's angina.[98] Some interesting work has been done on this subject. It has been shown that animals with cervical suppuration did not stop breathing under intravenous anæsthesia if denervation of the carotid sinus had first been performed. The theory has been advanced that the very rapid onset of anæsthesia such as obtains with the intravenous barbiturates does not at first affect the hypersensitive nerve endings of the carotid sinus and local trauma causes impulses to reach the respiratory centre with consequent paralysis. The more gradual onset of inhalation anæsthesia, on the other hand, desensitizes the nerve endings by the time the patient is ready for operation.[99] This theory is not necessary to explain the cause of death in patients suffering from respiratory obstruction so great that the accessory muscles are being used. These being of the voluntary type will cease acting if *any* type of general anæsthesia is induced quite possibly with fatal results. Intravenous anæsthesia should not be used for broncho-scopy unless a complete topical application of cocaine or other surface analgesic has been carried out (see Chapter XX) or unless curare is used. The method should also be avoided in cases of cystitis with a latent pyelitis.[100] It has been stated that intravenous barbiturates should be avoided in asthmatics as a severe attack may be induced.[101] In the author's opinion, this danger has been greatly exaggerated, at any rate in the case of thiopentone. It should be unnecessary to mention that intravenous anæsthesia alone should never be used if there is a possibility of fluids gaining access to the respiratory passages, but several deaths from asphyxia under these circumstances have been recorded.[64] The presence of shock is not an absolute contra-indication to intravenous anæsthesia as has been strikingly shown under Service and air-raid conditions. Nevertheless the injection should be given slowly and the patient watched most carefully. Extremely small doses are usually adequate (see Chapter XVII).

Intravenous Analgesia

Procaine is now often used as an analgesic and is given by the intravenous drip technique in concentrations of from $0 \cdot 2$ per cent. to 1 per cent. either in normal saline or in a 5 per cent. aqueous glucose solution. When given slowly in this way procaine is hydrolyzed in the blood stream into p-aminobenzoic acid and diethylamino ethanol by the enzyme procaine esterase. Both are passed in the urine, the former more rapidly than the latter.[119] If, however, the rate of injection is allowed to rise much above 20 mg. procaine per minute the blood concentration will steadily rise until toxic symptoms such as tachycardia, muscular twitching and convulsions develop.

Intravenous procaine has been used with success in a great variety of conditions, such as the relief of pruritus associated with jaundice,[102] for painful burn dressings,[103] for obstetrical analgesia[104] and for the control of severe asthmatical attacks.[105]   It has also been employed extensively for post-operative analgesia,[106] its advantage over the opiates being the relative freedom from respiratory depression. Patients will co-operate in breathing deeply as they are without pain and it is consequently reasonable to expect a decrease in respiratory complications following upper abdominal operations if the drug is used.   A simple technique is to substitute a $0 \cdot 2$ per cent. procaine solution (1 g. in 500 c.cm. normal saline) for the usual drip both already running at the end of the operation.   The use of intravenous procaine to stop arrhythmias in cardiac surgery is discussed in Chapter XXII and to speed up the rate of transfusions in Chapter XVII.

Toxic reactions are usually due to an excessive rate of drip as already mentioned.   If severe, an intravenous short-acting barbiturate should be given cautiously.   A few patients having intravenous procaine develop a type of tetany which appears to be due to a deficiency in vitamin C.[107]   A preliminary course of vitamin C with " glucose D " has therefore been recommended when possible.   It should be noted that local trauma often produces capillary permeability and an intravenous procaine drip will afford a local analgesia at the site of injection, a most convenient effect for the clumsy anæsthetist.

For further information on the subject, the reader is referred to the monograph recently published.[108]

Pethidine is also used as an intravenous analgesic and can also be employed as a supplement to nitrous oxide-oxygen anæsthesia, an average dose of 25 mg. being given every 30 minutes.[109]   It should be noted that pethidine is not miscible with thiopentone, a precipitate forming unless the needle and tubing are washed through with saline between alternate doses of the two drugs.[110] Caution should be observed when giving the first dose of intravenous pethidine as some patients are abnormally sensitive to its effects.[111]

Intramedullary Anæsthesia

The bone marrow (usually of the tibia or sternum) has been used since 1941 for the administration of a variety of fluids.[112]   Intrasternal anæsthesia using a dilute solution of a barbiturate such as $0 \cdot 5$ per cent. thiopentone, can be maintained by some apparatus similar to that shown in Fig. 67.   The continuous technique is preferable to the fractional one. The needle is usually inserted in the mid-line opposite the second intercostal space and penetrates the outer plate of the sternum. Aspiration of material resembling blood signifies that the needle point is correctly placed.[113] Two possible dangers are (1) sepsis with subsequent osteomyelitis (about 1 in 150 cases[114]) and (2) penetration of the inner plate of the sternum with possible mediastinitis. The method is of value if intravenous anæsthesia is indicated but for technical reasons is impossible. Intramedullary fluid replacement is referred to under " shock ".

Rectal Analgesia

In order to obviate the technical complications of intravenous procaine given as a post-operative analgesic, the drug has been given by the rectal route and found to be effective. A solution of 2 g. procaine hydrochloride with 0·5 g. vitamin C is made up with a pint of normal saline and given as a rectal drip running at 80 drops per minute when the patient is returned to bed. 1 or 2 pints can be given according to the severity of the operation and the condition of the patient and this can be repeated on the following day. Analgesia persists for several hours.[115] Rectal alcohol is mentioned in Chapter II.

References

1. ROOD, F. *Brit. Med. Jour.*, 1911, Oct. 11.
2. BLOMFIELD, J. *Med. Ann.*, 1930, p. 34.
3. FARKIN, E. *Arch. f. klin. Chir.*, 1928, April, p. 218.
4. DONALD, J. *Anesth. & Anal.*, 1928, May-June, p. 151.
5. LAMBERT, R. K. *Lancet*, 1926, Jan. 16, p. 121.
6. KILLIAN, H. *Anesth. & Anal.*, 1935, Jan.-Feb., p. 26.
7. CONSTANTIN, J. D. *Lancet*, 1929, *i.*, p. 1247 ; and 1930, *i.*, p. 1393.
8. LANDAU, A. *Presse Méd.*, 1931, **39**, p. 523.
9. ZONDEK, B., *et al. Zentralb. f. Gynäk.*, 1933, March 25, p. 674.
10. SELYE, H. { *Jour. Pharmacol. & Exp. Therap.*, 1941, **71**, p. 236. *Jour. Pharmacol. & Exp. Therap.*, 1941, **73**, p. 127. *Anesth. & Anal.*, 1943, Mar.-Apl., p. 105.
11. JARMAN, R. *Pro. Roy. Soc. Med.* (An. Sec.), 1948, Nov. 5.
12. BAETZNER, W. *Deut. med. Woch.*, 1933, Jan. 13, p. 48.
13. SHARMAN, A. *Glasgow Med. Jour.*, 1934, March, p. 104.
14. DALLEMAGNE, M. J. *Liége Méd.*, 1938, **31**, p. 197.
15. PASK, E. A. *Lancet*, 1941, March 29, p. 411.
16. POLDERMAN, *et al. Jour. Pharmacol. & Exp. Therap.*, 1943, **78**, p. 400.
17. ADRIANI, J. *Pharmacology of Anæsthetic Drugs*, 1941.
18. JARMAN, R., and ABEL, A. L. *Lancet*, 1936, Feb. 22, p. 422.
19. STEVENS, E. J. *Anesthesiology*, 1945, July, p. 376.
20. MALLINSON, F. B. *Lancet*, 1944, Oct. 7, p. 473.
21. LUNDY, J. S. *Ann. Surg.*, 1939, Nov. 5, p. 878.
22. HEWER, C. L. *Brit. Med. Jour.*, 1938, May 14, p. 1068.
23. MALLINSON, F. B. *Brit. Jour. Anæsth.*, 1941, Jan., p. 102.
24. ADRIANI, J. *Jour. Lab. & Clin. Med.*, 1939, July, p. 1066.
25. REYNOLDS, C., *et al. Anesth. & Anal.*, 1938, Nov.-Dec., p. 357.

26. VAIZEY, J. M.   *Brit. Jour. Anæsth.*, 1938, Jan., p. 55.
27. HEARD.   *Canad. Med. Ass. Jour.*, 1936, Aug., p. 628.
28. BURSTEIN, C. L., and ROVENSTEIN, E. A.   *Anesth. & Anal.*, 1938, July-Aug., p. 195.
29. MACINTOSH, R. R., and SCOTT, R.   *Lancet*, 1946, May 25, p. 767.
30. CARRINGTON, H. C., and RAVENTOS, J.   1946 (in Press).
31. HALTON, J.   *Lancet*, 1946, May 25, p. 771.
32. HILDEBRANDT, E.   *Münch. med. Woch.*, 1935, Aug. 23, p. 1348.
33. SCHMITT.   *Schmerz. Narkose u. Anæsth.*, 1936, Dec., p. 153.
34. SCHRANK, H., and DALHEIN, L.   *Deut. med. Woch.*, 1936, Feb. 21, p. 311.
35. MENSING, K.   *Deut. med. Woch.*, 1936, June 12, p. 970.
36. THALHEIMER.   *Anesth. & Anal.*, 1937, March-April, p. 61.
37. HELRICH, M., *et al.*   *Anesthesiology*, 1950, Jan., p. 33.
38. GAIN, E. A., *et al.*   *Canad. Med. Ass. Jour.*, 1951, Jan., p. 32.
39. CHALLIS, J. H. T.   *Brit. Med. Jour.*, 1937, Aug. 21, p. 386.
40. MULDAVIN, L. F.   *Brit. Med. Jour.*, 1938, Jan. 1, p. 45.
41. MACINTOSH, R. R., and PASK, E. A.   *Lancet*, 1941, July 5, p. 10.
42. GORDH, T.   *Anesthesiology*, 1945, May.
43. ROBERTSHAW, F. L.   *Brit. Med. Jour.*, 1949, July 9, p. 96.
44. ARCHIBALD, W. C.   *Brit. Dent. Jour.*, 1934, Feb. 1.
45. JARMAN, R., and ABEL, A. L.   *Lancet*, 1934, March 10, p. 510.
46. VOSS, E. A.   *Deut. med. Woch.*, 1933, No. 25.
47. MAGILL, I. W.   *Lancet*, 1942, Aug. 1, p. 126.
48. FREEDMAN, A.   *Lancet*, 1945, Sept. 1, p. 276.
49. WRIGHT, A. D.   *Lancet*, *i.*, p. 1040.
50. EVERSOLE, U. H.   *Jour. Amer. Med. Ass.*, 1941, Nov. 22, p. 1760.
51. GORDON, R. A.   *Brit. Med. Jour.*, 1941, July 5, p. 18.
52. MACINTOSH, R. R., and PASK, E. A.   *Lancet*, 1941, July 5, p. 10.
53. BUNYAN, J.   *Brit. Jour. Anæsth.*, 1938, Jan., p. 62.
54. MACINTOSH, R. R., and PASK, E. A.   *Lancet*, 1940, Nov. 23, p. 650.
55. CARRAWAY, B. M.   *Anesth. & Anal.*, 1931, Sept.-Oct., p. 259.
56. MALLINSON, F. B.   *Brit. Med. Jour.*, 1940, Jan. 27, p. 123.
57. VEAL, J. R., and REYNOLDS, C.   *Anesth. & Anal.*, 1939, May-June, p. 56.
58. ORGANE, G., and BROAD, R. I. B.   *Lancet*, 1938, Nov. 19, p. 1170.
59. PICKRELL, K. L., and RICHARDS, R. K.   *Ann. Surg.*, 1945, April, p. 495.
60. *Recommendation of Anæsthetics Committee of M.R.C. & R.S.M. on Evipan.*
61. HUNTER, A. R.   *Lancet*, 1943, Jan. 9, p. 46.
62. MALONEY, A. H.   *Amer. Jour. Surg.*, 1936, Dec., p. 572.
63. KLAGES, F.   *Der. Chirurg.*, 1933, Mar. 10.
64. { POULIQUEN, E.   *Mém. Acad. Chir.*, **63**, 20, p. 1217.
     { DAVISON, T. C.   *Anesth. & Anal.*, 1943, Jan.-Feb., p. 52.
65. FAYKISS, F.   *Zentralb. f. Chir.*, 1936, Aug. 1, p. 1819.
66. Annotation.   *Lancet*, 1949, Feb. 12, p. 285.
67. WIDLAKE, F., and CLUNIE, T.   *Jour. Trop. Med. and Hyg.*, 1937, April 15.
68. JOHNSTONE, I. L.   *Brit. Med. Jour.*, 1935, April 13, p. 761.
69. LANDAU, E., and WOOLEY, E.   *Brit. Med. Jour.*, 1934, Feb. 3, p. 192.
70. LAMSON, P. D., *et al.*   *Science*, 1949, **110**, p. 690.
71. VOSS, E. A.   *Deut. med. Woch.*, 1933, No. 25.
72. { WITTS, L. J., and WILLCOX, W.   *Pro. Roy. Soc. Med.* (Secs. of Med. and Therap.), 1935, Dec. 10.
     { VAIZEY, J. M.   *Brit. Jour. Anæsth.*, 1938, Jan., p. 53.
73. ANSCHÜTZ.   *Deutsche Gesellschaft für Chirurgie*, Berlin, 1933, April.
74. PETERKIN, C. A.   *Brit. Med. Jour.*, 1934, March 10, p. 456.
75. HUNTER, A. R.   *Lancet*, 1943, Jan. 9, p. 46.
76. ELDER, C. K., and HARRISON, E. M.   *Jour. Amer. Med. Ass.*, 1944, May 13, p. 116.

77. { PAYNE, R. T. *Lancet*, 1939, April 8, p. 816.
    { HEWSPEAR, D. *Lancet*, 1945, Sept. 4, p. 361.
78. COHEN, S. *Lancet*, 1948, Sept. 4, p. 361.
79. MACKINTOSH, R. R., and HEYWORTH, P. S. A. *Lancet*, 1943, Nov. 6, p. 571.
80. ANSCHÜTZ. *Deutsche Gesellschaft für Chirurgie*, Berlin, 1933, April.
81. MENEGAUX, G., and SECHEHAYE, L. *Jour. de Chir.* (Paris), 1934, **44**, p. 361.
82. *South Africa Med. Jour.*, 1936, Nov. 14.
83. MORTON, L. G. *Austral. & N.Z. Jour. Surg.*, 1942, **12**, p. 119.
84. *Jour. Amer. Med. Ass.*, 1937, April 3, p. 1172.
85. NIEDERLAND, W. *Schmerz, Narkose Anæsthesie*, 1936, Oct., p. 137.
86. DOOLEY, H. J. *Illinois Med. Jour.*, 1936, April, p. 352.
87. LYLE, T. K., and FENTON, F. C. *Brit. Med. Jour.*, 1934, Sept. 29, p. 589.
88. THOMAS, C. J. *Anesth. & Anal.*, 1944, Jan.-Feb., p. 13.
89. SLOT, G., and McDADE, R. S. *Lancet*, 1933, Nov. 4, p. 1035.
90. SPERBER, P. *New Eng. Jour. Med.*, 1936, **215**, p. 1065.
91. FRANKEL, F. *Brit. Med. Jour.*, 1940, Jan, 6, p. 14.
92. KUNTZE, W. *Münch. med. Woch.*, 1934, No. 25.
93. PICARD, H., and BENSIMON, T. *Lancet*, 1946, May 25, p. 767.
94. ASHWORTH, H. K. *Pro. Roy. Soc. Med.* (An. Sec.), 1946, Feb. 1.
95. RESCHE. *Zentralb. f. Chir.*, 1935, July 20, p. 1703.
96. KEUSENHOFF, W. *Fortsch. d. Therap.*, 1935, *ii.*, p. 705.
97. HUDSON, H. W. *New Eng. Jour. Med.*, 1937, May 27, p. 916.
98. PATTERSON, R. L. *Anesth. & Anal.*, 1941, July-Aug., p. 225.
99. WEESE. *Zbl. Chir.*, 1939, **22**, p. 1233.
100. WILLCOX, W. *Brit. Med. Jour.*, 1934, Mar. 10, p. 416.
101. DUNPHY, J. E., *et al. Surgery*, 1937, Feb.
102. LUNDY, J. S. *Clinical Anesthesia*, 1942. Philadelphia.
103. GORDON, R. A. *Canad. Med. Ass. Jour.*, 1943, Dec., p. 478.
104. JOHNSON, K., and GILBERT, C. R. A. *Anesth. & Anal.*, 1946, July-Aug., p. 133.
105. DOS-GHALI, *et al. Presse Méd.*, 1943.
106. BRITTAIN, G. J. C. *Anæsthesia*, 1949, Jan., p. 30.
107. JARMAN, R. *Pro. Roy. Soc. Med.*, (An. Sec.), 1948, Nov. 5.
108. GRAUBARD, D. J., and PETERSON, M. C. " Clinical Uses of intravenous procaino." 1951. Oxford.
109. MUSHIN, W. W., and RENDEL-BAKER, L. *Brit. Med. Jour.*, 1949, Aug. 27, p. 472.
110. SUMMERS, F. H. *Lancet*, 1950, Dec. 9, p. 774.
111. ZUCK, D. *Brit. Med. Jour.*, 1951, Jan. 20, p. 125.
112. TOCANTINS, L. M., and O'NEILL, J. F. *Surg. Gyn. & Obst.*, 1941, **73**, p. 281, and *Ann. Surg.*, 1945, Aug., p. 266.
113. MUSHIN, W. W. *Pro. Roy. Soc. Med.* (An. Sec.), 1945, Mar. 2.
114. MASSEY, L. W. C. *Brit. Med. Jour.*, 1950, July 22, p. 197.
115. SWERDLOW, M. *Anesth. & Anal.*, 1950, May-June, p. 169.
116. KEELE, C. A. *Pro. Roy. Soc. Med.* (An. Sec.), 1952, Feb. 1.
117. BRODIE, B. B., *et al. Jour. Pharmacol.*, 1950, **98**, p. 85.
118. MAYNERT, E. W., and VAN DYKE, H. B. *Pharmacol. Rev.*, 1949, *i*, p. 29.
119. BRODIE, B. B., *et al. Anesth. & Anal.*, 1950, **29**, p. 29.

CHAPTER XI

MUSCLE RELAXANTS

Curare—D.M.E.—Gallamine triethiodide—Decamethonium iodide—" Win. 2747."—Myanesin—Dihydro-β-erythroidine—Tachycurine—Succinyl-choline iodide and chloride—Brevedil—Magnesium sulphate.

It has already been noted (Chapter I) that most general anæsthetics in heavy dosage produce muscular relaxation as will local analgesics used to paralyse motor nerves.

Certain drugs, however, produce general muscular relaxation as their main effect and some of these are becoming used for this purpose, the accompanying general narcosis being kept at a very light plane. This practice which has become widespread during the past five years, undoubtedly tends towards ideal operating conditions with minimal toxic effects. The first and best known of these relaxing agents is curare.

CURARE

History. Curare, also known as wourari, wourali, urari and urirarery, was first described as an arrow poison by Sir Walter Raleigh to Queen Elizabeth on his return to England from his voyage to the Orinoco in 1584.[1]

In 1800, Humboldt found that certain Indian tribes in South America were smearing on their arrow-heads and blow-pipe darts a syrup obtained from a creeper which was later named *strychnos toxifera*.

In 1812, Charles Waterton in his book "Wanderings in South America" gave a detailed description of the paralysis which ensued when an animal was hit by an arrow poisoned with curare, as the concoction was now called, and in 1814 he and Brodie stated that the paralysis was probably due to a toxic action on the neuro-muscular mechanism.

The first scientific research work on the substance was carried out about fifty years later by the French physiologist Claude Bernard[2] who, in his classical series of experiments, proved that the poison acted on the myoneural junction.

Therapeutic use of curare in the human subject was then held up for a long time owing to the toxic effects, notably bronchospasm,[3] which occurred fairly frequently when using unknown and differing mixtures of alkaloids, but even as early as 1878 success was claimed in the treatment of tetanic spasms.[4]

At last in 1935 a pure alkaloid was isolated in England by H. King of The National Institute of Medical Research and named d-tubocurarine chloride.[5] This was found to be a quaternary ammonium compound. (It might be noted in passing that the corresponding l-alkaloid has only $\frac{1}{35}$ of the physiological activity.)

Since that date progress has been rapid. In August, 1939, the drug was first used in London at the Middlesex Hospital to lessen the risk of trauma from electro-convulsive therapy in mental patients.[6] It was then tried out with great success as a muscle relaxant during light general anæsthesia, the first large series of cases being described in Canada by Griffiths and Johnson[7] and in England by Gray and Halton.[8]

Action. (1) *On Nervous and Muscular Systems.* Tubocurarine has negligible lipoid-solubility so that it probably does not penetrate cells.[60] When curare is injected intravenously it takes about 90 seconds to act. This is greater than the " arm-brain circulation time " and would in itself suggest a peripheral rather than a central effect.

The current theory of muscular contraction is that when an impulse travelling along a motor nerve arrives at the myoneural junction, acetylcholine is released from the nerve ending and depolarizes (or renders electrically negative) the muscle end-plate. This " current of depolarization " excites the adjoining muscle fibre and propagation of this excitation wave along the membrane of the muscle fibre causes contraction of the contractile elements.

In the meantime the released acetylcholine has been hydrolyzed by the enzyme cholinesterase present in the nerve ending and end plate into inactive choline and acetic acid so that when the muscle fibre emerges from its refractory period, it will not become excited again until a fresh nerve impulse arrives. Curare and some of the other relaxants block the normal depolarizing action of acetylcholine and are consequently antagonized by the anti-cholinesterases such as neostigmine (q.v.).[9]

All voluntary muscles are affected by large doses of curare, becoming paralysed and flaccid but they are not all acted upon to the same extent : for example, those of the eyes, pharynx and larynx are particularly susceptible.

Curare also paralyses sympathetic ganglia and it is possibly this action which minimizes traumatic shock even if a severe stimulus is inflicted on a lightly anæsthetized patient.

When used in very small dosage to conscious patients, it is said that curare and some other relaxants have a " lissive " effect. This means that they diminish muscle spasm without impairing voluntary muscle power. This action may be exploited in the treatment of spastic states, often combined with physiotherapy.[10]

In ordinary dosage curare has no effect on the cerebral cortex[11] and as no anæsthetic or analgesic action is present, a light general narcosis must be maintained. In this connection a case has been reported of a curarized patient regaining consciousness and sensitivity to pain during the course of an abdominal operation but being quite unable to indicate the fact.[12] In very large doses, curare does have a central as well as a peripheral action and consciousness may be lost.

(2) *On Respiratory System.* It has already been stated that curare does not affect all muscles to the same extent. If sufficient dosage is given for abdominal relaxation, the intercostal muscles will almost certainly be paralysed and the breathing will become diaphragmatic. Direct recordings of the effect of a given dose of curare on the contractions of the diaphragm and of a voluntary muscle have shown that the former is less susceptible than the latter whether stimulated naturally or artificially through the phrenic nerve. The " therapeutic index " of curare,[13] i.e. the ratio of the dose required to arrest breathing to that needed to abolish muscle tone has been estimated at about 1·4. It is therefore obvious that it may prove impossible to secure complete relaxation with efficient natural breathing and if curare is used the anæsthetist must be prepared to use assisted or controlled respiration.

Bronchospasm, although rare, does occur even with pure preparations of tubocurarine. It is probably due to histamine release[14] and in the author's opinion is practically never encountered unless thiopentone is being administered at the same time.

(3) *On Gastro-intestinal Tract.* Although it is usually stated that curare has no effect on smooth muscle, it would seem likely that since the intestinal musculature contracts by acetylcholine action, it would be affected by the drug. In most animals curare inhibits intestinal peristalsis[15] but in man the effect is variable. The stomach and gut are usually quiescent but occasionally they exhibit increased movements.[8] The intestines are rarely contracted as often seen during spinal block.

(4) *On Cardio-vascular System.* In normal dosage curare usually causes a slight rise in blood-pressure[16] and occasionally the rise is spectacular.[17] The cause is obscure as the original suggestion of a rise in carbon dioxide tension from depressed respiration is demonstrably false. Forced hyperventilation with an absorber does not bring down the pressure to its original level. Occasionally a fall in blood pressure follows an injection of curare. This is thought to be due either to sympathetic ganglia paralysis or to the release of histamine or to both factors. In experimental arterial injections this effect is readily demonstrated.[18] No clinical changes in the cardiac rhythm and no typical electro-cardiographic changes have been noted. The injection of large doses of curare into the circuit of the heart-lung preparation in the dog has no effect on cardiac output, arterial pressure or coronary flow. It does, however, cause a slight fall in venous pressure which would indicate an improvement of the cardiac condition.[19]

Increased bleeding from wounds is occasionally observed in curarized patients. This has been ascribed to the release of heparin.

Elimination. Curare is eliminated fairly rapidly, partly by destruction in the liver and partly by being passed unchanged in the urine.

Antidotes. Neostigmine (prostigmine) is the theoretical antidote but its use (by injection) should seldom be necessary unless the operation has been completed and the patient is still curarized. As already explained neostigmine is an anti-cholinesterase and thus allows acetylcholine to have an abnormally long effect. Animal experiments, however, indicate that neostigmine is by no means a complete neutralizing agent for large doses of curare[20] and in the human subject collapse has followed its use.[21] If really indicated, a full dose of the drug should be given, e.g. 5 mg. intravenously.

This is usually preceded (by at least 2 minutes) by intravenous atropine gr. 1/100 in order to minimize the undesirable parasympathomimetic side-effects such as salivation, diarrhœa and

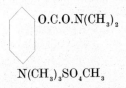

$$O.C.O.N(CH_3)_2$$

$$N(CH_3)_3SO_4CH_3$$

pulmonary œdema, but it should be remembered that, at least theoretically, the combination might cause ventricular fibrillation.[22] Furthermore although the immediate effect of neostigmine may be dramatic, the patient may afterwards relapse into curarization.[59]

Preparations and Dosage. Crude curare is classified quite unscientifically by the containers in which it is packed. Thus three varieties are recognized : (1) Calabash or gourd curare, (2) pot or jar curare, and (3) tube curare which is placed in bamboo tubes. It has been said that these varieties of crude curare contain differing proportions of curarine and allied alkaloids such as protocurarine, protocurine and curine. As, however, the properties and even the identities of these substances are uncertain, it is unprofitable to pursue the subject further.

There are several therapeutic preparations available at the present time.

(*a*) " **Tubarine** " (B.W.) is most commonly used in Great Britain and is claimed to be identical with the pure alkaloid isolated by King. It replaces the former product " **curarine chloride** " (B.W.) which was a white powder which had to be dissolved and sterilized. Tubarine is a sterile solution containing 10 mg. per c.cm. and is supplied in 1·5 c.cm. ampoules and 5 c.cm. rubber capped bottles. The ordinary preparation forms an insoluble precipitate when mixed with thiopentone but " **tubarine miscible** " is also available for mixed injections.

(*b*) **d-tubocurarine chloride** (Duncan) is a solution of the same potency as tubarine. It contains glycerine and alcohol and can be mixed with thiopentone.

(*c*) " **Myostatin** " is a similar preparation to tubarine.

(*d*) "**Intocostrin**" (Squibb) is an American preparation of a yellow sterile solution containing 20 mg. of " curare extract " per c.cm. with 0·5 per cent. chlorbutanol added as a preservative. It is supplied in rubber capped bottles of 5 c.cm. and 10 c.cm. capacity and is a purified extract from the plant *chondodendron tomentosum*. As this is not a pure solution of d-tubocurarine chloride, its action is more variable than that of the British product[7] and the dosage is higher, 2 to 3 c.cm. (40 to 60 mg.) being an average initial dose, i.e. it has about one-fourth the potency of tubarine.[23]

It is unfortunate that no international agreement has yet been reached to standardize the potency of curare preparations and it is at present imperative to distinguish between them.

All curare solutions keep best in a refrigerator but if they become cloudy they should be discarded.

Indications. Curare can be given in most cases where complete muscular relaxation is required for some time. The most obvious scope for its use is in upper abdominal or thoraco-abdominal surgery, where there is a remarkable absence of shock from severe trauma such as peritoneal traction. A possible reason for this has already been mentioned. Curare appears to cross the placental barrier from mother to fœtus very slowly if at all,[60] although it has been shown in animals to pass in the reverse direction.[24] There, therefore, seems no reason to withhold its use in obstetrics, e.g. in Cæsarian section. Curare is also useful during thoracotomies to facilitate controlled respiration and to avoid the cough reflex which may be so troublesome when the surgeon is working near the hilum of the lung under cyclopropane anæsthesia or local analgesia. If short periods of relaxation only are required, e.g. for bronchoscopy or in electro-convulsive therapy, it is preferable to substitute a shorter-acting agent such as gallamine, or succinylcholine, for curare.

Contra-indication. Curare should be avoided in patients suffering from myasthenia gravis except for the minute test dose sometimes used for diagnosing this condition.

Technique of Administration. Curare has no effect by mouth and is usually given intravenously, but when this is impossible the intramedullary route can be used. For a very prolonged effect, e.g. for controlling the spasms of tetanus, curare can be given intramuscularly dissolved in wax and peanut oil.

The original and still sound method of giving curare for the average long abdominal operation is to establish the patient in a steady but light plane of general narcosis and then to give an initial intravenous dose of (say) 10 mg. If relaxation is insufficient in three minutes, a supplementary dose of 5 mg. is given. If the respiratory exchange becomes insufficient, assisted or fully controlled respiration is instituted. No curare should be given within 30 minutes of the completion of the operation and if the muscles tighten during peritoneal closure, a small dose of intravenous thiopentone will always relax them temporarily. In many cases an intravenous drip will be set up and the injection can conveniently be made into the rubber tubing as near the needle as possible. Otherwise a Gordh's needle (q.v.) or one of its modifications is satisfactory. As a general rule, endotracheal anæsthesia is desirable

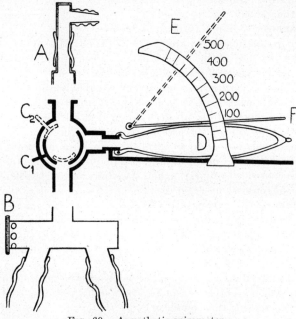

FIG. 69. Anæsthetic spirometer.
(C. T. Barry. *Lancet.*)

with curare, not so much for fear of laryngospasm or bronchospasm, but as a safeguard against gastric regurgitation since the cardiac sphincter is completely relaxed. A cuff or pack is, of course, essential for this purpose.

It is not always easy to decide when an additional dose of curare is indicated and it is worth noting that an increase in the tidal respiratory volume generally occurs just before the return of muscle tone. Inspection of the rebreathing bag gives a rough indication of the tidal volume, or, by means of a 2-way tap, it is possible to divert one expiration into a 600 c.cm. bag and estimate its disten-sion.[25]   A more refined type of simple spirometer is illustrated.   A by-pass is plugged in between the facepiece or endotracheal tube fitting A and the expiratory bag mount B containing a rotating drum moved by a lever C.   In this way one expiration can be diverted into a 600 c.cm. bag D which moves a hinged perspex plate F over a calibrated dial.[26]

An alternative technique which has become popular is to give a preliminary dose of 5 mg. curare to the conscious patient.   This should produce no obvious effect beyond a mild ptosis but occasion-ally patients are met with who appear to have a true idiosyncrasy to the drug although not suffering from myasthenia gravis.   Should a normal response occur, a further 10 mg. dose is given followed immediately by 0·5 g. thiopentone.   Complete relaxation, uncon-sciousness and depression of respiration will follow.   An artificial airway or tracheal tube is then passed and anæsthesia maintained with the desired method accompanied at first by assisted or controlled respiration.[27]   This technique, colloquially termed a " crash induction ", is spectacular and rapid, but is not devoid of risk.   In the first place, it is possible for the needle to slip out of the vein before the thiopentone has been given, and if difficulty in reinsertion is experienced the patient will have the unpleasant sensation of becoming curarized without losing consciousness. Secondly the anæsthetist must be sure that the stomach is empty or regurgitation from a relaxed cardiac sphincter may occur before tracheal intubation can be carried out.   This danger is, of course, aggravated in such conditions as acute intestinal obstruction.[28]

The nature of the general narcosis accompanying curarization varies to some extent with the operation.   The author prefers nitrous oxide and oxygen (about 70/30) with minute additions of ether, trichlorethylene or cyclopropane.   If a non-volatile agent is required, pethidine seems preferable to thiopentone except for closing the abdomen at the end of the operation.   If the latter drug is employed for long, there is a tendency towards jerky respiration and hiccough and the blood-pressure curve seems to show greater deviation from normal.   Whatever method is used, adequate oxygenation is of paramount importance.

After-effects.   The only after-effects attributable to curare so far reported are paresis of some of the ocular muscles which may persist for a few days.[11, 26]   Further information on curare will be found under " abdominal surgery ".

DI-METHYL ETHER OF D-TUBOCURARINE IODIDE

The preparation of the di-methyl ether derivative of tubocurarine chloride (D.M.E., **metubine**) was first described by H. King in 1935,[29] and its pharmacology has now been worked out in animals,[30] and in man.[31] It has now been established that D.M.E. acts in the same way as the parent drug and is antagonized by the anticholinesterases, such as neostigmine.

Dimethyl ether of
D-tubocurarine iodide

The chief differences between the two preparations are that D.M.E. is 2 to $2\frac{1}{2}$ times as potent and that sympathetic ganglia paralysis and histamine release are no greater in spite of the increased potency.

D.M.E. is available in 3 c.cm. ampoules containing 6 mg. of the drug. After considerable clinical use it is the general opinion that D.M.E. has a slightly shorter period of causing diaphragmatic paralysis than curare and that the inflation of collapsed lungs and lobes was slightly easier during thoracotomy, this effect being probably due to less histamine release with correspondingly less bronchiole constriction. It would seem therefore that D.M.E. may have a slight advantage over curare, but owing to the fact that the complicated molecule has four optical isomers, it is difficult to be certain that all samples are identical.[32]

GALLAMINE TRIETHIODIDE

Gallamine triethiodide (**flaxedil** and " **R.P.3697** " is tri (β-diethylaminoethoxy) benzene triethyliodide, and was first

synthesized in France in 1947.[33]   It is a white amorphous powder
with a melting point of 145-150° C. and a molecular weight of 891.
It is supplied in a 4 per cent. solution in water for intravenous
injection (i.e. 40 mg. per c.cm.).   This is miscible with thiopentone.

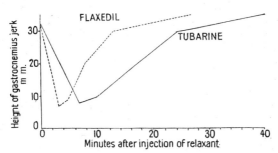

Gallamine triethiodide

The first long series of cases with gallamine was reported in
this country[34] in 1949, and it has now been shown that in general
it has a curare-like effect, but is about one-fifth as potent, 80 mg.
being equivalent to about 15 mg. curare.   The duration of action
is about half that of curare as is well shown in the accompanying
graph.[35]

Fig. 70.   Chart comparing duration of action of gallamine
(flaxedil) and curare. (Doughty and Wylie, *Pro. Roy.
Soc. Med.*)

For this reason, gallamine is useful for short procedures requir-
ing relaxation, e.g. laryngoscopy and bronchoscopy.   It has also
been used with success in softening electrical convulsions,[36] in some
such intravenous cocktail as

thiopentone	..	0·25 g.
gallamine	..	60 to 80 mg.
atropine	..	gr. 1/100.

Gallamine appears to have less effect than curare on paralysing
sympathetic ganglia but it tends to cause tachycardia.   It is

antagonized by neostigmine and should not be used on patients suffering from myasthenia gravis.

DECAMETHONIUM IODIDE

Decamethonium iodide ("**C.10,**" **syncurine** and **eulissin**) is bistrimethylammonium decane diiodide $[N(CH_3)_3(CH_2)_{10}N(CH_3)_3]2 \cdot 1$ supplied as a solution containing 2 mg. per c.cm. Its effects were studied by the Anæsthetics Committee of the Royal Society of Medicine and Medical Research Council, and it was found to be a stable non-irritating solution miscible with thiopentone. Its potency (by weight) is about five times that of d-tubocurarine, 3 mg. usually producing a short period of complete muscular relaxation in the fit adult.[37]

It has now been established that decamethonium acts in an entirely different way to curare and can be regarded as an acetyl-choline which cannot be hydrolyzed, i.e. prolonged depolarization occurs with consequent neuromuscular block.[9] As a result of this action, the anticholinesterases, such as neostigmine, have no antagonizing action. A further difference is that patients with myasthenia gravis have an *increased* tolerance for decamethonium.[58] It was at first thought that lower members of the same series (e.g. pentamethonium and hexamethonium) could be used as antidotes to decamethonium. It was soon realized, however, that in effective doses these drugs caused profound falls in blood pressure from their action of blocking autonomic ganglia and were useless for the purpose (see Chapter XVI).

Decamethonium has about the same length of action as gallamine and can be used for the same purposes. The author has not found it as reliable while undesirable side-effects are common, e.g. bradycardia and fall in blood pressure.[61]

" WIN. 2747 "

This substance, 2-5-bis-(3-diethylamino propylamino) benzo-quinone-bis-benzyl chloride, was synthesized in America[67] and some clinical work suggested that it might be useful as a muscle relaxant in man.[66]

Two investigations in animals and man in Great Britain have shown that WIN. 2747 is undoubtedly an effective relaxant acting for a rather shorter time than curare but that it has various unpleasant side-effects, chiefly of a vago-mimetic type. Its pharmacological effects appear to be partly of the curariform and partly of the decamethonium type and no effective antidote is known.[68]

MYANESIN

Myanesin (**atensin, lissephen, mephenesin**) is β-dihydroxy-γ-(2 methyl phenoxy) propane and consists of colourless crystals with a melting point of 70° C. It is put up as a 10 per cent. solution (1 g. in 10 c.cm.) which is miscible with thiopentone.

O. CH₂.CHOH.CH₂OH

CH₃

Strychnine and picrotoxine antagonize myanesin to some extent and it was at first thought to act as a depressant on the spinal cord.[38] As, however, it relieves pain of thalamic origin, it seems more probable that its effect is on the basal ganglia.[39] Myanesin has been observed to check epileptic fits in 30 seconds, so that it almost certainly has a central rather than a peripheral effect[40] (cf. curare's time of 90 secs.).

An intravenous injection of from 5 to 10 c.cm. in the average fit adult usually produces muscular relaxation with little intercostal or diaphragmatic impairment.[41] Myanesin has, however, lost popularity owing to various complications which may occur such as thrombophlebitis,[42] haemolysis followed by haemoglobinuria,[43] and renal failure.[44] It may be that the hypertonicity of the solution or the composition of the solvent may play a part in these sequelæ, but however this may be, the use of the drug is now practically confined to oral administration (as an elixir) for spastic states such as tetanus.

DIHYDRO-β-ERYTHROIDINE

This substance has been extracted from the sub-tropical tree " Flame of the Forest ", and has been used for some time in the treatment of spastic conditions[45] and for preventing fractures in leptazol convulsive therapy.[46]

It appears to act like curare on the myoneural junction but differs in that it is effective when taken by mouth and that it causes a *fall* in blood pressure.

In a series of 215 administrations dihydro-β-erythroidine gave good muscular relaxation for operations with an average total intravenous dose of 240 mg.[47]

TACHYCURINE

Tachycurine ("**3621.S**") is a synthetic relaxant acting for about one-fifteenth of the time taken by curare. This very short duration is due to rapid hydrolysis. No known antidotes are effective. A 2 per cent. solution has been used with success in man, 60 mg. being equivalent to about 5 mg. of tubocurarine chloride. Up to 400 mg. in 30 minutes has been given without toxic effects. It would seem that tachycurine might be useful for short procedures such as endoscopy, but occasionally muscular tremors and salivation are troublesome. The solution is miscible with thiopentone.[48]

SUCCINYLCHOLINE IODIDE

This agent has been used as a relaxant and is said to cause a consistent rise in blood pressure and no histamine release. It is non-miscible with thiopentone.[49] In a study of 1,000 administrations in man a single dose of from 60 to 80 mg. was found sufficient for intubation, but prolonged relaxation was best attained by a continuous drip of 1 mg. per c.cm. normal saline at a rate of from 40 to 60 drops per minute.[50]

SUCCINYLCHOLINE CHLORIDE
(scoline, anectine, celocurine, lysthenon)

This is similar to but more stable than the iodide[50] and has the structural formula

$$CH_2COOCH_2CH_2N(CH_3)_3Cl.$$
$$|$$
$$CH_2COOCH_2CH_2N(CH_3)_3Cl.$$

The solution contains 50 mg. per c.cm. and the dose varies from 2 c.cm. in a large muscular adult to $0\cdot5$ c.cm. in a child.

The action of succinylcholine is that of depolarization and it can be regarded as a short-acting decamethonium (q.v.). Neostigmine should therefore *not* be used as an antidote.[57]

Although the drug is hydrolyzed by alkalis, it can be mixed with thiopentone if the mixture is injected immediately. It is, however, a poor technique as the preliminary wave of muscular contraction is painful and may occur before consciousness is lost. A better method is to start with a "sleep-dose" of thiopentone and then to inject succinylcholine. The lungs should be inflated with oxygen as respiration will probably cease for some minutes. Since its introduction the drug has been used with great success for such procedures as intubation, examination under anæsthesia, E.C.T. and manipulations.[62]

It was soon found, however, that in a few patients the action of succinylcholine was considerably prolonged over the usual 3 to 4 minutes.[63] The current theory to account for this is that the drug acts by inhibition of the " true " or acetyl-cholinesterase of the red corpuscles at the myoneural junction and that the duration of its effect depends on the speed of its destruction into succinic acid and choline by the " pseudo " cholinesterase of the plasma.[64] Abnormally low levels of the latter enzyme have been found in patients affected for a long time by succinylcholine.

The drug has also been given in diluted form as an intravenous drip during prolonged operations with the idea of maintaining a constant degree of relaxation.[65]

" BREVIDIL " DRUGS

The " brevidil " drugs are short-acting relaxants unstable in solution and are supplied in powder form for dissolving in water immediately before intravenous injection.

" **Brevidil M** " is succimethonium bromide, or more exactly bis(β-dimethylaminoethyl) succinate-bismethobromide, and is supplied in ampoules of 60 mg., this being the average full adult single dose.

" **Brevidil E** " is succiethonium bromide and is less potent and even shorter in action. It is supplied in ampoules of 150 mg.

MAGNESIUM SULPHATE

Some years ago it was claimed in America that magnesium sulphate and ether had a synergistic action but this was later denied.[52] It has also been stated that actual anæsthesia can be produced by magnesium sulphate[53] but that muscular relaxation occurs before this and the effect has been made use of (as in the case of curare) to mitigate the trauma of electro-convulsive therapy.[54] Besides being a relaxant of voluntary muscle, magnesium sulphate is said to have anti-histamine and broncho-dilator effects.[55]

Tests in this country have so far proved inconclusive but some relaxation was usually obtained with intravenous doses of from 20 to 25 c.cm. 25 per cent. magnesium sulphate.[56]

From a consideration of this chapter it will be seen that there is a very large choice of relaxant drugs at the present time, but it should be emphasized that many of them have not been thoroughly worked

out. In the writer's opinion all reasonable needs can be met by
using tubocurarine for prolonged relaxation, gallamine for shorter
cases, and succinylcholine chloride for procedures lasting for a
few moments. The actions of the agents in common use can be
tabulated thus.

	Duration of Effect		
	Long	*Medium*	*Short*
1. Drugs which prevent the normal depolarizing action of acetylcholine. Antagonized by prostigmine.	Tubocurarine D.M.E.	Gallamine (Flaxedil)	
2. Drugs which cause prolonged depolarization not antagonized by prostigmine		Decamethonium (C.10)	Succinylcholine chloride (Scoline)

References

1. RALEIGH, SIR WALTER. "Hakluyt's Voyages." III. p. 649.
2. BERNARD, C. *Bull. gen de Therap.*, 1865, **69,** p. 23.
3. WEST, R. *Lancet*, 1938, Feb. 19, p. 432.
4. COLE, L. *Lancet*, 1934 and 1935.
5. KING, H. *Nature*, London, 1935, **135,** p. 469.
6. PALMER, H. 1948, Aug. Personal communication.
7. GRIFFITHS, H. R., and JOHNSON, G. E. *Anesthesiology*, 1944, **5,** p. 166.
8. GRAY, T. C., and HALTON, J. *Pro. Roy. Soc. Med.* (An. Sec.), 1946, Mar.1.
9. { BAILEY, P. J. *Anæsthesia*, 1949, Apr., p. 52.
   { PATON, W. D. M., and ZAIMIS, E. J. *Lancet*, 1950, Nov. 18, p. 568.
10. RANSOMOFF, N. S. *Bull. N.Y. Acad. Med.*, 1947, **23,** p. 661.
11. KELLGREN, J. H., *et al.* *Brit. Med. Jour.*, 1946, Dec. 14, p. 898.
12. WINTERBOTTOM, E. H. *Brit. Med. Jour.*, 1950, Jan. 28, p. 247.
13. GRAHAM, J. D. P., and HEATHCOTE, R. *Brit. Jour. Anæsth.*, 1950, Jan., p. 17.
14. WEST, R. *Pro. Roy. Soc. Med.* (Sec. Exp. Med. and Therap.), 1949, Mar. 8.
15. GROSS, E. G., and CULLEN, S. C. *Anesthesiology*, 1945, May, p. 231.
16. PRESCOTT, F., *et al.* *Lancet*, 1946, July 20, p. 80.
17. OSTLERE, G. *Brit. Med. Jour.*, 1947, Apr. 5, p. 448.
18. GROB, *et al.* *Bull. Johns Hopkins Hosp.*, 1947, **80,** p. 299.
19. GRAY, T. C., and GREGORY, R. A. *Anæsthesia*, 1948, Jan.
20. PICK, E. P., and UNNA, K. *Jour. Pharmacol. & exp. Therap.*, 1945, Jan., p. 59.
21. { MACINTOSH, R. R. *Brit. Med. Jour.*, 1949, i., p. 852.
    { CLUTTON-BROCK, J. *Ibid.*, p. 1007.
22. JOHNSTONE, M. *Brit. Heart Jour.*, 1951, **13,** p. 47.
23. Memo. Anæsthetics, C.I.E., M.R.C. & R.S.M. 1947.
24. YOUNG, M. *Lancet*, 1949, June 18, p. 1052.
25. HARBORD, R. P. *Brit. Jour. Anæsth.*, 1948, **21,** p. 94.
26. BARRY, C. T. *Lancet*, 1951, Jan. 27, p. 214.
27. GRAY, T. C. *Pro. Roy. Soc. Med.*, (An. Sec.), 1948, Apr. 2.

28. MORTON, H. J. Y., and WYLIE, W. D.   *Anæsthesia*, 1951, Oct., p. 190.
29. KING, H.   *Jour. Chem. Soc.*, 1935, p. 1381.
30. COLLIER, M. O. J.   *Lancet*, 1950, June 3, p. 1293.
31. WILSON, H. B., *et al.*   *Lancet*, 1950, June 3, p. 1296.
32. MOGEY, G. A., and TREVAN, J.   *Brit. Med. Jour.*, 1950, July 22, p. 216.
33. BOYET, D., *et al.*   *C.R. Acad. Sci. Paris*, 1947, **223**, p. 597.
34. MUSHIN, W. W., *et al.*   *Lancet*, 1949, i., p. 726.
35. DOUGHTY, A. C., and WYLIE, W. D.   *Pro. Roy. Soc. Med.* (An. Sec.),
    1951, Jan. 5.
36. { THOMPSON, O., and MORTON, A.   *Brit. Med. Jour.*, 1951, Apr. 21, p. 857,
    { SMITH, R., and THOMAS, D. L.   *Brit. Med. Jour.*, 1951, Apr. 21, p. 860.
37. { PATON, W. D., and ZAIMIS, E. J.   *Nature*, 1948, **162**, p. 810.
    { ORGANE, G.   *Lancet*, 1949, May 7, p. 773.
38. BERGER, F. M., and BRADLEY, W. { *Brit. Jour. Pharmacol. & Chem.*,
                                     { 1946, Dec., p. 265.
                                     { *Lancet*, 1947, Jan. 18, p. 97.
39. STEPHEN, C. R., and CHANDY, J.   *Canad. Med. Ass. Jour.*, 1947, **59**,
    p. 463.
40. HUNTER, A. R., and WATERFALL, J. M.   *Lancet*, 1948, Mar. 6, p. 366.
41. MALLINSON, F. B.   *Lancet*, 1947, Jan. 18, p. 98.
42. GRIFFITH, H. R., and CULLEN, W. C.   *Anesth. & Anal.*, 1048, July-Aug.
43. PUGH, J. I., and ENDERBY, G. E. H.   *Lancet*, 1947, Sept. 13, p. 387.
44. { HEWER, T. F., and WOOLMER, R. F.   *Lancet*, 1947, Dec. 20, p. 909.
    { GOODIER, T. E. W., and GOODHART, C. E.   *Lancet*, 1949, Jan. 29, p. 183.
45. BURMAN, M. S.   *Arch. Surg. & Psych.*, 1939, Feb., p. 307.
46. ROSEN, S. R.   *Psychiat. Quart.*, 1940, July, p. 477.
47. DRIPPS, R. D., and SERGENT, W. F.   *Anesthesiology*, 1947, May, p. 241.
48. OTTOLENGHI, R.   *Internat. Congress Ass. London*, 1951, Sept.
49. THESLEFF, S.   *Ibid.*
50. VON DARDEL, O.   *Ibid.*
51. MYERHOFFER.   *Ibid.*
52. SHACKELLAND, L. F., and BLUMENTHAL, R. R.   *Anesth. & Anal.*, 1933,
    May-June.
53. MELTZER and AVER.   *Jour. Amer. Med. Ass.*, 1916, **67**, p. 1131.
54. YASHIN, H. E.   *Arch. Neurol. Psychiat.*, 1941, **46**, p. 81.
55. HAUREY.   *Jour. Labor. & Clin. Med.*, 1940, **26**, p. 310.
56. ORGANE, G., and ENGLISH, I. C. W.   *Brit. Med. Jour.*, 1947, Feb. 15
57. BOVET, D., *et al.*   *Rendiconti Institute Superiore de Sanita*, 1949, **12**,
    p. 106.
58. CHURCHILL-DAVIDSON, H. C.   *Pro. Roy. Soc. Med.* (An. Sec.), 1951,
    Dec. 7.
59. SPEIRS, R. B.   *Pro. Austral. Soc. An.* (N.S.W. Sec.), 1951, Aug. 9.
60. BULLER, A. J., and YOUNG, I. M.   *Jour. Physiol.*, 1949, **109**, p. 412.
61. GUERRIER, S. M., and MASON, J. C.   *Brit. Med. Jour.*, 1952, June 21,
    p. 1329.
62. ADAMSON, D. C., and KINSMAN, F. M.   *Anæsthesia*, 1952, July, p. 166.
63. { GOULD, R. B.
    { HURLEY, M. J., and MONRO, A. B.   } *Brit. Med. Jour.*, 1952, i.
    { HEWER, C. L.   } Correspondence.
    { HARPER, J. K.
    { LOVE, S. H. S.   *Anæsthesia*, 1952, April, p. 113.
64. EVANS, F. T., *et al.*   *Lancet*, 1952, June 21, p. 1229.
65. BOURNE, J. C., *et al.*   *Lancet*, 1952, June 21, p. 1225.
66. HOPPE, J. O.   *Jour. Pharmacol.*, 1950, **100**, p. 333.
67. { ARROWOOD, J. G.   *Anesthesiology*, 1951, **12**, p. 753.
    { FOLDES, F. F.   *Ann. New York Acad. Sci.*, 1951, **54**, p. 503.
68. { DUNDEE, S. W., *et al.*   *Anæsthesia*, 1952, July, p. 134.
    { HUNTER, A. R.   *Ibid.*, p. 145.

CHAPTER XII

GENERAL ASPECTS OF LOCAL ANALGESIA

Indications—Contra-indications—Mode of Action—Mortality—General and Local Toxic Effects.

In spite of many prophecies to the contrary, the vogue of pure local analgesia has diminished rather than increased in Great Britain during the past few years. The reason for this lies not so much in any inherent disadvantage of the method as in the growing insistence of the general public upon unconsciousness, not only during operation, but for an appreciable period before and after it. The psychological aspects of local analgesia are referred to in Chapter XXVI.

On the other hand, the combination of local analgesia with light general anæsthesia is now making considerable progress. This is largely due to its study being taken up seriously by anæsthetists rather than being regarded as a minor side-line by surgeons.[1]

Indications. Local analgesia may be used alone in minor operations when it is undesirable for the patient to lose consciousness, e.g. if he has had a recent meal, if he is coughing up sputum, or if an anæsthetist is not available. The method is also used in major surgery, usually in combination with light general anæsthesia, in order to secure muscular relaxation without the aid of toxic volatile drugs, intravenous barbiturates or specific relaxants, to diminish capillary oozing, and to minimize " reflex " shock (q.v.).

Contra-indications. Local analgesia should be avoided in children (apart from young babies)[2] in uncoöperative patients and in cases where the injection would have to be made through septic areas or scar tissue.[3] Certain local analgesics should not be used if they have to come into contact with drugs of the sulphonamide group (see Chapter XIII).

Mode of Action. Local analgesics in common use are highly lipoid-soluble alkaloids. The non-irritant, water-soluble salts of these alkaloids are used for injection. The slight alkalinity of the tissue fluids is believed to hydrolyze these salts and the resulting alkaloid bases are taken up by the lipoids in nerve tissue, e.g. procaine $HCl + NaHCO_3 \rightarrow$ procaine base $+ NaCl + H_2CO_3$. Another factor is probably the ionization of the alkaloidal salt which produces an ion of the analgesic base having a positive charge, e.g. procaine HCl→ procaine$^+$ + Cl$^-$. This is taken up by a nerve structure having a negative electrical charge.[4] The effect produced upon the nerve is complete depression without previous stimulation. The depression is not, however, uniform. For example, in mixed nerves the sensory fibres are affected before the motor ones, the order for loss of function being firstly vaso-constriction, then temperature followed by pain and touch and lastly joint and pressure sensation. In animals this order corresponds to the thickness of the myelin sheath of the various fibres.[5] (See also under spinal analgesia.)

It has been demonstrated by Donaggio that an early primary degeneration occurs in nerve fibres in contact with an analgesic solution. This change starts in the axis cylinder and extends to the myelin sheath. The process is normally reversible and its degree can be taken as an index of the local toxicity of the agent employed. If this is done, cocaine, procaine and stovaine show up best. The first-named agent is, however, unsuitable for injection purposes on account of its high general toxicity.[6]

It should be pointed out that " degeneration " in the accepted sense is difficult to reconcile with the rapid onset of analgesia and the fact that blocked nerves do not have a reduced oxygen consumption (G. S. Dawes). It is believed, however, that definite changes, e.g. a lowering of surface tension, occur in cell membranes.[7]

At one time it was thought that dissolving the drugs in oil prolonged their action when injected, but this has now been shown to be false.[8] The elimination of local analgesics is considered later.

Mortality. It is extremely difficult to assess the relative mortality rates of local and general anæsthesia as up to the present it has been impossible to collect statistics from strictly comparable series (see Chapter XXVIII). In an exhaustive survey of nearly 50,000 unselected and consecutive operations performed under every variety of general and local anæsthesia, it was shown that the immediate death rate under local methods was more than double that under general anæsthesia ($0 \cdot 001301$ per cent. as against $0 \cdot 00614$ per cent.).[9] It is quite possible, however, that local analgesia was used in worse risks than the other series. From a study of 21,000 case reports, a Continental surgeon gives it as his considered opinion that the general adoption of local analgesia does not in itself diminish the operative mortality rate.[10]

The mortality from spinal analgesia is discussed in Chapter XV.

Immediate Toxic Effects

It has already been pointed out that local analgesics are protoplasmic poisons possessing special affinity for nerve tissue. The injection of large amounts of solution into the general circulation will naturally affect the brain and vital centres. The potency of local analgesics is in approximately direct ratio to their concentration, but the toxicity is in geometrical ratio to their concentration (Farr).

The relative toxicities of the various local analgesics discussed in the next chapter are usually measured experimentally by injecting them intravenously at a constant rate. The results vary with the type of animal used and cannot be regarded as applying exactly to man. Any figures of toxicity quoted should therefore be regarded with reserve.

Cases of collapse from local analgesics can be divided into three main groups.

Overdose. It is not difficult to give a patient an overdose of a toxic drug such as cocaine even if it is simply applied to mucous surfaces. The almost universal adoption of procaine, nupercaine, amethocaine and xylocaine for infiltration and nerve block has provided a fairly wide margin of safety, and overdosage in adults is rare although by no means unknown. It is worth noting that the minimum lethal dose of cocaine and its substitutes is raised by basal narcosis with the barbiturates but is lowered by ether anæsthesia.[11] The toxic symptoms produced by overdosage of local analgesics are excitement, restlessness, rapid and deep respiration, dilated pupils, rapid, feeble pulse, followed in severe cases by unconsciousness, convulsions and death. If convulsions have actually occurred (they resemble ether convulsions, q.v.) a short-acting barbiturate should be injected intravenously.[12] Recovery has followed the inadvertent hypodermic injection of 3 gr. of cocaine hydrochloride after treatment with intravenous hexobarbitone.[13]

Normal Dosage in a Susceptible Patient. Cocaine is very highly toxic to some patients, and death has occurred from the mere application of trifling amounts of solution to mucous surfaces.[14] An allergic factor is sometimes present. For example, cocainization of the nasal septum in asthmatics may initiate a violent paroxysm, and this can even prove fatal.[15] Idiosyncrasy to the cocaine substitutes is less common but undoubtedly occurs[16]; for example, typical gradual procaine poisoning ending in death has resulted from the injection of only 16 c.cm. of 2 per cent. solution.[17] Particulars of six fatalities from procaine investigated by the Laryngological Section of the American Medical Association suggest that some at least fall into this category.

Inadvertent Intravenous Injection. The introduction of the solution into a vein seems to afford the most reasonable explanation of the tragic cases of *sudden* collapse and death.[18] It has been estimated that the intravenous lethal dose of a local anæsthetic is about one-tenth of its subcutaneous lethal dose (Farr). (For the technique of intravenous analgesia, see Chapter X). Analgesics injected into the tissues are gradually absorbed into the blood stream and are then either excreted directly by the kidneys or are converted into inert substances by the liver (Eggleston and Hatcher). For example procaine is hydrolyzed (partly by an enzyme in the blood termed " procaine esterase " and partly by a similar enzyme in the liver) into p-amino benzoic acid and diethyl-amino-ethanol. The direct and rapid injection of the drug into the blood stream, however, does not give time for these changes to take place and the effect may be serious if the rate of injection greatly exceeds 20 mg. per minute, e.g. a fatality occurred when 25 c.cm. of 2 per cent. procaine was injected into a vein by mistake during a brachial plexus block.[19] Recent work suggests that the cardiac effects are bundle branch block, slowing of conduction through the A-V node, ventricular tachycardia and finally ventricular fibrillation.[20] It is probable that the addition of adrenaline increases the liability to cardiac failure, and it has been suggested that here, too, the actual cause of death is ventricular fibrillation as in the chloroform-adrenaline fatalities. It is probable that a simultaneous injection of atropine should diminish the effects of adrenaline poisoning.[21] The correlation of these findings with the known action of procaine in diminishing or abolishing cardiac arrhythmias produced by direct trauma in thoracic surgery (q.v.) is not entirely clear. The practical deductions from the foregoing considerations are that the needle point should be kept moving during injections, and that the aspiration test should always be performed before injecting a large quantity of solution into one area, e.g. in nerve blocks. Some anæsthetists inject the solution only during movements of withdrawal of the needle. Others inject during the entry of the needle, believing that the issuing fluid will push away any small vessel from the point. In the writer's opinion, the important matter is to see that the needle point is always moving. If cardiac failure should occur, the only hope of recovery is to institute immediate treatment on the lines described in Chapter XVII.

Local Toxic Effects

Freshly prepared local analgesic solutions made up in sterile isotonic form should give rise to very little tissue irritation. If, however, an excessive amount of adrenaline is added, dangerous vaso-constriction may occur, especially in patients suffering from vaso-motor or trophic disturbances. It has been shown, for example, that 1 in 20,000 adrenaline solution readily produces tissue necrosis.[22]   Extensive sloughing may follow local analgesia in debilitated patients[23] and may even precipitate a fatal issue.[24] Gangrene appears specially likely to follow local analgesia for operations on the fingers, a survey of the literature producing twenty-nine references. It is concluded that for such operations, if a local method can be avoided so much the better. If not, no adrenaline should be added to the solution, a tourniquet should not be used and massage should be instituted as soon as possible.[25]

Continual application of analgesic solutions to tissues eventually causes irritation and procaine dermatitis is a recognized occupational disease of dentists.[26]

Solutions should preferably be freshly prepared from drugs supplied in sterile powder form in glass ampoules. Ready-made solutions tend to deteriorate on keeping and, if the container is not air-tight, an increase in concentration occurs from evaporation which may lead to an inadvertent overdose being given.[27]   Procaine, in particular, tends to oxidize thus lowering the pH, i.e. increasing the acidity. This is well illustrated by the investigation of 800 procaine solutions offered for sale. The pH was found to vary from $3 \cdot 9$ to $7 \cdot 5$. If ready-made solutions must be used, it is worth noting that they keep best in all-glass ampoules and worst in rubber-capped bottles. Vacuum packing apparently has no effect in retarding oxidation.[28]   It is essential that the injected solution should be isotonic. The writer knows of two instances of extensive tissue necrosis where the saline used as solvent proved to be hypertonic.

Remote Toxic Effects

Occasionally diseases of the central nervous system follow operations performed under local analgesia, but no convincing explanation has yet been offered to account for them. For example, a case of bulbar paralysis following a nerve-block for a dental operation has been recorded, as have two cases of transverse myelitis following local analgesias for thoracoplasty.[29]   Such cases are sufficiently rare to justify the doubt that they may have been *post sed non propter hoc.*

References

1. Editorial, *Brit. Med. Jour.*, 1943, June 5, p. 700.
2. SINGTON, H. *Brit. Med. Jour.*, 1923, Nov. 3, pp. 801, *et seq.*
3. MARSHALL, C. J. *Clin. Jour.*, 1936, June, p. 221.
4. BIETER, R. N. *Amer. Jour. Surg.*, 1936, Dec., p. 500.
5. HEINBECKER, P., *et al.* *Pro. Soc. Exper. Biol. & Med.*, 1932-3, **30**, p. 304.
6. RUGGLIERI, E., *et al.* *Gior. Ital. di Anestesia e di Analgesia*, 1938, Sept.
7. GARDNER, J. H., and SEMB, J. *Jour. Pharmacol. & Exper. Ther.*, **54**, p. 309.
8. KELLY, M. *Lancet*, 1947, May 24, p. 710.
9. BORTONE, F. *Anesth. & Anal.*, 1932, Nov.-Dec., p. 256.
10. BAZY, L. *Bull. et Mém. Soc. Nat. de Chir.*, 1932, Dec. 17, p. 1523.
11. BARBOUR, H. C. *Amer. Jour. Surg.*, 1936, Dec., p. 441.
12. LUNDY, J. S., and TUOHY, E. B. *Amer. Jour. Surg.*, 1936, Dec., p. 511.
13. DALY, H. J. *Anesth. & Anal.*, 1937, Sept.-Oct., p. 293.
14. ROSS, J. S., and FAIRLIE, H. P. " Handbook of Anæsthesia," 3rd edit.
15. WALDBOTT, G. L. *Jour. Amer. Med. Ass.*, 1932, Dec. 3.
16. MAXSON, L. H. *Anesth. & Anal.*, 1934, Jan.-Feb., p. 30.
17. AUSTEI, E. T. *Jour. Amer. Med. Ass.*, 1932, Aug. 25, p. 555.
18. CADE, S. *Pro. Roy. Soc. Med.* (An. Sec.), 1934, Dec. 12, p. 16.
19. DE PABLO, J. S., and DIEZ-MALLO, J. *Ann. Surg.*, 1948, **128**, p. 956.
20. LONG, J. H., *et al.* *Anesthesiology*, 1949, July, p. 406.
21. DOUBLEDAY, F. N. *Pro. Roy. Soc. Med.* (Odont. Sec.), 1925, Feb. 23.
22. SERAFIN, F. J. *Jour. Amer. Med. Ass.*, 1928, **91**, p. 43.
23. ABEL, A. L. *Practitioner*, 1936, April, p. 509.
24. SLOT, G. *Pro. Roy. Soc. Med.* (An. Sec.), 1935, Feb. 1.
25. KAUFMAN, P. A. *Arch. Surg.*, 1941, May, p. 929.
26. LADEN, E. L., and WALLACE, D. A. *Jour. Invest. Dermat.*, 1949, **12**, p. 151.
27. JAMES, H. R. " Regional Analgesia for Intra-abdominal Surgery," 1943, J. & A. Churchill.
28. GROSSMAN, L. I. *Jour. Amer. Cent. Ass.*, 1937, Sept., p. 1538.
29. SCHMIDT, W., and BILLIG, E. *Brun's Beitr. z. Klin. Chir.*, 1935, Oct. 23, p. 441.

CHAPTER XIII

DRUGS USED IN LOCAL ANALGESIA

THE drugs in common use as local analgesics are cocaine, cocaine derivatives and quinine derivatives. The most popular analgesics in Great Britain at the present time are cocaine, procaine, nupercaine, amethocaine and xylocaine. These will now be considered in some detail.

Cocaine was the first local analgesic introduced, in 1884 by Carl Coller, and is a derivative of the base ecgonine with the structural formula

$$
\begin{array}{c}
\qquad\quad \text{H} \qquad \text{H} \quad \overset{\displaystyle O}{\overset{\|}{}} \\
\text{H}_2\text{C}\!-\!-\!-\!\text{C}\!-\!-\!-\!\text{C}\!-\!\text{COCH}_3 \\
\qquad\quad | \qquad\quad | \;\; \overset{O}{\overset{\|}{}} \\
\qquad \text{H}_2\text{C.N} \quad \text{H.COC}\!-\!\text{C}_6\text{H}_5 \\
\text{H}_2\text{C}\!-\!-\!-\!\text{C}\!-\!-\!\text{CH}_2
\end{array}
$$

(The discovery that coca leaves when chewed appeased hunger and delayed fatigue was made by the Peruvians in dim antiquity, but was unknown to the civilized world until the Spanish conquest in the sixteenth century. An interesting account of this history is given in the reference.[1])

The hydrochloride is generally used in fresh solution as decomposition occurs on boiling. Cocaine combines the effects of analgesia with strong vaso-constriction. It is a powerful surface analgesic, and its use is now practically confined to this class of work. For example, it is frequently employed in a 4 per cent. solution for instillation into the eye and in a 10 per cent. to 20 per cent. solution for nasal and laryngeal work (q.v.). Certain patients appear to be specially susceptible to cocaine poisoning ; for example, death has occurred from the cocainization of the urethra with a 5 per cent. solution (Greig). The toxicity of the drug precludes its use for injection work, an analysis of fourteen deaths in America showing the very real dangers involved.[1] The potency of injected cocaine is about 1·5 relative to procaine and its toxicity 4·2. The tendency to a " drug habit " which cocaine induces constitutes a further powerful argument against its general use. The preparation

known as " **Locosthetic** " contains 0·75 per cent. cocaine hydrochloride with adrenaline chloride, 1 in 50,000. " **Neurocain** " is
cocaine hydrochloride compressed into tiny cylinders for " pressure "
dental analgesia (q.v.). It must not be confused with novocaine.
" **Surfacaine** " is a fluid containing cocaine with sufficient antiseptic
to make it self-sterilizing.

Procaine (**allocaine, ethocaine, kerocaine, néocaine, novocaine,
planocaine, scurocaine, sevicaine** and **syncaine**) is the hydrochloride
of para-aminobenzoyldiethyl-aminoethanol with the formula

$$
\begin{array}{c}
NH_2 \\
C \\
HC \quad CH \\
HC \quad CH \\
C \\
O\,C-O-CH_2CH_2N(C_2H_5)_2
\end{array}
$$

and was introduced in 1905 by Einhorn. In the pure state procaine
exists as colourless crystals melting at 156° C. and is readily soluble
in water. It has a toxicity of one-fifth to one-seventh that of
cocaine, and can be sterilized by boiling. As procaine is a vaso-
dilator[2], a 0·5 per cent. solution is usually combined with 1 in
250,000 adrenaline. This combination is very effective, and until
the introduction of nupercaine, amethocaine and xylocaine was used
almost exclusively for infiltration. For this reason procaine is used
as a standard of comparison as regards toxicity and potency. The
toxic effects of the drug have been described in Chapter XII.
The maximum permissible volumes for injection (excluding spinal
block) in a fit male are usually given as :

0·5% solution	..	..	200 c.cm.
1% solution	..	..	75 c.cm.
2% solution	..	..	25 c.cm.

The use of the stronger solutions is usually confined to nerve
blocking. Procaine has a negligible surface action on the unbroken
skin but often causes dermatitis (e.g. in dentists).

As mentioned in the previous chapter, procaine solutions tend to
deteriorate on keeping, and cases have been reported in which old
solutions have caused dizziness and even unconsciousness.[3]

The preparations known as **spinocaine, gravocaine** and **duracaine**
contain procaine as the analgesic principle and are referred to in

Chapter XV. **Neotonocain** tablets are a combination of procaine and adrenaline in varying strengths, while **parsetic** is a solution of 2·25 per cent. procaine with 1 in 30,000 adrenaline.

Various procaine solutions containing enough antiseptic to make them " self-sterilizing " are now on the market. **Novutox** contains 2 per cent. procaine, 1 in 200,000 adrenaline, thymol and " capryl-hydrocupreinotoxin HCl " in Ringer's solution.[4] **Waite's local analgesic** contains procaine and adrenaline, but in this case the incorporated antiseptics are ortho- and para-mono-iodo-phenol. **Arecan** solutions also contain procaine and adrenaline in various strengths with enough antiseptic to keep them sterile. These solutions are useful in that they are " self-sterilizing ", but a word of warning is necessary to avoid placing reliance in antiseptics when injecting infected tissues. An investigation carried out with three characteristic organisms, viz. B. subtilis, Staph. pyogenes aureus and B. paratyphosus B., showed that " the bactericidal action of local analgesic fluids in the strength ordinarily employed is so slight as to be negligible, and these solutions should not be injected into inflamed or septic tissues in the hope of their proving innocuous ".[5] As a matter of fact, some of these so-called " self-sterilizing " solutions, when kept in rubber-capped bottles for some time, have proved to be infected and spinal meningitis has occurred from organisms carried through the theca from the subcuticular wheal. **Proctocaine** contains 1·5 per cent. procaine with 5 per cent. benzyl alcohol and 6 per cent. butyl-p-amino benzoate in vegetable oil. It is used to inject the peri-anal subcutaneous tissues in such conditions as painful fissures and pruritus ani. Care must be taken to avoid injection into septic areas. The original claim that the action of proctocaine was extremely prolonged (7 to 28 days) has not been substantiated[6] as any lasting effect is due to destruction of nerve fibres by benzyl alcohol.

The chief disadvantages of pure procaine are its comparatively evanescent effect (three-quarters to one hour) and its poor surface action. It has been shown that the anti-bacterial properties of the sulphonamide group of drugs are suppressed by local analgesics containing the p-amino benzoic acid grouping, e.g. procaine, anæsthesin, butyn, larocaine, orthoform and tutocaine. It has been estimated that one molecule of p-amino benzoic acid counteracts the action of 200 to 500 molecules of sulphapyridine. It follows, therefore, that these local analgesics should not be used if the wounds are to be impregnated with a sulphonamide preparation to combat infection[7] or if the sulpha-drug is being given by mouth.

The antagonistic action is so marked that if, for example, procaine be used for pleural aspiration, the remaining chest fluid may contain sufficient of the drug to inhibit the action of sulpha-pyridine and thus permit bacterial growth.[8] The effects of penicillin are *not* counteracted by any of the local analgesics and in fact **procaine-penicillin** (a true salt formed by the equimolecular combination of procaine and sodium or potassium penicillin G) is used as a suspension in oil to give a prolonged effect with minimal pain when injected.[9]

Nupercaine (**cinchocaine** B.P.C. formerly **percaine,** and known in Russia as **sovkain** !) differs from the cocaine-procaine group in being a derivative of quinoline, its actual structure being butyl-oxycinchoninic acid diethylethylendiamide hydrochloride with the formula :

$$CONH.CH_2CH_2N(C_2H_5)_2HCl$$

Nupercaine forms colourless, tasteless crystals, having a melting-point of $97°$ C. It is readily soluble in water and alcohol, and may be repeatedly boiled for sterilization. Nupercaine must be kept in alkali-free glass containers, and syringes, needles, etc., must be boiled in water free from sodium bicarbonate. Its ready decomposition by alkali renders the addition of a trace of hydrochloric acid desirable to solutions which must be stored. The discovery of the analgesic properties of nupercaine was made by Karl Meischer and published by Uhlmann[10] in 1929. It was quickly realized that this drug possessed very remarkable properties, and its introduction has profoundly modified the technique of spinal analgesia (see Chapter XV). The main characteristics of nupercaine are its extreme potency and duration of action. It has been estimated that the toxicity of nupercaine is twenty-five times that of procaine, but this is more than counterbalanced by the fact that its minimal effective concentration is about one-fortieth.[11] Nupercaine is extremely effective for surface application,[12] and with amethocaine and xylocaine has largely replaced cocaine for this purpose.[13] Some idea of its potency can be gained by the fact that a dilution of 1 in 125,000 has a pronounced effect on a rabbit's cornea.[14] For infiltration work a concentration of 1 in 1,500 to 1 in 2,000 is usual, combined with adrenaline. From work in Russia it would appear that the very dilute solution of 1 in 10,000 is fairly effective.[15] It must not, however, be assumed that nupercaine can be given with impunity, as in excessive doses toxic effects will occur as with any of the other local analgesics. The maximum permissible dosage for infiltration in a fit male adult is said to be :

1 in 2,000 nupercaine	..	250 c.cm.
1 in 1,000 nupercaine	..	120 c.cm.
1 in 500 nupercaine	..	35 c.cm.

Nupercaine poisoning has been described many times,[16] sometimes with fatal results.[17] For example, death has followed infiltration with 12 c.cm. of 2 per cent. nupercaine used in error.[18] The drug has practically no irritating effect on tissues and little delay in healing has been observed after its use.[19] After-pain is definitely reduced when compared with procaine owing to the longer effect of nupercaine.

Amethocaine (Anethaine, Butethanol, Decicaine, Dikaine, Pantocaine, Pontocaine " Regional D." and **Tetracaine**) was introduced by Bayers about 1930 and is the hydrochloride of para-butylamino benzoyl dimethylamino ethanol with the formula

$$NH.C_4H_9$$

$$OC.-O-CH_2CH_2N(CH_3)_2.HCl$$

It occurs as a white crystalline powder with a melting-point of 147° C. It is readily soluble in water or saline and the resulting solution can be sterilized by boiling.[20] When once prepared, the fluid will remain sterile for some time as it is lethal to non-sporing organisms.[21] Amethocaine has a fairly good surface effect when combined with adrenaline,[22] and its duration is longer than that of procaine but not so long as that of nupercaine. When used in a 1 per cent. solution for ophthalmic work it has been found to cause no rise in intra-ocular pressure[23] or dilatation of the pupil. It has been suggested that the drug could be used in first aid posts for the relief of pain from mustard gas burns of the eye.[24] The same concentration of amethocaine is used for surface analgesia in oto-rhino-laryngological work[25] and for spinal block (q.v.). A combination of amethocaine and procaine has been used both for infiltration and for spinal block and it is claimed that the mixture enhances the desirable effects of both drugs while minimizing their disadvantages.[26] When used alone for infiltration work a 1 in 1,000 amethocaine solution is commonly employed.[27] The drug is about twenty times as potent and as toxic as procaine[28] and can produce very severe toxic effects[29] to counteract which nikethamide is recommended. Many fatalities have followed the administration of from 0·2 g. to 0·5 g. of the drug either by injection into tissues or mere spraying on the throat.[30] At least twelve fatalities have been reported during bronchoscopy and gastroscopy and a further three during preparation for urethral instrumentation.[31] Preliminary sedation with a barbiturate should always be used as a prophylactic measure. It is held by one authority that it is safe to regard the maximum dose as 2 mg. per lb. body weight with an upper limit of 300 mg.[32] This, of course, does not apply to intrathecal injections.

Other drugs which have been used at one time or another to produce local analgesia will now be listed alphabetically.

Acoine, or di-para anisyl monophenethyl quinidine hydrochloride.

Alypin (Amydricaine hydrochloride), or tetra methyl diamino benzoyl ethyl dimethyl carbinol hydrochloride. It is about ten times as toxic and one-third as potent as procaine.

Anæsthesin (Anesthone, Benzocaine B.P.), or the ethyl ester of para amino benzoic acid. This is sometimes used in powder form as a surface analgesic for painful wounds. It has one-tenth the toxicity of cocaine.[28]

Apothesine, or the cinnamic ester of γ-diethyl amino alcohol hydrochloride.

Borocaine, or β-eucaine borate, is useful for surface analgesia and has to some extent displaced cocaine for this purpose,[33] mainly for ophthalmic,[34] nasal[35] and urethral work.[36] It is not, however, a vaso-constrictor.

Bromsalizol (a 4 per cent. solution of monobromhydroxybenzyl alcohol in peanut oil) apparently has a prolonged and selective effect on sympathetic fibres.

Butacaine (Butyn) is the sulphate of p-amino benzoyl dibutyl amino propanol and has been used for ophthalmic and nasal surgery.[37] It can be boiled for sterilization,[38] and is about nine times as toxic and three times as potent as procaine.

Diothane, the hydrochloride of piperidinopropanedioldiphenyl urethane, appears to be even less toxic than procaine. It has a slight bactericidal action,[39] and, although analgesia develops slowly, it exists for a longer time than with any other drugs except nupercaine, quinine and urea. Diothane has been used with success in ophthalmic[40] and urological surgery.[41]

Eucaine, or benzoyl-vinyl-diacetone alkamine, was used extensively before the advent of procaine. It can be boiled without decomposition and is practically non-irritant to tissues. β-**eucaine hydrochloride** and **lactate (benzamine lactate)** have also been used. The borate has already been mentioned under borocaine.

Holocaine (Phenocaine), or para diethoxyethenyl diphenyl amidine hydrochloride. It is about twice as toxic as cocaine.[28]

Intracaine (β-diethylamino ethyl-p-ethoxy benzoate hydrochloride) is slightly more toxic than procaine, but is efficient in lower concentrations (0·5 per cent. intracaine corresponds to 0·75 per cent. procaine). It has little irritative effects on tissues. A case of intracaine poisoning following the inadvertent intravenous administration of the drug was saved by means of hexobarbitone, thus illustrating once again the antagonistic actions of the barbiturates and the cocaine derivatives.[42]

Larocaine (para-aminobenzoyl, 2-2-dimethyl-3-diethyl-amino-1-propanol hydrochloride) has a good surface action, and is used for this purpose in about the same concentration as cocaine. The toxicities of the two drugs are also about the same.[28] Larocaine can be sterilized by boiling, and is used for infiltration work in a 0·25 per cent. solution. Its effects are said to be rather more prolonged than those of procaine and tissue irritation is not marked.[43]

Locaine (β-benzoyl-β-phenyl ethyl dimethylamine hydrochloride) has a shorter action than procaine, and may cause some tissue irritation on injection. It has, however, quite a good surface effect.[44]

Lucaine (P.T.19) β(2 piperidyl) ethyl orthoaminobenzoate hydrochloride seems to be the most promising member of the various new piperidine derivatives recently investigated.[45] Used as a spinal analgesic, lucaine is about five times as potent (by weight) as procaine and its action lasts about twice as long.[46] The drug appears to have more effect on the sensory side and less on the motor one than most other spinal analgesics.[47]

Monocaine (mono-isobutyl amino ethyl para-amino benzoate) has been used as the hydrochloride and the formate. The former has been employed for infiltration and is about as toxic as procaine but with a slightly longer action.[48] The formate has been tried for spinal block in doses of from 50 to 150 mg. in a 5 per cent. solution in cerebrospinal fluid.[49]

Neothesine (Metycaine) is γ-2-methyl piperidine-propyl benzoate hydrochloride, and was synthesized by McElvain.[50] It appears to be slightly more potent than procaine[51] and to have a better surface effect.[52] For example, a 2 per cent. solution instilled into the conjunctival sac usually produces good analgesia in one minute. The usual strenth for injection purposes is 1 per cent.[53] Neothesine has been used in a 10 per cent. solution for spinal analgesia, the maximum dose being regarded as 200 mg.[54] It is said to be about three-quarters as toxic as cocaine.[28]

Orthocaine (Aminobenz, Orthoform) is an insoluble powder sometimes used to alleviate the pain of inflamed surfaces.

Panthesine (" S.F. 147 ") is the N-diethyl-leucinol ester of p-amino-benzoic acid, i.e. it has the same aromatic nucleus as procaine but a longer side chain. The absolute toxicity of panthesine is greater than that of procaine, but this is offset by the fact that only half the concentration is necessary, e.g. 0·25 per cent. for infiltration combined with adrenaline. The advantages claimed over procaine are (a) that panthesine has a better surface effect and (b) that it acts for a longer time. The drug is stable in solution and can be sterilized by boiling.[55]

Phenolaine is dimethyl-diethyl-diphenyl-monobenzoic amine, and is a heavy brown liquid with a strong antiseptic action. It is used in strengths of 2 to 4 minims to the ounce of normal saline combined with adrenaline.

Quinine and urea hydrochloride was introduced by Thibault[56] in 1904, and is made by the addition of urea to a solution of quinine in hydrochloric acid. The analgesic properties of the compound were discovered accidentally during its hypodermic use in the treatment of malaria. The crystals are dissolved in water and used in a strength of 0·25 per cent. to 1 per cent. This solution can be boiled and provides an exceptionally long period of analgesia[57] (sometimes up to six days). Unfortunately, however, the irritation to the tissues delays healing and the preparation is now seldom used. At one time imperfect sterilization led to several cases of tetanus following the injection.

Quinine hydrochloride and urethane has been used for packing septic wounds in a 0·75 per cent. solution. This fluid is definitely bactericidal and has a very prolonged analgesic effect. It is particularly useful in the post-operative treatment of rectal wounds.[58]

Scuroform (Butoform) is N-butyl-p-amino benzoate and is

practically insoluble in water. The drug has been used in a saturated oily solution (8 per cent.) or in a glycero-alcoholic-solution (10 per cent.) for surface analgesia.

Stovaine (Amylocaine) is ethyl-dimethyl-amino-propanol benzoate hydrochloride, and was first prepared by Fourneau (*Anglicé*, " stove ") in 1904. Stovaine has an irritant effect on tissues, and is consequently unsuitable for infiltration analgesia. It has been used extensively, however, for spinal block, especially in France. A 10 per cent. solution in isotonic saline is a favourite preparation. (Chaput's formula, see spinal analgesia.)

Tropacocaine is the hydrochloride of benzoyl pseudo tropeine and has a toxicity about half that of cocaine and a shorter action. It is said to be the only local analgesic apart from cocaine which occurs in the natural state. It is obtained from Java Coca. Tropacocaine has been used for spinal block in doses of 5 to 15 cg. in adults, according to the desired extent of analgesia.[59]

Tutocaine or para amino benzoyl dimethyl amino methyl butanol hydrochloride. It is about as potent as procaine but three times as toxic.

Xylocaine (Lidocaine, Lignocaine) is w-diethylamino-2-6-dimethyl acetanilide and is probably the most promising of the newer local

$$\langle\rangle \begin{array}{c} CH_2 \\ \\ CH_2 \end{array} NH.CO.CH_2N(C_2H_5)_2$$

analgesics. It is used in the same concentration as procaine but has a slightly longer action and appears to be less toxic.[60] Opinion on this point is not, however, unanimous,[61] and deaths have occurred from absorption of the drug.[69] Xylocaine is more stable than procaine to boiling acids and alkalis so that it can be sterilized more easily. A preparation with adrenaline has been evolved which is said to be completely stable for prolonged periods. When used as a 2 to 4 per cent. solution, xylocaine has a good surface action on mucous membranes. If instilled into the eye no dilatation of the pupil occurs.[62] In the writer's experience, xylocaine causes less vaso-dilatation than procaine and gives a more certain and intense analgesia.

Drugs Employed for Vaso-constriction

It has already been noted that all local analgesics except cocaine cause vaso-dilatation. It is customary, therefore, to incorporate a vaso-constrictor in all solutions used for infiltration and field blocking. The advantages then secured are : (*a*) a relatively ischæmic operative field ; (*b*) a more prolonged effect of the analgesic drug from its delayed escape from the injected area ; and (*c*) diminished toxic effects from the analgesic drug owing to its slower absorption. The actual vaso-constrictors in common use will now be mentioned.

Adrenaline (epinephrin, exadrin, suprarenin and **surrenin)** was first used as a vaso-constrictor in local analgesia by Braun in 1903,[63] and is still the agent most commonly employed. Adrenaline is the secretion of the medulla of the adrenal gland but it is made commercially by chemical synthesis. Its structural formula is

$$HO \text{—} \text{benzene ring} \text{—} CHOH.CH_2NH.CH_3$$
$$HO$$

being 1-3-4 dihydroxyphenyl-2-methylaminoethanol. The laevo-rotatory isomer is used as the dextro-rotatory variety is less active. If combined with procaine solution, the usual concentration is 1 in 250,000. In order to be stable, all local analgesics containing adrenaline must have a pH of 4. They are therefore acid and can dissolve metals in contact with them. When dissolved in saline only, the strength of 1 in 500,000 is sufficient to produce good vaso-constriction. Such solutions are commonly used in infiltration for toxic goitre (q.v.) as stronger concentrations tend to cause tachycardia. No local analgesic effect, of course, will be produced. Adrenaline is usually put up in glass ampoules in a concentration of 1 in 1,000. The drug is unstable and cannot be re-sterilized by boiling. When kept in contact with air the solution changes colour to pink and finally to brown. All coloured solutions should be discarded. It is worth noting that intramuscular adrenaline appears to have a slight general analgesic effect and has in fact been used to relieve the pain of leprosy.[64] The systemic effects of adrenaline are considered in Chapters XV and XVII.

Epinine is a synthetic product with an action similar to that of adrenaline. It is rather more stable than the latter substance and is used in about ten times the strength.

Cobefrin (corbasil, dipheprolamin) 3-4-dihydroxy-phenyl-amino-propanol is related chemically to adrenaline and is used in about ten times its strength. It is stated to have one-twelfth the pressor activity of adrenaline and one-fifty-third its toxicity.[65] It is said that the sudden collapse with fall of blood pressure which sometimes

occurs in adrenaline-sensitive patients is practically unknown.   Its
structural formula is

$$HO - \bigcirc - CO.CNOH.CH_3$$

Ephedrine, although useful as a general vaso-constrictor to
maintain blood pressure in spinal analgesia (q.v.) is of little service
for local effects.[66]   Its structural formula is

$$\bigcirc - CHOH.CH(NH.CH_3)CH_3$$

being 1-phenyl-2-methylaminopropanol.   Ephedrine itself has a
slight local analgesic action.[67]

Use of Hyaluronidase in Local Analgesia

The addition of hyaluronidase to solutions of local analgesics
will increase the area of tissues affected[68] but it is most important
to add an adequate dose of a vaso-constrictor drug or general
absorption will occur rapidly (see Chapter XII) with increased
risk of toxic reactions.   On the whole it is doubtful whether the
idea is a good one.

References

1. { CHRISTENSEN, E. M.   *Anæsthesia,* 1947, Jan.
   { *Jour. Amer. Med. Ass.,* 1920, **75,** p. 315.
2. MACDONALD, A.   *Lancet,* 1937, April 24, p. 1016.
3. PRESTON, T. W.   *Brit. Med. Jour.,* 1938, June 4, p. 1236.
4. { BERGIN, E.   *Deut. med. Woch.,* 1919, **58,** p. 1835.
   { ARMATTOE, R.   *Brit. Med. Jour.,* 1943, Feb. 3, p. 191.
5. MACPHEE, G. C.   *Brit. Dent. Jour.,* 1932, Nov. 15, p. 565.
6. KELLY, M.   *Lancet,* 1947, May 24, p. 710.
7. KELTCH, A. K., *et al.*   *Pro. Soc. Exper. Biol. & Med.,* 1941, Jan., p. 533.
8. BOROFF, D., *et al.*   *Pro. Soc. Exper. Biol. & Med.,* 1941, **47,** p. 182.
9. JONES, P. F., and SHOOTER, R. A.   *Brit. Med. Jour.,* 1948, Nov. 27,
    p. 933.
10. UHLMANN, T.   *Narkose und Anæsthesie,* 1929, **6,** p. 168.
11. ISRAELS, M. C. G., and MACDONALD, A. D.   *Brit. Med. Jour.,* 1931,
     Nov. 28, p. 986.
12. WALKER, K.   *Brit. Jour. Urol.,* 1930, **2,** p. 129.
13. POPPER, O.   *Brit. Med. Jour.,* 1930, *i.,* p. 669.
14. BROWN, G. G.   *Med. Jour. Australia,* 1931, May 16.
15. SYNOVICH, I. M.   *Khirurgiya,* 1940, **9,** p. 70.

16. { THOMSEN, E.   *Ugeskrift. f. Laeger*, 1930, Sept. 10, p. 922.
     { WITH, S.   *Ugeskrift. f. Laeger*, 1930, Sept. 10, p. 295.
     { GRIFFITH, H. R.   *Anesth. & Anal.*, 1938, Sept.-Oct., p. 299.
17. KÜHMEL.   *Ugeskrift. f. Laeger*, 1930, Sept. 10, p. 924.
18. *Brit. Med. Jour.*, 1939, Oct. 28, p. 888.
19. LAKE, N. C., and MARSHALL, C. J.   *Brit. Med. Jour.*, 1930, March 15.
20. FUSSANGER, R., and SCHAUMANN, O.   *Arch. f. Exper. Path. v. Pharm.*, 1931, April 25, p. 53.
21. MICHELI, E.   *Giorn. Ital. Anestesia Analgesie*, 1935, **1**, p. 424.
22. PFITZNER, H.   *Zentralbl. f. Chir.*, 1931, May 2, p. 1116.
23. MARX, E.   *Klin. Monatsblatt f. Augenheilkunde*, 1932, **89**, p. 209.
24. STALLARD, H. B.   *Lancet*, 1939, Sept. 2, p. 576.
25. RIECKE, H. G.   *Zeitschr. f. Laryng. Rhinol. v. Otol.*, 1932, **22**, p. 457.
26. WIGGIN, S. C., and TARTAKOFF, J.   *New Eng. Jour. Med.*, 1938, Jan. 27, p. 170.
27. DODD, H.   *Brit. Med. Jour.*, 1940, Sept. 14, p. 345.
28. PITKIN, G. P.   " Conduction Anesthesia," 1946.
29. KNEPPER.   *Munch. med. Woch.*, 1937, Oct. 1, p. 1572.
30. { BRACK.   *Deut. med. Woch.*, 1935, Feb. 8, p. 220.
     { DOANE, J. C., and COHN, E. M.   *Anesthesiology*, 1945, July, p. 421.
31. JACKSON, C. A.   *Brit. Med. Jour.*, 1949, Jan. 15, p. 99.
32. JAMES, N. R.   " Regional Analgesia for Intra-abdominal Surgery," 1943.   J. & A. Churchill.
33. COPELAND, A. J., and NOTTON, H. E. F.   *Brit. Med. Jour.*, 1925, Sept. 26, p. 547.
34. BUTTER, T. H., and GILLAN, R. U.   *Brit. Med. Jour.*, 1926, Jan. 16, p. 83.
35. WILLIAMS, E. W.   *Lancet*, 1926, Jan. 2, p. 16.
36. COYTE, R.   *Brit. Med. Jour.*, 1926, Jan. 16, p. 84.
37. *Jour. Amer. Med. Ass.*, 1922, Feb. 4, p. 343.
38. ADRIANI, J.   " Pharmacology of Anæsthetic Drugs," 1941.
39. BANDLER, C. G.   *Amer. Jour. Surg.*, 1933, **19**, p. 251.
40. KRAUSE, A. C.   *Anesth. & Anal.*, 1933, July-Aug., p. 179.
41. McKIM, C. F., *et al.*   *Jour. Urol.*, 1933, March.
42. ROVENSTINE, E. A., and CULLEN, S. C.   *Anesth. & Anal.*, 1939, March-April, p. 86.
43. RICH, B. S.   *Med. Record*, 1936, Nov. 4, p. 419.
44. FERBER, E. W.   *Jour. Amer. Dent. Ass.*, 1936, May, p. 788.
45. HUNT, W. H., and FOSBINDER, R. J.   *Anesthesiology*, 1940, Nov., p. 305.
46. FINER, G. H., and ROVENSTINE, E. A.   *Anesthesiology*, 1947, Nov., p. 619.
47. CULL, W. A., and SCHOTZ, S.   *Anesthesiology*, 1950, May, p. 353.
48. ABRAMSON, D. L., and GOLDBERG, S. D.   *Jour. Pharmacol. & Exp. Therap.*, 1938, Jan., p. 69.
49. BORDICK, D. L., and ROVENSTINE, E. A.   *Anesthesiology*, 1942, Sept., p. 514.
50. McELVAIN, S. H.   *Jour. Amer. Chem. Soc.*, 1927, Nov.
51. WOODBRIDGE, P. D.   *Anesth. & Anal.*, 1932, July, p. 177.
52. CORMACK, J. W.   *Indianapolis Med. Jour.*, 1931, Oct.
53. LUNDY, J. S.   *Ann. Surg.*, 1939, Nov. 5, p. 878.
54. ROMBERGER, F. T., and RATCLIFF, F. W.   *Indianopolis Med. Jour.*, 1931, Oct.
55. WILD, W.   *Revue Mensuelle de Stomatologie*, 1929, **39**, No. 3.
56. *Jour. Arkansas Med. Soc.*, 1907, Sept. 15.
57. MOYNIHAN, Lord.   " Abdominal Operations."
58. KILBOURNE, N. J.   *Surg. Gyn. & Obst.*, 1936, March, p. 590.
59. ALS-NIELSON.   *Hospitalstidende.*, 1932, Nov. 10, p. 6 (Denmark).
60. GORDH, T.   *Anæsthesia*, 1949, Jan., p. 4.
61. HUNTER, A. R.   *Brit. Jour. Anesth.*, 1951, July, p. 153.
62. CARNEGIE, D. M., and HEWER, A. J. H.   *Lancet*, 1950, July 1, p. 12.

63. BRAUN, H.   *Arch. f. Klin. Chir.*, 1903, **69,** p. 541.
64. WHEATLEY.   *Ann. Rep. Med. Dept. Straits Settlements*, 1927, **18,** p. 71.
65. TAINTER, M. L.   *Arch. internat. de pharm. et de therap.*, 1931, **41,** p. 365.
66. LUNDY, J. S., and TUOHY, E. B.   *Amer. Jour. Surg.*, 1936, Dec., p. 511.
67. SCHULTZ, F. H.   *Anesthesiology*, 1940, **1,** p. 69.
68. { KIRBY, C. K., *et al.*   *Surgery*, 1949, **25,** p. 101.
     { THORPE, S. N.   *Lancet*, 1951.   Jan. 27, p. 210.
69. Annotation.   *Brit. Med. Jour.*, 1952, Feb. 2, p. 280.

CHAPTER XIV

RECENT ADVANCES IN THE TECHNIQUE OF LOCAL ANALGESIA

THE technique of local analgesia is now fairly standardized and can be classified as follows :

Surface or Permeation analgesia.
Infiltration analgesia.

Regional analgesia.
- (a) Field block.
- (b) Nerve-block or Conduction analgesia.
  - (1) Intraneural.
  - (2) Paraneural.

Miscellaneous.
- (1) Refrigeration analgesia.
- (2) Intravenous local analgesia.
- (3) Intra-arterial local analgesia.

These various techniques will now be considered separately.

Surface application is mainly limited to the mucous surfaces of the eye, nose, larynx and urethra, the drugs generally used being cocaine, nupercaine, amethocaine and xylocaine. Some details of recently-developed techniques of surface analgesia for nose and throat operations are given in Chapter XX.

It has recently been shown that the mere **swallowing** of from 50 to 100 c.cm. of 1 per cent. procaine would relieve spasm of the pyloric sphincter for some hours and that this simple procedure can be repeated indefinitely if necessary.[1]

For the repair of lacerated wounds, a " **procaine pack** " can be used. Gauze strips soaked in 1 per cent. procaine are packed into the wound and allowed to remain for about eight minutes. This avoids spreading infection from the injection of solution.[2]

Infiltration analgesia aims at paralysing the nerve endings at the actual site of operation. A very fine needle is first of all introduced into the skin and an intradermal wheal is raised. Through this insensitive area a longer needle is passed, and by keeping almost parallel with the skin the subcutaneous tissues are infiltrated along and beyond the line of the proposed incision. If the deeper layers of tissue are to be incised, they must also be infiltrated, the exact procedure being determined by the nature of the operation.

Some anæsthetists use a continuous intradermal wheal and then infiltrate the tissues beneath it. This practice is not to be recommended as the tension of fluid in the skin may lead to subsequent necrosis. The writer has seen several such instances.

In order to see what tissues have been infiltrated, **coloured solutions** can be used, e.g. indigo-carmine can be added until a fairly deep coloration results.[3]

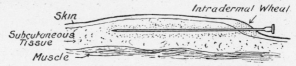

FIG. 70.   Diagrammatic section showing principle of infiltration.

The hæmatoma-injection method for setting fractures is a special form of infiltration analgesia and is considered later in this chapter, as is " spreading infiltration " for abdominal surgery and " transverse section analgesia " for limb injuries.

Field blocking consists in creating walls of analgesia encircling the operative field. The solution is distributed in certain definite planes so that it will paralyse all the nerves crossing them, although no attempt is made to localize individual nerves.

Field blocking can be accomplished in three different ways :

(*a*) The creation of walls of analgesia perpendicular to the skin surface and involving the entire thickness of the tissues in which the nerves lie. These walls meet at their extremities and form a polygon described round the operative field.

(*b*) The creation of oblique walls of analgesia involving only part of the tissues but meeting below like a cup.

(*c*) The creation of a single wall of analgesia is sufficient in certain areas of the body depending on the nerve supply to the operation area.

Nerve blocking consists in the " physiological section " of the sensory nerves supplying the operative field at a point remote from that field. The block may be :

(*a*) *Intraneural*, i.e. injection into the nerve sheath. This is generally used where permanent analgesia is desired, e.g. the injection of alcohol into the Gasserian ganglion for trigeminal neuralgia or the injection of cut nerves in amputation stumps. The intraneural injection of 5 per cent. procaine followed by absolute alcohol into intercostal nerves has been employed in the treatment of pulmonary tuberculosis and herpes zoster.[4]

(*b*) *Paraneural*. The analgesic solution is deposited in close proximity to the nerves. Examples of this are splanchnic and spinal blocks (q.v.).

Refrigeration Analgesia. The freezing of small areas of skin with an ethyl chloride spray has been practised for a long time and probably originated from the observation that frost-bitten tissues were analgesic. This proceeding is unsatisfactory as the subsequent thawing process may be extremely painful and any tissues actually frozen will die. An ethyl chloride spray may, however, be useful therapeutically in relieving localized pain produced by such conditions as sprains, pleural friction, etc.[5]

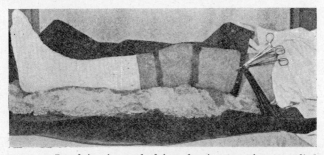

Fig. 71.   Leg lying in crushed ice, showing tourniquet applied.
Skin markings show line of incision and line of saw cut.
(After F. M. Allen, *Medical Annual*.)

More recently, amputations have been performed under a somewhat different type of refrigeration analgesia. The site of the tourniquet is selected and packed round with ice bags. The tourniquet can be applied painlessly after some time and the limb distal to it is then packed with crushed ice on rubber sheeting or is immersed in a pail of ice-water for $1\frac{1}{2}$ to $2\frac{1}{2}$ hours. There is a definite risk of infection from contaminated ice and a fatal case of gangrene has been recorded in which the organism was actually recovered from the ice.[6] Particular care should therefore be taken to sterilize the skin thoroughly after drying. The tissues are not frozen but are cooled to between $+5°$ C. and $+15°$ C. at which temperature organisms cease to grow. (Under no circumstances must salt be mixed with the ice or a temperature of $-5°$ C. may be reached at which point the tissues freeze and die immediately.)[7] Painless amputation can now be performed as conduction of impulses in a nerve trunk fails at or below $25°$ C. to $30°$ C. in warm-blooded animals.[8] From personal observation the writer is convinced that shock and after-pain are diminished (especially if post-operative refrigeration is continued) but it is said that healing may be delayed.[9] The method described is efficient but messy. In America various electrically cooled types of apparatus are in use and permit of accurate temperature regulation.[10]

It is interesting to recall that Napoleon's famous military surgeon, Baron Larry, amputated limbs painlessly in a temperature of —19° C. during the retreat from Moscow in 1812.

Refrigeration has a definite therapeutic value in treating limbs with incipient gangrene. The probable explanation of this paradox is that the tissue metabolic rate is lowered so much that the impaired circulation may prove adequate for the time being.

The actual physiology of survival of tissues at +10° C. is probably that, although at this temperature hæmoglobin will not release its oxygen, metabolism is so reduced that the minute amount required is obtained from that dissolved in plasma.[7] At this temperature, tissues will live for between 15 and 17 days. Curiously enough, at +15° C. the survival time is only four days. No certain explanation of this phenomenon is known but it has been suggested that at +10° C. both anabolism and catabolism cease whereas in cooling to that temperature, anabolism ceases first, so that between 10° C. and 27° C. it is the accumulated products of catabolism which limit the time of survival.[11]

Intravenous Local Analgesia. This method was introduced by August Bier in 1908 and can only be used for operations on the extremities.

For example, an intravenous analgesia for an adult upper limb will require about 10 c.cm. of 2 per cent. procaine solution, and the tourniquet must not be removed for thirty-five minutes or the drug may reach the general circulation with disastrous results.[12]

Intravenous general analgesia has been described in Chapter X.

Intra-arterial Local Analgesia. This technique was first used in animals by Alms in 1886 and in man by Goyanes in 1908 (in Spain).

Intra-arterial injections can be made into either full or empty vessels, but cannot be used on patients suffering from endarteritis obliterans[13] or acute inflammatory lesions.[14] Here again the method can only be used for limb operations and it has made little progress in Great Britain.

Apparatus for Injection of Analgesic Solutions

A 10 to 20 c.cm. eccentric syringe fitted with a needle-lock and finger grips (e.g. Labat's) is adequate for most work.

For extensive infiltrations, a **continuous-flow syringe** saves time as the upward motion of the piston automatically refills the barrel

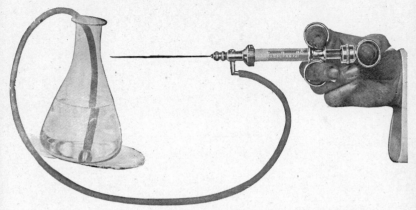

FIG. 72. " Dunn " continuous flow syringe with tube near needle lock.

through a non-return valve. Adapters can be obtained for converting the standard Labat syringe to the continuous-flow type.

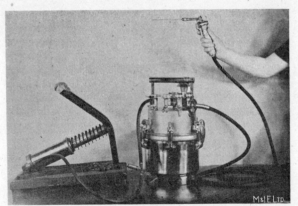

FIG. 73. Infiltrator with foot pump attached (N. R. James).

In addition, syringes of smaller capacity specially designed for this type of work are available. Two varieties are in use : (*a*) those in which the tube for solution is attached near the needle lock (e.g. the American " Dunn " glass-piston syringe and the British " Vann " syringe with metal piston), and (*b*) those in which the tube is fixed to a hollow piston rod as in the "Pitkin" syringe. It should be observed that unless the rubber tube be pinched the aspiration test cannot be carried out with these syringes. In each case the flexible

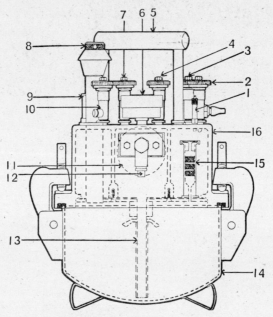

Fig. 74.   Section through Infiltrator to show construction.
(N. R. James, *Pro. Roy. Soc. Med.*)

1. Schrader connection for foot pump for use when compressed gases are not available. 2. Pressure intake control valve when compressed gases are available. 3. Filter sump outlet valve. 4. Supply control valve No. 1 for analgesic solution. 5. Lifting handle. 6. Combined vacuum and pressure gauge. 7. Supply control valve No. 2 for analgesic solution. 8. Swing-over filler cap for recharging machine with analgesic solution. 9. Pressure safety valve. 10. Steam inlet control valve for sterilization. 11. Ball-float for operating automatic safety trap to ensure that the compressed gas cannot be injected when the supply of the solution is exhausted. 12. Automatic valve to maintain vacuum after steam sterilization. 13. Solution uptake pipe from reservoir. 14. Stainless steel reservoir polished to mirror finish. 15. Compressed gas intake filter fitted with ultra-fine replaceable fabric filtration cartridges. 16. High tensile bronze casting.
All components unless of stainless steel are chromium plated. Dimensions (overall) : Height, 14 in.   Diameter, 10½ in.

tube is attached to a sinker, which is placed in the flask of solution as shown in the figure.

Instead of using syringes, some anæsthetists now employ needles fitting into a pistol-grip control connected by a pipe-line to an

" **infiltrator** " which delivers the solution under a pressure of about 50 lb. per sq. in.[15] (see Fig. 71). This pressure is obtained either from a motor tyre pump[16] or from the reducing valve of an oxygen cylinder.[17] In these machines special provision must be made for performing the aspiration test and a trap must be provided so that it is impossible to inject air into the tissues if the supply of fluid becomes exhausted. Sterilization can be effected by blowing steam through the entire apparatus.

In America, a needle-less injector or " **hypospray** " has been evolved.[18] The liquid to be injected is contained in a metal ampoule or " metapule " having at one end an orifice with a diameter of 3/1000 in. or 0·012 mm. The sterile ampoule is placed in the instrument and the orifice is firmly pressed against the patient's sterilized skin at the selected site. A powerful spring (125 ·lb. pressure acting on a plunger 0·5 cm. in diameter) is now released and the fluid is forced through the skin in a jet 1/136th of the bore of a 20 gauge needle. It is said that very little pain is caused but the instrument must be kept perfectly still or the skin puncture will be converted into a slit. Whether the cost and complication of this jet injector outbalance the absence of a needle puncture remains to be seen. Viscous solutions cannot be injected with this apparatus.

The detailed account of the individual methods necessary for various operations is outside the scope of this book. Certain methods are, however, described in subsequent chapters, while it is proposed to mention here briefly certain common techniques and others which have been developed comparatively recently.

Local Analgesia for the Reduction of Fractures

Local analgesia has been used for the reduction of fractures since 1885;[19] and Böhler of Vienna has developed a technique which presents some advantages over general anæsthesia in certain cases.[20] This has been used to a limited extent in this country.[21]

Technique. A 2 per cent. solution of procaine in normal saline, without adrenaline, is used. The site of fracture is accurately located by X-rays. An intradermal wheal is raised and the point of the needle passed down to the site of the fracture. The object of the procedure is to inject solution into the hæmatoma between the ends of the bones ; 5 c.cm. of solution are injected and the piston of the syringe withdrawn. The easy injection and the withdrawal of bloodstained fluid will confirm the correct position of the needle point, and an injection of some 20 to 50 c.cm. of fluid is made according to the site and nature of the fracture. The needle is then removed, gentle pressure being kept on the site of puncture for five minutes, and the necessary manipulation carried out. With this technique failure to secure adequate analgesia only occurs in about 6 per cent. of cases. The main advantages of the method are the co-operation of the conscious patient and the possibility of effecting reduction single-handed.[22] It is said that the addition of hyaluronidase to the solution diminishes the time of onset and increases the intensity of analgesia.[23]

Contra-indications. The hæmatoma-injection method should not be used in young children nor when a skiagram locating the site of fracture has not been obtained, nor in the case of open fractures. Neglected cases of some days' duration are also unsuitable for this method, as are those in which unusual or prolonged force may be necessary to effect reduction.[24] Levi considers that some of the failures may be due to the unsuspected loculation of the hæmatoma.[25]

"Transverse Section Analgesia"

This term has been applied by Russian workers to a form of infiltration for injuries to the limbs. A ring of analgesia is formed by infiltrating all the tissues from the skin to the bone with a 0·5 per cent. solution of procaine some distance proximal to the injury. It is said that shock is relieved, that any necessary manipulation can be carried out and that the healing of the wound is accelerated.[26]

Therapeutic Uses of Infiltration Analgesia

Local analgesia by infiltration methods is now being used as a therapeutic measure for the relief of pain. It has been demonstrated (by Head and Mackenzie) that hyperæsthetic zones of skin and underlying muscle exist in morbid conditions of viscera, the nerve supply of which communicates in or near the spinal cord with the zonal nerves. If these zones are mapped out and infiltrated with an analgesic solution, relief of pain usually occurs and may be permanent. For example, in 200 cases of *chronic adnexal disease* the injections were successful in 80 per cent.[27] Encouraging results have also been obtained in *angina pectoris*[28] and *recurrent herpes*.[29] Lériche has extended the therapeutic use of infiltration in recent years and has obtained striking results by injecting analgesic solution into joints which have suffered from *articular* or *peri-articular injuries*. The injection should be made as soon as possible after

accident and may have to be repeated.[30] *Painful scars, amputation
stumps*[31] and areas of *fibrositis*[32] can also be treated successfully by
repeated infiltrations. It is said that *painful flat feet* can be relieved
at once by the injection of up to 15 c.cm. of 2 per cent. procaine

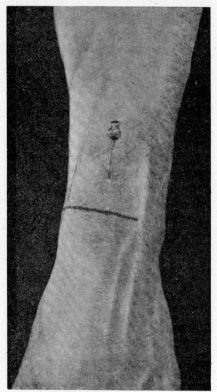

Hæmatoma-injection tech-
nique of local analgesia for
reduction of fractures.

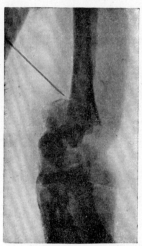

FIG. 75. Dorsum of forearm and hand.
The level of a Colles's fracture is indi-
cated, and the site for injection shown.
(*British Journal of Surgery.*)

FIG. 76. Skiagram showing
the position of the needle
while injecting a Colles's
fracture. (*British Journal
of Surgery.*)

into any tender areas followed by massage of the soles and a gentle
walk of a quarter of a mile.[33]

When the pain occasioned by all these varied conditions is
relieved by an analgesic injection it often does not return although
tenderness may persist for some weeks. Several ingenious theories

have been propounded to account for this curious fact but none is very convincing.

Therapeutic Use of Nerve Block

An example of the recent introduction of nerve blocking into therapeutics is provided by the peri-sympathetic injection of absolute alcohol in the treatment of *bronchial asthma*.[34] Attempts have been made to treat *shock* by suitable nerve blocking, e.g by brachial plexus block for arm injuries. The results, however, have been disappointing, as a further fall in blood pressure usually occurs. The procedure therefore appears to be unjustifiable.[35]

" Chemical Sympathectomy "

It has been shown that certain drugs, such as 6 per cent. phenol in water, have a selective effect on sympathetic fibres and destroy them permanently. This fact has been made use of in gynæcology, and " chemical sympathectomy " of the nerve supply to the reproductive organs is said to be beneficial in various diseases.[36]

Paravertebral Block

An interesting application of paravertebral block in *diagnosis* has recently been made. It has been shown that a right-sided block of T. 9, T. 10, and T. 11 will abolish pain due to a lesion of the gall bladder, but has no effect upon pain from adjacent viscera.[37] Similarly, left-sided injections of T. 8, T. 9, and T. 10 are said to relieve the pain caused by acute pancreatitis and to diminish the volume of pancreatic juice secreted.[38]

A bilateral block of L. 3 and L. 4 has been used as a *therapeutic measure* for the relief of pain due to diseases of the uterine adnexa,[28] and a block from C. 1 to T. 4 for angina pectoris.[39]

Cases of herpes zoster have been improved, but the method does not appear to be of much value in tabetic gastric crises.

Paravertebral block, especially in the cervical region, has been the cause of several fatalities. It has been proved (by using methylene blue) that if the needle point happens to lie in a nerve or spinal ganglion, a solution under ordinary pressure penetrates within the perineural sheath into the subarachnoid space or else into the substance of the spinal cord along the posterior nerve root.[40] This, in the author's opinion, provides a much more convincing explanation of the cause of death than the theories advanced previously. It must also be remembered that misplaced needles not infrequently give rise to pneumothorax.

Splanchnic Block

It has been recognized for many years that a large proportion of the shock occurring during operations on the upper abdomen is due to traumatic impulses passing from the viscera via the

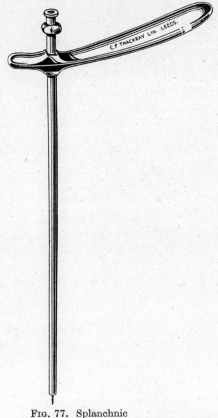

Fig. 77. Splanchnic needle and cannula for Braun's technique. (Upcott.)

splanchnic nerves to the central nervous system.[41] Splanchnic block aims at cutting off this path and has been used extensively in upper-abdominal surgery both in this country[42] and abroad.[43] Since splanchnic block is automatically included in high spinal analgesia (no splanchnic fibres being given off above T.4) the separate nerve block has been largely discontinued. A brief summary of the methods employed may, however, be given.

Anatomy. The solar plexus is formed by the splanchnic nerves from the thoracic sympathetic chain (derived from fibres from T. 5 to T. 10) which pass down on each side and enter the abdomen by piercing the crura of the diaphragm and join the semilunar ganglia. These lie immediately internal to the suprarenal bodies, at the level of the first lumbar vertebra, and are interconnected by numerous filaments which pass in front of the aorta chiefly round the origin of the cœliac axis artery. The solar plexus receives fibres from the secondary plexuses around the abdominal viscera.[44]

Technique. The solar plexus can be approached by three routes :

Anteriorly. The needle is inserted vertically 1 cm. below and 0·5 cm. to the left of the tip of the ensiform cartilage. This method is not devoid of risk and is seldom practised.

Braun's Method. The abdominal incision is made under general anæsthesia or field block. The hand is introduced and the aorta gently retracted with the finger. Procaine is then injected in close contact with the lateral aspects of the body of the first lumbar vertebra. This method is highly recommended by Finsterer, of Vienna, using not more than 70 c.cm. of 0·5 per cent. procaine solution.[45] If desired, a blunt-ended cannula can first be passed along the finger and when in position a syringe is attached to a special long needle which is passed down the cannula as shown in Fig. 77.[46]

Posteriorly. Kappis' Method. The patient is placed on his side with a small pillow under his loin so that the vertebral column is straight. The spinous process of the first lumbar vertebra is then identified and a point taken 7 cm. external to it. This spot is usually just below the lower border of the twelfth rib and in no case must the injection be made above this rib. A 12-cm. needle is now introduced at an angle of 45° to the median plane (see Fig. 79), and its point should strike the side of the body of the first lumbar vertebra. The needle is then partially withdrawn and re-introduced in a slightly more forward direction until its point is felt to slide tangentially past the body of the vertebra. It is then pushed 1 cm. further and, *the aspiration test being negative*, 20 to 30 c.cm. of sterile 1 per cent. procaine solution are injected.[40] For long operations, 50 c.cm. of 1 in 2,000 amethocaine solution can be substituted.[47] The patient is then turned over to his opposite side and the procedure repeated. If the patient's back slightly overhangs the edge of the table, it is possible to perform bilateral splanchnic block without altering his position.[47] Experimental injections made in the post-mortem room with methylene blue show that this technique does soak the splanchnic area efficiently. If the operation is to be performed under local analgesia only, an anterior field block or a paravertebral block must also be performed (see Chapter XXIII). Posterior splanchnic block is a reasonably safe procedure if carried out with all precautions. In a series of 2,475 operations using this technique there were eight deaths (Takats).

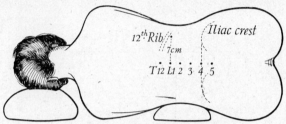

FIG. 78. Patient in position for right posterior splanchnic injection. · is site of puncture.

The main disadvantages of splanchnic block are : (i) a considerable fall in blood pressure ; the pressure curves show a marked resemblance to those obtained during spinal block as would be expected ; (ii) occasional post-operative backache ; (iii) the relatively large amount of analgesic solution required,[48] and (iv) an increased tendency to post-operative ileus.[49]

Therapeutic Splanchnic Block. Posterior splanchnic block has been used with varying success in the treatment of *cardio spasm* and of idiopathic *hyperpiesia*.[50] Very prolonged sympathetic blocks can be obtained by using the drug known as bromsalizol (see Chapter XIII).

An alternative technique for abdominal surgery has been described as " creeping " local analgesia, which is really a modification of **mesenteric block.**[51] The abdominal wall having been infiltrated as usual and incised, the transverse mesocolon is injected with procaine and an œdematous area formed. A further injection is made at the edge of this, and so on, until the duodenum is embedded in fluid. The lesser omentum and the mesentery of the hepatic flexure can be treated in the same way, and the adjacent viscera subsequently manipulated relatively painlessly. This method of

" **spreading infiltration** " necessitates great gentleness in handling, and the time consumed is so great that it now has little vogue in this country, although it is still used on the Continent, especially in Russia.[52]

Another possible alternative to splanchnic block is the wholesale **introduction of solution into the peritoneal cavity.** After the incision

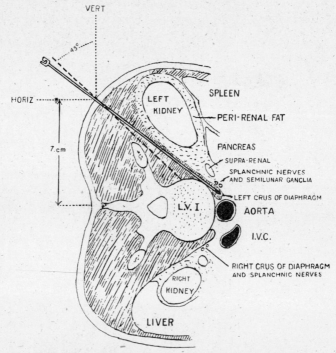

FIG. 79. Transverse section, showing needle in position for left posterior splanchnic injection. The preliminary or trial position of the needle is shown by the dotted line.

through skin and muscle has been made under general anæsthesia or field block, a 2-inch incision is made through the peritoneum and 200 c.cm. of 0·25 per cent. procaine or 0·15 per cent. amethocaine[53] are poured through it into the abdominal cavity. After ten minutes' interval the incision is enlarged, the excess of fluid is removed and the operation proceeded with. The obvious danger is paralysis of the intestines, but this is said to be successfully overcome by the injection of pituitrin and eserine.[54]   A case of immediate death has been reported after flooding the peritoneal cavity with 150 c.cm. of 1 in 3,200 nupercaine solution.[55]

Brachial Plexus Block

A brachial plexus block renders all the structures of the upper extremity insensitive except the skin of the upper part of the arm which is supplied by the cervical plexus. If the incision is to be in this area it will be necessary to use infiltration in addition.

The indications for brachial plexus block are for operations on the upper extremity when the surgeon or the patient desires consciousness to be retained, e.g. in ambulatory cases or when an accident has followed a recent meal. The block is also used as part of the local technique for upper stage thorocoplasty and for treating vasospasm due to intra-arterial thiopentone (q.v.).

The patient lies with his head and shoulders on a pillow. His affected shoulder is depressed and his head turned towards his sound side. The supra-clavicular approach is generally used. The subclavian artery is located and an intradermal wheal is raised immediately lateral to the palpating finger. If the artery cannot be felt, the wheal is raised one-third of an inch above the mid-point of the clavicle. A 22 S.W.G. needle is then inserted through the wheal in a backward, inward and downward direction aiming towards the spinous process of T. 3. If any paræsthesia of the arm occur, 20 to 30 c.cm. of solution should forthwith be injected. If not, the needle should be pushed on until it hits the first rib and by re-insertion at slightly different angles the point is moved along the upper surface of the rib until the pulsation of the subclavian artery can be felt. If the aspiration test is negative, 10 c.cm. of solution are now injected and a further 10 c.cm. with the needle point slightly more lateral. The danger of inadvertent intravenous injection should not be minimized as a fatality resulted from 25 c.cm. of 2 per cent. procaine given in this way.[56] Several injections may have to be made to secure a complete block. 2 per cent. procaine solution will cause muscular paralysis as well as sensory loss. 1 per cent. procaine usually leaves sufficient muscular power for the patient to move tendons for identification during suture. For prolonged operations amethocaine or nupercaine will be necessary.

For fuller details the reader is referred to the excellent monograph on the subject.[57]

Stellate Ganglion Block

It has recently been recognized that stellate ganglion block can produce remarkable improvement in the paralysis due to embolism

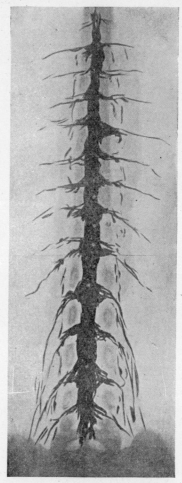

Fig. 80.   Skiagram of peri-dural
space filled with radio-opaque
fluid.   (*Anesth. & Anal.*)

and thrombosis of the cerebral vessels probably by abolishing spasm
of the affected vessels.[86]   The pain of angina pectoris and of
dissecting aortic aneurysm can also often be relieved by this means.
A fairly simple and reliable technique has now been worked out
for this procedure.[87]   The patient lies supine with his head turned
away from the side to be blocked.   A subcuticular wheal is raised

just above the clavicle and lateral to the sternal head of the sterno-mastoid and through it a 7·2 cm. needle is inserted directly back-wards until its point impinges on bone which should be the body of C.7. The needle is then withdrawn for 0·5 cm. and after a negative aspiration test for blood or C.S.F., 5 c.cm. of 2 per cent. procaine solution are injected. The rapid development of Horner's syndrome signifies success. Other techniques are described in the reference given.[88]

Extra-dural Spinal Block (Epidural Analgesia)

The peri-dural space is occupied by loose areolar tissue and easily displaceable blood vessels and its extent is indicated by the subjoined skiagram. Superiorly, the space ends at the foramen magnum by the fusion of the dura with the periosteum. Below there is a communication with the sacral canal, and laterally with the paravertebral tissue through the various foramina. Strictly speaking it should be called the " inter-dural space " as it is formed by a splitting of the dura, one sheath of which lines the spinal canal

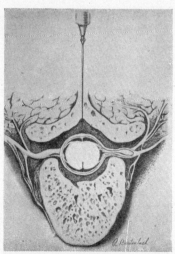

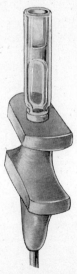

Fig. 81. Semi-diagrammatic section through lower dorsal region showing position of needle in peri-dural space. (Harger *et al.* *Amer. Jnl. of Surg.*)

Fig. 82. Odom's indicator con-nected to needle (magnified). (*Amer. Jnl. of Surg.*)

while the other encloses the cord, nerve roots and cerebrospinal fluid.[58]

Analgesic fluid can be deposited within this space at the appropriate level between two spinous processes. The possibilities of the method were first demonstrated on dogs by Cathelin in 1901[59] and applied to the human subject by the Spanish surgeon Fidel Pagés in 1920.[60] Since then the technique has had some vogue in Italy and in America for abdominal surgery but is generally considered less reliable than subarachnoid block. It has been used in this country for thoracoplasty.[61]

By injecting a 2 per cent. solution of procaine in lipiodol into the peridural space and taking a series of skiagrams, it has been shown that the fluid diffuses through the intervertebral foramina along the peri-neural sheaths and thus blocks the nerve roots (see Fig. 80). On analysing the cerebrospinal fluid, procaine was consistently absent, so that the drug does not percolate into the subarachnoid space as had at one time been suggested.[62]

Technique.   Until recently it has been somewhat difficult to make sure that the point of the needle was actually in the peri-dural space, but in 1928 it was shown that a negative pressure of from 1 to 18 mm. Hg normally exists there.[63]   Three theories have been propounded to account for this :   (1) that the advancing needle point produces a cone in the dura mater thus creating an artificial space ;   (2) that the negative pressure only exists when the spine is flexed by separation of the vertebral arches with consequent increase in the peri-dural space[64] ;   (3) that the negative pressure within the thoracic cage on inspiration is transmitted via the paravertebral space to the peri-dural space.[65]   However this may be, the presence of negative pressure can be turned to practical account by filling the lumbar puncture needle with normal saline, omitting the stilette and inserting the needle with a drop of fluid hanging from its proximal end.   When the needle reaches the correct position, the hanging drop is sucked in and the injection can be started.   The meniscus in the glass indicator illustrated gives an even more obvious check on the position of the distal end of the needle.[66]   Some anæsthetists prefer a small glass U-tube as a manometer.[67]   An even clearer way of demonstrating the difference in pressure is to use a small rubber balloon attached to a male record mount.[68]   The lumbar puncture needle is pushed through the skin for about one inch and the record mount is then firmly inserted into its hub.   A hypodermic needle is then pushed through the neck of the balloon to distend it with air from a syringe.

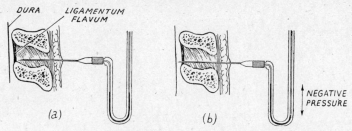

FIG. 83. Diagrammatic sagittal section showing needle attached to U-shaped manometer before and after entering peri-dural space. (Macintosh and Mushin.)

The lumbar puncture needle is advanced and collapse of the balloon indicates when the extra-dural space is entered.

The nature of the solution varies with different workers,[69] but a reliable technique is to use up to 50 c.cm. of a mixture of 1 per cent. procaine and $0 \cdot 2$ per cent. amethocaine. The aspiration test being negative, 10 c.cm. of this mixture are first injected and after a pause of five minutes the patient is asked to move his legs. If he can do so, it is certain that the subarachnoid space has not been entered inadvertently and the rest of the solution is injected slowly. At least fifteen minutes must then elapse before the operation is started.[70] In Great Britain, 50 c.cm. of $0 \cdot 2$ per cent. nupercaine in half-normal saline has been used with success. This solution is slightly hypobaric (S.G. $1 \cdot 0035$) so that with the patient slightly tilted head downwards, it will tend to diffuse away from the medulla if the dura has accidentally been punctured.[64] It is said that a sharply defined zone of *unilateral analgesia* can be obtained by injecting $7 \cdot 5$ c.cm. to 15 c.cm. of 3 in 1,000 amethocaine mixed with an equal volume of 5 per cent. gelatin solution with the patient lying on his affected side.[71] Extra-dural block differs from

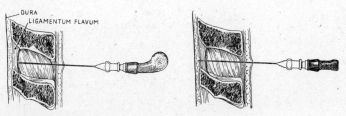

FIG. 84. Diagrammatic sagittal section showing balloon distended before and collapsed after needle has entered extra-dural space. (Macintosh from *Anæsthesia*.)

subarachnoid block in that the motor fibres are little affected. The fall in blood pressure is also less and post-analgesic headache is said to be almost non-existent.

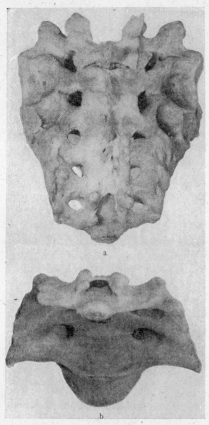

Fig. 85.   Average female sacrum viewed (*a*) from behind and (*b*) from below to show sacral hiatus.   (Trotter, from *Surg. Gyn. & Obstet.*)

A combination of extra-dural and subarachnoid blocks has been described by Soresi under the title " **epi-subdural analgesia** ".   The chief advantages claimed are reliability, prolonged analgesia and freedom from post-operative pain.[72]

The peri-dural space can also be approached from the sacral

canal, this procedure being known as **extra-dural sacral or caudal block.** The sacral hiatus having been localized, an 8 cm. needle is introduced at an angle of 20° to the plane of the back and, having pierced the tough ligament, is directed horizontally and parallel to the back till about 5 cm. of its length lies within the sacral canal. The introduction of 30 c.cm. of 2 per cent. procaine will, in the average adult, permit of operations upon the bladder, rectum, genitalia and perineum.[73] The method has had some vogue for suprapubic prostatectomy, especially in Canada,[74] and has been used for mitigating the pains of labour,[75] and therapeutically in the treatment of sciatica.[76] Difficulty may be experienced, especially in fat patients, in finding the exact position of the sacral cornua, which varies considerably. Furthermore, it is essential that the aspiration test be negative as large amounts of procaine have been accidentally injected into a vessel or into the cerebrospinal fluid with disastrous results. The commonest faults in position are that the needle slips dorsal to the sacrum or that the tip pierces the periosteum lining the caudal canal. The most dangerous error is for the needle to pass to one side of the root of the coccyx and to enter the peri-rectal tissues or the rectum itself. If such a needle be withdrawn and reinserted correctly, fatal sepsis may ensue[77] (see Fig. 86 c). Normally the dural sac terminates opposite the second segment of the sacrum but in exceptional cases it may extend farther down. In post-mortem examinations of over 1,000 male and female sacral canals the chief abnormalities from normal were : (1) in nearly 50 per cent. the canal reached a higher level than the lower third of S. 4. This reduces the distance between the highest possible position of the sacral needle and the inferior limit of the subarachnoid space ; (2) in about 25 per cent. deficiencies existed in the dorsal wall of the sacral canal which could permit exit of the needle point into the soft tissues ; (3) in about 5 per cent. the antero-posterior diameter of the sacral canal was 2 mm. or less, in which case the introduction of a 19 gauge needle is virtually impossible ; and (4) occasionally the lumen of the canal is entirely obliterated.[78] It will be obvious that sacral puncture is not devoid of pitfalls and it seems probable that "low" subarachnoid spinal block is both safer and more reliable for operations, such as those mentioned.

Caudal block is much easier to perform in animals and is much used in bovine obstetrics.[79]

Fractional caudal block has recently been tried using a malleable needle, a continuous-flow syringe and a 1·5 per cent. solution of

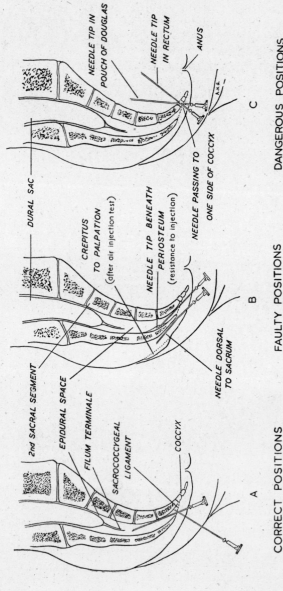

CORRECT AND INCORRECT POSITIONS OF NEEDLE

DURAL SAC

NEEDLE TIP IN POUCH OF DOUGLAS

NEEDLE TIP IN RECTUM

ANUS

2ND SACRAL SEGMENT

EPIDURAL SPACE

FILUM TERMINALE

SACROCOCCYGEAL LIGAMENT

COCCYX

CREPITUS TO PALPATION (after air injection test)

NEEDLE TIP BENEATH PERIOSTEUM (resistance to injection)

NEEDLE DORSAL TO SACRUM

NEEDLE PASSING TO ONE SIDE OF COCCYX

A

B

C

CORRECT POSITIONS   FAULTY POSITIONS   DANGEROUS POSITIONS

Fig. 86.   Caudal Block.   (A. H. Galley from *Anæsthesia*.)

neothesine. The assembled apparatus is shown in Fig. 87. An initial dose of 30 c.cm. is given and about 20 c.cm. every thirty to forty minutes subsequently.[80]   1 per cent. procaine has also been

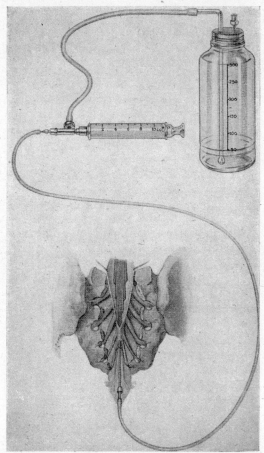

FIG. 87. Assembly of malleable needle, tubing, syringe and container for fractional caudal block. (Southworth, J. L., *Annals of Surgery*.)

tried as a continuous drip.[81] The chief complications with this technique appear to be collapse, sepsis, inadvertent subarachnoid block,[82] prolonged backache afterwards, and broken needles. To avoid the latter bugbear, an alternative method has been devised.

A large (13 gauge) needle is inserted into the caudal canal and a ureteric catheter is passed up through it. The needle is then withdrawn.[83] (See also under obstetrics.) In America the technique has been developed using very fine needles and extremely narrow bore plastic tubing. At the time of writing, however, this material cannot be obtained in Great Britain.

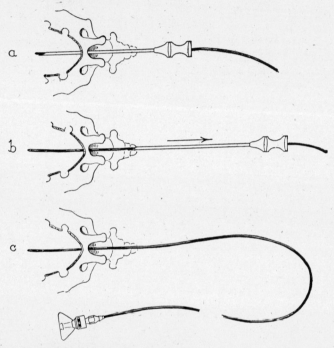

FIG. 88.   Fractional caudal block obtained by means of ureteric catheter.
(*a*) Large needle inserted with catheter inside, the top being flush with the needle bevel.
(*b*) Needle being withdrawn over catheter.
(*c*) Catheter in position.   (C. Adams *et al.*, *Jour. Amer. Med. Ass.*)

Apart from surgical analgesia, fractional caudal block can be of great value as a therapeutic measure in acute nephritis and eclampsia. The block will relax the spastic vessels and decrease the systolic and venous pressures. Furthermore the kidneys and suprarenals can temporarily be denervated by carrying the block higher. By careful and constant attention the process can, if necessary, be continued for several days.[84]

Strictly speaking, **sacral block** is the term applied to the combined procedures of caudal and trans-sacral blocks. This method is not much used at the present time in Great Britain owing to the large number of injections necessary, the time consumed and the uncertainty of perfect analgesia. It has, however, considerable vogue in America.[85]

References

1. ROKA, G., and LAJTHA, L. *Brit. Med. Jour.*, 1950, May 20, p. 1174.
2. FRITZ, M., and TANNER, E. K. *Anesth. & Anal.*, 1936, Nov.-Dec., p. 291.
3. DODD, H. *Brit. Med. Jour.*, 1940, Sept. 14, p. 345.
4. BUTTAFARRI, G. *Policlinco Sez. Prat.*, 1936, Apr. 6, p. 619.
5. MACDONALD, N. *Brit. Med. Jour.*, 1943, Feb. 13, p. 202.
6. KIRZ, E. *Brit. Med. Jour.*, 1944, Nov. 18, p. 662.
7. HELLIWELL, P. J. *Anæsthesia*, 1950, Apr., p. 58.
8. LARGE, A., and HEINBECKER, P. *Ann. Surg.*, 1944, Nov., p. 707.
9. ALLEN, F. M., *et al. Jour. Internat. Coll. Surg.*, 1942, Mar.-Apr., p. 125.
10. PITKIN, G. P. " Conduction Anesthesia," 1946. J. P. Lippincott Co., p. 854.
11. LAKE, N. C. *Lancet*, 1917, **2**, p. 560.
12. *Brit. Jour. Surg.*, 1931, April, p. 641.
13. GOINARD, P. *Bull. et Mém. Soc. Nat. de Chir.*, 1934, Dec. 29, p. 1362.
14. GOINARD, P. *Rev. de Chir.*, 1936, Feb., p. 109.
15. KIRSCHNER, M. *Surg. Gyn. & Obst.*, 1932, Sept., p. 328.
16. JAMES, N. R. { *Lancet*, 1943, June 12, p. 738.
{ *Pro. Roy. Soc. Med.* (An. Sec.), 1944, May 5.
17. WILLWAY, W. *Lancet*, 1937, Oct. 9, p. 856.
18. Annotation. *Lancet*, 1949, June 4, p. 966.
19. CONWAY, N. *Med. Jour.*, 1885.
20. BÖHLER, L. " Treatment of Fractures," 1929.
21. HOSFORD, J. P. *Brit. Jour. Surg.*, 1931, **18**, No. 72.
22. { STEWART, C. E. *Med. Jour. Australia*, 1931, Sept. 12, p. 330.
{ CAROTHERS, R. C. *Jour. Amer. Med. Ass.*, 1931, Aug. 22.
23. THORPE, J. N. *Lancet*, 1951, Jan. 27, p. 210.
24. PLATT, H. *Brit. Med. Jour.*, 1932, Aug. 13, p. 290.
25. LEVI, D. *Practitioner*, 1930, Dec., p. 738.
26. BEKKERMAN, L. S., and NEYMARK, A. I. *Soviet Medicine*, 1941, **4**, p. 25.
27. KRISS, B. *Zentralbl. f. Gynäk.*, 1932, Aug. 13, p. 1986.
28. PICCARD, H. *General Practice*, 1935, **11**, No. 4, p. 192.
29. TZANCK and SIDI. *Bull. Soc. Franç. de Derm. et de Syph.*, 1934, Nov., p. 1694.
30. DUMONT, A. *Scalpel, Liége*, 1937, Jan. 16, p. 78.
31. POZZAN, A. *Arch. ital. Chir.*, 1936, **46**, 1, p. 1.
32. PERKINS. *Practitioner*, 1939, Nov., p. 510.
33. HIPPS, H. E., and NEELY, H. *Naval Med. Bull.*, *Washington*, 1945, **44**, p. 262.
34. LEVIN, G. L. *Lancet*, 1934, Aug. 4, p. 249.
35. MAHAFFEY, H. *Anesth. & Anal.*, 1939, July-Aug., p. 200.
36. BINET, A. *Gynéc. et Obstét.*, 1933, May, p. 393.
37. ROSENTHAL, E. *Policlinico*, 1930, Dec., p. 592.
38. POPPER, H. L. *Zentralbl. f. Chir.*, 1933, Sept. 2, p. 2050.
39. MANDL, F. *Wien. klin. Woch.*, 1935, Apr. 19, p. 490.
40. FALK, P. *Arch. Ohr. Nos. Kehl. Neith.*, 1936, Dec., p. 254.
41. PANNETT, C. A. *Brit. Jour. Surg.*, 1915, **15**, pp. 248-259.
42. HILLMAN, O. S. *Pro. Roy. Soc. Med.* (An. Sec.), 1924, Dec. 12, p. 10.
43. FINSTERER, H. *Brit. Med. Jour.*, 1926, Aug. 14, pp. 290 *et seq.*

44. HEWER, C. L. *St. Bart's Hosp. Rep.*, 1925, p. 37.
45. FINSTERER, H. *Brit. Med. Jour.*, 1932, Aug. 27, p. 400.
46. UPCOTT, H. *Brit. Med. Jour.*, 1937, Mar. 20, p. 614.
47. JAMES, N. R. " Regional Analgesia for Intra-abdominal Surgery," 1943. Churchill, London.
48. { APPERLY, R. E. *Pro. Roy. Soc. Med.* (An. Sec.), 1924, Dec. 12, p. 13.
     { MEEKER, W. R. *Arch. Surg.*, 1925, Mar.
49. EDWARDS, F. R. *Brit. Med. Jour.*, 1936, Nov. 7, p. 939.
50. TYLER, E. A. *Anesth. & Anal.*, 1936, Jan.-Feb., p. 44.
51. { WISHJEWSKY, A. *Surg. Gyn. & Obst.*, 1930, May, p. 897.
     { RENDLE SHORT, A. *Med. Ann.*, 1931, p. 9 (abstract).
52. VISHNEVSKY, A. V. *Acta. med.*, *U.R.S.S.*, 1938, **1**, p. 148.
53. WEGENER, R. *Münch. med. Woch.*, 1937, Feb., pp. 26, 342.
54. BANKOFF, G. *Lancet*, 1934, Feb. 10, p. 287.
55. *Rep. of Austral. Soc. of An.*, 1937, May 3.
56. DE PABLO and DIEZ-MALLO, J. *Ann. Surg.*, 1948, **128**, p. 956.
57. MACINTOSH, R. R., and MUSHIN, W. W. " Local Anæsthesia Brachial Plexus Block," 1944. Oxford.
58. GALLEY, A. H. *Anæsthesia*, 1949, Oct., p. 154.
59. CATHELIN, F. *Compt. rend. Soc. de Biol. Paris*, 1901, vol. 53.
60. PAGÉS, F. *Rev. de san. milit.*, 1921, **11**, p. 351.
61. DURRANS, S. F. *Anæsthesia*, 1947, July, p. 106.
62. ODOM, C. B. *Anesth. & Anal.*, 1940, March-April, p. 106.
63. HELDT and MOLONEY. *Amer. Jour. Med. Sci.*, 1928, **175**, p. 371.
64. DAWKINS, C. J. M. *Pro. Roy. Soc. Med.* (An. Sec.), 1945, Jan. 5.
65. MACINTOSH, R. R., and MUSHIN, W. W. *Anæsthesia*, 1947, July, p. 100.
66. ODOM, C. B. *New Orleans Med. & Surg. Jour.*, 1937, Jan., p. 349.
67. PITKIN, C. P. " Conduction Anesthesia," 1946. J. P. Lippincott Co., p. 683.
68. MACINTOSH, R. R. *Anæsthesia*, 1950, April, p. 98.
69. DOGLIOTTI, A. M. *Anesth. & Anal.*, 1933, March-April, p. 59.
70. ODOM, C. M. *Amer. Jour. Surg.*, 1936, Dec., p. 553.
71. DENECKE, K. *Zentralbl. f. Chir.*, 1937, Jan. 16, p. 130.
72. SORESI, A. L. *Anesth. & Anal.*, 1937, Nov.-Dec., p. 306.
73. LUNDY, J. S. *Amer. Jour. Surg.*, 1928, **2**, p. 262.
74. MITCHELL, W. E. M. *Lancet*, 1933, Aug. 12, p. 348.
75. BOURQUE, N. O. *Med. Record*, 1935, Dec. 4, p. 497.
76. SARBATORESCU, C. *Jour. Amer. Med. Ass.*, 1936, July 11, p. 144.
77. GALLEY, A. H. *Anæsthesia*, 1949, Oct., p. 154.
78. TROTTER, M., and LETTERMAN, G. S. *Surg. Gyn. & Obst.*, 1944, **78**, p. 419 ; p. 551.
79. EDWARDS, J. T. *Pro. Roy. Soc. Med.* (Comp. Med. Sec.), 1933, Jan. 25.
80. { HINGSON, R. A., and EDWARDS, W. B. *Anesth. & Anal.*, 1942, Nov.-Dec., p. 301.
     { SOUTHWORTH, J. L., *et al.* *Ann. Surg.*, 1943, Mar., p. 301.
81. GLUCK and ROCHBERG. *Amer. Jour. Obst. & Gyn.*, 1943, **45**, p. 645.
82. SMALL, M. S. *Jour. Amer. Med. Ass.*, 1943, July 3, p. 671.
83. ADAMS, C., *et al.* *Jour. Amer. Med. Ass.*, 1943, May 15, p. 152.
84. WOOLMER, R. F. *Pro. Roy. Soc. Med.* (An. Sec.), 1949, **42**, p. 12.
85. CAMPBELL, W. C. *Pro. Staff. Mtgs.*, *Mayo Clin.*, 1935, Oct. 19, p. 667.
86. LERICHE, R. *Brit. Med. Jour.*, 1952, Feb. 2, p. 231.
87. APGAR, Y. *Anesth. & Anal.*, 1948, **27**, p. 23.
88. { DAVIES, R. M. *Anæsthesia*, 1952, July, p. 151.
     { BRYCE-SMITH, R. *Anæsthesia*, 1952, July, p. 154.

CHAPTER XV

THE PRESENT POSITION OF SPINAL ANALGESIA

In this chapter " spinal analgesia " will be taken to mean the commonly used technique of subarachnoid spinal block. The alternative extra-dural method has been discussed in the previous chapter.

The method of producing analgesia in the lower part of the body by blocking the nerve trunks of the cauda equina was first attempted about 1896 by Bier using cocaine,[1] but it was not brought into general use until 1906, when Barker employed the less toxic drug stovaine.

Anatomy and Physiology

The **level at which the spinal cord terminates** has been the subject of recent investigations which have shown our previous conceptions to be erroneous. Out of 240 adult cadavers, no less than 49 per cent. of the cords ended at the levels of the lower third of L. 1 and the upper third of L. 2. Exceptionally the cord reached the lower third of L. 3. It therefore follows that a lumbar puncture should not be made higher than the L. 2-L. 3 interspace and should preferably be in the space below this.[2]

Normal cerebrospinal fluid is clear, colourless and contains up to 5 lymphocytes per c.cm. The glucose content is about 70 mg. per cent., protein 20 mg. per cent. (half being albumin and half globulin), sodium chloride 0·75 per cent. and a trace of urea. The total **volume** probably lies between 60 and 150 c.cm., and its **specific gravity** varies from 1·004 to 1·010, the fluid obtained by cisternal puncture being slightly lighter than that obtained by lumbar puncture.[3] The latter fluid contains less sugar but more protein than the former, and the average S.G. in 150 normal patients was found to be 1·00697. In certain diseases the S.G. may lie outside the limits given above.[4] For example, in hydrocephalus it may be below 1·004 and in uræmia higher than 1·010. The **reaction** is slightly on the alkaline side of neutrality, its pH being usually 8·1. This may, however, vary (see below). The normal **cerebrospinal pressure** in the recumbent position is from 110 to 140 mm. H_2O. It is worth noting that the spinal fluid pressure measured in centimetres of water is approximately equal to the diastolic blood pressure measured in centimetres of mercury (Aceves). The spinal pressure is about 20 cm. H_2O higher in the sitting position and appears to rise during sleep, but, contrary to previous belief,[5] is thought to fall if narcotic doses of the barbiturates are given. In slight overdosage with these drugs, the pressure may become zero or even negative. It is now thought that the cerebrospinal pressure is controlled by a central hypothalamic mechanism.[6]

The **rate of absorption of injected fluids** is high. For example, 580 c.cm. have been introduced into the subarachnoid space of a dog within two hours.[7]

The chief **effects of injecting an analgesic solution** into the subarachnoid space are blocks of the contained nerves. The vasomotor and sensory nerves are blocked before the motor ones and recover after them. It has recently been shown that if a sufficiently dilute analgesic solution (e.g. $0 \cdot 2$ per cent. procaine) is injected, it is possible to block fibres conveying vasomotor and sudo-motor impulses and sensitivity to pinprick while the remaining sensory (and all motor) fibres remain functioning normally. This method **of differential spinal block** can be used for diagnosing various peripheral vascular disorders.[8] In general it can be said that the degree of difficulty in paralysing nerve fibres corresponds roughly with the thickness of their myelin sheaths.

In order to explain partial or complete failure in the development of analgesia when the technique appears to be faultless, some authorities suppose the existence of a condition known as " **rachi-resistance** ". Sebrechts considers that " rachi-resistant " individuals are sympatheticotonic in type and that the condition may be familial.[9] The opposite condition of "**rachi-sensitivity**" is supposed to occur in certain toxæmias, jaundice, high blood-urea concentration and pregnancy. It is conceivable that these variations may be due to differences in the permeability of the sheaths of the spinal nerve roots to analgesic drugs.[10] It cannot be said, however, that this theory is generally accepted, and failures of spinal analgesia can usually be explained by anatomical peculiarities or technical errors.[11] For example, if any blood has mixed with the C.S.F. in the syringe the blood proteins may " fix " the analgesic drug and render it ineffective.[12] Another possible explanation is that the pH of C.S.F. varies considerably and in certain cases may be high enough to precipitate the base from the analgesic solution.[13]

The **elimination** of substances injected into the theca has been the subject of considerable speculation. Recent work suggests that the venous channels are the direct route of drainage and (in the cat) the azygos vein carries the highest concentration of such substances.[14] Of the body tissues, only the spinal roots concentrated the analgesic above the level in the C.S.F. at the site of injection and only the liver and kidney concentrated it above the level in the circulating blood. Final elimination appears to be in the urine.[15] The radioactive tracer technique has proved useful in this field of investigation by introducing Br.[82] into the procaine molecule. The resulting dibromoprocaine is radioactive and the fate of the brominated benzine rings can be traced.

After spinal analgesia (with procaine and amethocaine) the **globulin** content of the cerebrospinal fluid shows a trifling rise, while the **albumin** increases steadily until by the eighteenth day it is nearly doubled.[16]

Behaviour of Hyperbaric Solutions

Until comparatively recently all injected solutions were heavier than C.S.F. since the drugs employed had to be used in a fairly high concentration in order to be effective. When such a solution is injected, its behaviour can be visualized as that of a globule of mercury which will travel to the most dependent part of the dural sac. For low blocks the lumbar puncture is therefore preferred in the sitting position, the patient afterwards reclining against pillows. For higher blocks (up to T. 6) the patient, after injection in the sitting or lateral position, lies on his back in a 8° Trendelenburg position with his head and neck raised. It is dangerous to lower the head for at least fifteen minutes or upward spread towards the phrenic nerve roots may occur. This is a great disadvantage for high blocks, as a head-down tilt is the best corrective against fall in blood pressure. For this reason the hypobaric method is preferable for high blocks. If a unilateral block is required, the lumbar puncture will have to be made with the patient on his affected side. This will necessitate turning him over later if the operation is to be performed in the lateral position.

The actual solutions in use are many and diverse. **Cocaine** was soon recognized as being too dangerous and was replaced by **tropacocaine** and later by **stovaine**. The latter drug in a 10 per cent. solution (**Chaput's formula**, S.G. 1·080) is still popular and is used in doses of from 0·2 to 0·5 c.c. It is also known as " **Stovaine Billon** ". **Barker's solution** (stovaine 5 per cent. and glucose 5 per cent., S.G. 1·023) is now seldom employed. For some curious reason Chaput's solution is sometimes called " light stovaine " and Barker's solution " heavy stovaine ". Both are, of course, strongly hyperbaric.

At the present time **procaine** is extensively used. Probably the most satisfactory technique is to use crystals of the drug dissolved in the cerebrospinal fluid and re-injected. The dose varies from 50 to 200 mg., according to the desired height of analgesia. Various solutions containing procaine are procurable. For example, **gravocaine** (S.G. 1·109) is a heavy solution of procaine which also contains strychnine, which seems an undesirable and unnecessary addition.[17] In order to prolong the period of analgesia, the addition of adrenaline (to about 1 in 100,000) to the procaine solution has been tried with success.[18]

" **Heavy nupercaine** " (1 in 200 in 6 per cent. glucose, S.G. 1·024 at 15° C.) is useful for longer analgesia. One c.cm. is usually sufficient for perineal blocks for such operations as perurethral prostatectomy and 2 c.cm. should give complete abdominal analgesia.

Hyperbaric amethocaine solutions can also be used for prolonged analgesia. " **Spinal D** " consists of 1 per cent. amethocaine with dextrose and has a S.G. of 1·025. It is, however, hypertonic and it is thought by some that this is undesirable.[19] Another solution termed " **Spinal D isotonic** " is available and consists of amethocaine 0·029 (0·4 per cent.), dextrose 0·239 (4·6 per cent.), water to 5 c.cm. The S.G. is 1·018 and the pH 5·0. It has been stated that the addition of 3 mg. neosynephrine (see Chapter XVII) to the amethocaine solution will produce a spinal analgesia lasting from 3 to 3½ hours.[20]

Fractional Spinal Block

Another method of prolonging the effect is to use **fractional spinal block.** The lumbar puncture is performed with the patient lying on his side on a special rubber mattress, 5 inches thick, having a gap cut in it beneath the lumbar part of the spine. A 20 c.cm. syringe filled with some such solution as 3·3 per cent. procaine is then connected to the needle by 3 feet of rubber tubing, 2·5 to 3 c.cm. of fluid are injected and the patient is turned on to his back. The needle is left *in situ* and protrudes into the gap in the mattress. As the analgesia wears off, more solution can be injected without disturbing the patient.[21]

Various modifications of this technique have been tried, e.g. a strongly hyperbaric solution of 5 per cent. procaine in glucose (S.G. 1·026).[22]

The most recent work on the subject suggests that the use of a dilute (1 per cent.) solution of procaine renders fractional spinal block a safer method.[23] This is confirmed by the discovery that solutions weaker than 1·25 per cent. procaine do not completely paralyse the phrenic nerve roots so that a greater margin of safety is assured.[24]

The results of 1,000 consecutive cases of fractional spinal analgesia have now been reported. The incidence of headache was 2·8 per

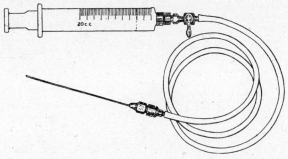

FIG. 89. Syringe and needle connected to tubing by Luer-Lok connections for fractional spinal analgesia. (Nicholson *et al.*)

cent., urinary retention 3·4 per cent., and pulmonary complications 3·4 per cent. The deaths which occurred were not considered to be attributable to the method.[25]

A report on another series of 1,200 administrations gave similar results.[26]

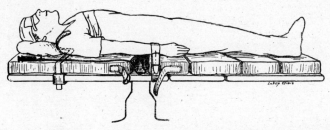

FIG. 90. Patient in position for abdominal operation under fractional spinal analgesia. Needle in place and shoulder braces and wrist restraints adjusted. Note gap in mattress and syringe lying at side of pillow.

The chief drawbacks of the fractional spinal technique are needle breakage (see later) and displacement of the needle point from the subarachnoid space during the positioning of the patient. These risks can be minimized by using a large (15 gauge) lumbar puncture needle and passing through it a No. 4 ureteric catheter so that its tip lies 4 to 5 cm. beyond the needle point pointing towards the head. The needle is then removed leaving the catheter in position.[27] The principle is similar to the fractional caudal block technique (q.v.).

Continuous Spinal Block

A similar set-up as for fractional block is used and an initial dose for an upper abdominal operation in a fit adult of about 6 c.cm. of a mixture of 2·5 per cent. procaine and 2·5 per cent. dextrose in normal saline is injected. This represents 150 mg. of procaine. A 5° Trendelenburg tilt is maintained until the desired level of analgesia is reached, the solution being, of course, hyperbaric. After 20 minutes a drip of 0·5 per cent. procaine at about 8 drops per minute is started. This rate may have to be altered to keep the level of analgesia constant and to provide adequate relaxation. It is said that there is less risk of infection than with fractional block as there is no syringe to detach after the injection has begun.[28]

Total Spinal Block

In the past, analgesia of the whole body has frequently been attempted by intrathecal injection, but the method has been regarded as dangerous owing to an extreme fall in blood pressure and the risk of respiratory paralysis.[29] The technique has, however, been revived in order to produce an ischæmic field for such operations as thoraco-lumbar splanchnicectomy and sympathectomy for essential hypertension.[30] After induction of anæsthesia with intravenous thiopentone, a lumbar puncture is performed in the second lumbar space and 150 to 250 mg. procaine dissolved in 3 to 4 c.cm. C.S.F. are injected. The patient is then turned on to his back in a steep Trendelenburg position until an appreciable fall in blood pressure occurs. An airway is inserted, 100 per cent. oxygen is given by mask and he is then turned into the " lateral jack-knife position " ready for operation, the pelvis being at the highest point. Unconsciousness is maintained either with thiopentone or cyclopropane. Controlled respiration may be necessary especially if the pleura is opened. Phrenic paralysis is unusual owing to the fact that the vaso-motor fibres are affected by dilute analgesic solutions before motor and sensory ones (see above). After operation a 20° head-down tilt is maintained for at least eight hours. The blood pressure is often unrecordable but the optimum figure is usually regarded as 70 mm. Hg. More details about controlled hypertension are given in the chapter devoted to it, but the

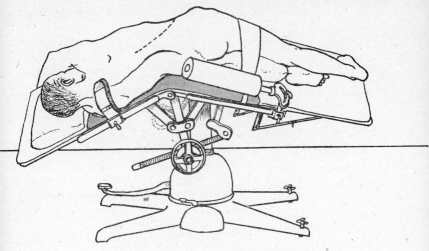

Fig. 91. Lateral jack-knife position.
(Griffiths and Gillies, *Anæsthesia*.)

inexperienced anæsthetist will be well advised to treat total spinal block with the greatest respect and caution.

Behaviour of Isobaric Solutions

It might be thought that a solution of the same S.G. as C.S.F. would be ideal for spinal block as the extent of the analgesia could be controlled by the volume injected and the patient could be placed in any position without further spread of effect. Unfortunately, however, as mentioned before, the S.G. of normal C.S.F. varies between the wide limits of 1·004 and 1·010, so that the chances of any standardized solution being isobaric in any given case are remote. It follows, therefore, that before injecting alleged isobaric solutions a test must be undertaken to determine if in fact the injection will be hypo-, iso- or hyperbaric. Neglect of this precaution has led to fatalities from respiratory failure.

The two solutions in common use which are most likely to be isobaric are **Querella's solution** which is buffered isotonic 1 in 200 nupercaine (S.G. 1·006) and 1 per cent. **amethocaine** which has a S.G. of 1·0068. In the latter case a test solution has been devised by Hans Clarke. This is a mixture of xylol and chlorobenzene in such proportions as to have a S.G. equal to that of the amethocaine solution. When a drop of C.S.F. is placed in a test-tube of this solution it will sink if it is heavier than 1 per cent. amethocaine and float if it is lighter.[31]   The recommended dose is 1 mg. per 10 lb. (4·5 kg.) body weight + 5 mg. up to a maximum of 25 mg. amethocaine.[32]   Analgesia is prolonged with amethocaine but takes some time to develop.   It is said that this delayed effect is minimized if the drug is given in a very finely divided and soluble " niphanoid " form.

In the opinion of the writer, it is better to employ definitely hyper- or hypobaric solutions than to test supposedly isobaric ones.

Behaviour of Pseudo-hypobaric Solutions

In order to overcome the disadvantages for high blocks of hyperbaric solutions already mentioned, artificially lightened solutions were introduced.

" **Spinocaine** " contains 14·5 per cent. alcohol, procaine (0·1 gm. in 1 c.c.), gliadin and strychnine, the S.G. being 1·0005.

" **Light duracaine** " also contains alcohol, procaine and gliadin and has a S.G. of 1·002.

Although these solutions are hypobaric in vitro, when injected the alcohol diffuses very rapidly, causing much turbulence, and the heavier constituents are left, which spread like a hyperbaric solution by gravitational diffusion.   It cannot therefore be said that the claims for " absolute controllability " have been realized in these preparations.[33]

Behaviour of Hypobaric Solutions

The introduction of nupercaine has rendered practicable a true hypobaric solution.   The drug acts in such extreme dilutions that the S.G. of the solvent is not appreciably raised.   " **Light nupercaine** " (1 in 1,500 in 0·5 per cent. saline) has a S.G. of 1·0036 at 37° C., and when injected into C.S.F. assumes the shape of an elongated air bubble, the length being proportional to the volume of the injected fluid.   In cross section this bubble resembles the segment of a circle whose circumference will hug the *upper* boundary of the enclosing dural sac.   The width of the bubble is such that it will cover both posterior nerve roots or both anterior roots, or the anterior and posterior roots of one side, according as the patient's posture is changed.[34]

Howard Jones Technique

For *bilateral blocks* the lumbar puncture is performed on either side and the volume of solution injected is calculated in accordance with the desired height of analgesia. For example, upper abdominal operations such as gastrectomy or cholecystectomy require a block up to T. 4, and this should be obtained by the injection of 14 to 15 c.cm. Sub-umbilical operations such as hysterectomy or appendicectomy necessitate a block up to T. 9, which will require about 12 c.cm. of solution. These doses are calculated for a man of average build ; a tall man will require slightly more and a short woman a slightly less amount.

A somewhat more precise method for calculating dosage for a high block was recommended by Howard Jones. If P is the volume of nupercaine solution in cubic centimetres and D is the distance in inches between C. 7 and the intercristal line, then

$$P = D - 6 \text{ in women,}$$
$$P = D - 4 \text{ in men.}[35]$$

The patient is then turned on to his face and the table given a slight tilt with the head down. This position will soak the posterior roots and should be maintained for about five minutes. If this manœuvre be omitted an anterior root block only may take place, i.e. the patient will develop motor paralysis without analgesia. The patient is next turned on to his back and may now be placed in any degree of Trendelenburg or in the lithotomy position, but on no account must a " foot-down " slope be allowed for at least thirty minutes after injection. There is reason to believe that the nupercaine is " fixed " after this length of time, partly by its absorption by nerve tissue and partly by the precipitation of the insoluble nupercaine base owing to the alkalinity of C.S.F.

For *unilateral blocks* where the incision is to be made well away from the mid-line, the lumbar puncture should be made with the affected side uppermost. This position is maintained for five minutes and a hemi-analgesia with muscular paralysis should ensue. When possible unilateral blocks are preferable to bilateral ones as only half the number of vasomotor nerves are paralysed, and consequently there is less fall in blood pressure. The adaptation of this technique to thoracic surgery is discussed in Chapter XXII.

Modifications of the Technique for Hypobaric Solutions

Three modifications of the above technique have been suggested and are claimed to offer certain advantages.

Etherington-Wilson's Method. The same solution is used, but the lumbar puncture is made in the sitting position through the third lumbar space. The original dosage and timing was as follows :

> For a low block 10 c.cm. are injected and twenty seconds are allowed sitting up.
>
> For a medium block 12 c.cm. are injected and thirty seconds are allowed sitting up.
>
> For a high block 15 c.cm. are injected and forty seconds are allowed sitting up.

At the end of the allotted time the patient is placed in the dorsal position with a 15° head-down slope. This method was evolved from a study of the spread of coloured solutions in glass tubes,[36] but there are good grounds for mistrusting an exact parallel between this device and the conditions obtaining in the living dural sac.[37] This technique does not take into consideration the great variations in the S.G. of C.S.F.,[38] which must affect the rate of ascent of a solution of fixed S.G.,[39] and fatalities have occurred.[40] The method has, however, attained some popularity in Great Britain and America, and good results have been claimed for it.[41]

The technique has recently been modified and it is now said that more uniform results in high blocks can be obtained by using a fixed volume of solution (13 to 14 c.cm. in adults) and to calculate the sitting-up time in seconds by multiplying by five the distance in inches between the 4th thoracic spinous process and the 4th lumbar interspace. Medium blocks require three-quarters of this time and low blocks one-half.[42]

Sebrecht's Method. The same solution is also used in this modification, but the puncture is made with a special malleable needle which is left in place while the patient is turned over to the ventral position. Fractional doses of 5 c.cm. are given until the required level of analgesia is attained. Any slowing of the pulse is taken as an indication that a pause should be made before injecting more solution.[43] This technique has some vogue in Belgium.

Lake's Method. The usual hypobaric nupercaine solution is used but the lumbar puncture is performed with the patient lying prone with pillows packed under the lower part of his chest, giving a marked dorsal curve with the head flexed forwards. The table is tilted until the seventh thoracic spinous process lies uppermost, as seen against a horizontal black line painted on the wall of the theatre. After injection the patient is, as usual, turned on to his back with a slight head-down tilt. It is claimed that a smaller volume of fluid is used than with the orthodox technique, 9 c.cm.

being regarded as the maximum dose for a high abdominal operation in an adult male.[44]

It is the author's opinion that the original method described by Howard Jones is essentially sound and that the modifications suggested up to the present time afford no appreciable advantages, except possibly the third (Lake's technique).

It should be noted that in whatever way hypobaric nupercaine is used, the solution must always be heated to body temperature before injection.

Instruments for Spinal Block

The original wide-bore needle introduced by Barker is far too clumsy and should never be used. In the writer's opinion, Howard Jones' pattern is the most satisfactory. It is 9 cm. in length,

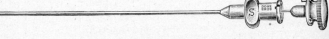

Fᵢɢ. 92.   Spinal needle and stilette (Howard Jones).

1·2 mm. in diameter and is made of stainless steel. The bevel is set at an angle of 45° to minimize the possibility of partially puncturing the theca. These needles are so fine and sharp that a preliminary local injection is sometimes omitted. It is usually better, however, to raise a subcuticular wheal with a fine hypodermic needle and the same analgesic solution as is to be injected intrathecally. It is worth noting that two cases of spinal meningitis were traced to an alleged " self-sterilizing " fluid which had been used for the preliminary injection and was subsequently found to contain living organisms.

A modification of the Howard Jones needle has two wings projecting at right angles at the junction of hub and shaft. This enables the anæsthetist to avoid touching either the nozzle of the syringe or the hub of the needle.[45]

In order to overcome any difficulty of using a fine spinal needle in patients with thick skins, and to minimize the risk of introducing infection, an instrument termed a " spinawl " has been invented. This is shaped like an enlarged drawing pin and has a triangular shaft $1\frac{1}{4}$ inches long, with cutting edges terminating in a fine point. It is easily introduced and leaves a tiny opening in the skin through which the fine spinal needle can be passed.[46]   An improvement on

the "spinawl" is the Sise introducer illustrated.   When this has
been inserted through the skin and fascia, an exceedingly fine
hardened gold needle (21-gauge) passed through the shaft punctures
the dura with a minute hole which
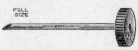
FULL
SIZE
practically excludes subsequent seepage.[47]
It is said that although these needles are
extremely fine the risk of breakage is
Fig. 93. Sise introducer.   small.[48]   If no introducer is available,
the skin can be snicked with a scalpel.

Breakage of Spinal Needles.   This accident is the anæsthetist's
nightmare and is commoner than is often supposed, the first case
(during simple lumbar puncture) having been reported as long
ago as 1889.   In a questionnaire, ninety-one American anæsthetists
reported a personal total of sixty-three such accidents.[49]   Two
types of fracture may occur.   Firstly, the break takes place during
insertion and is evident from the jamming of the stilette.   In this
event, the needle and stilette should be left in position as a guide
and an immediate attempt made to remove the broken fragment.
In the second type, the needle breaks because of some movement
of the patient after the stilette has been withdrawn.   In these
cases it is usually best to take a skiagram and attempt removal at
a later date.   It is worth noting that if the fragment is left,
symptoms may develop months after the event.   In order to avoid
this distressing accident, it is wise to discard spinal needles which
have been in use for a long time or have ever been severely bent
or corroded.   The method should be avoided in conscious patients
who will not coöperate by keeping still.

Indications for Spinal Analgesia

There is probably no subject upon which the views of both
surgeons and anæsthetists are more divergent than this.   Some
will never employ the method at all, while others use it upon every
possible occasion.   The popularity of spinal block has waned
during the past few years, partly because of the large numbers of
late complications reported and partly from the fact that curare
and other relaxants provide similar operative conditions with less
risk.   The actual relaxation provided is equal in the two cases but
spinal block ensures that the intestines are contracted whilst curare
does not.   If, for any reason, the use of a relaxant is undesirable
or if it is desired that the patient should retain consciousness, spinal
block can be reasonably used for the following conditions :
(i) Operations below the level of the diaphragm which are

liable to cause much shock or are likely to be very prolonged, or which require complete muscular relaxation for some time, particularly in patients who are suffering from or are liable to pulmonary disease. Such operations as partial gastrectomy, Gallie's operation for the repair of hernias, excision of the rectum, panhysterectomy and disarticulation through the hip joint may be cited as examples. Some surgeons favour spinal analgesia for prostatectomy,[51] while others consider that the liability to reactionary hæmorrhage when the blood pressure regains its normal level constitutes a grave disadvantage.

(ii) Paralytic ileus,[52] as opposed to mechanical obstruction. The theoretical objection against using spinal block for the latter condition is the possibility of rupturing a gangrenous loop of bowel from the increased peristalsis. The validity of this objection has recently been questioned, and there is no doubt that spontaneous reduction of hernias frequently occurs after the induction of spinal analgesia.[53] On the other hand, it must be remembered that a sudden massive action of the bowels may cause collapse and even death in elderly patients who are gravely ill. It is the opinion of the author and others,[54] that spinal analgesia should not be used in such cases.[55]

(iii) " Low " spinal blocks limited to S. 3 to S. 5 may be used for operations about the anus, perineum and urethra,[56] and seem destined to replace the alternative extra-dural caudal and trans-sacral methods as the results appear to be more certain and the technique is easier and safer.

(iv) High thoracic blocks are used to some extent in thoracic surgery for patients suffering from bronchiectasis (q.v.).

(v) Spinal analgesia, induced before electrical convulsive therapy, has been found useful in avoiding spinal injuries. Repeated injections have been made with very little change in the composition of the C.S.F.[57] This method has now been almost entirely super-seded by the intravenous injection of a short-acting relaxant.

Therapeutic Spinal Block

Spinal analgesia has been used with success in the treatment of *eclampsia*[58] and *anuria* following crush syndrome, incompatible blood transfusion and Weil's disease.[59] It has also been used for gastro-intestinal achalasia, e.g. *cardiospasm, mega-œsophagus* and congenital *megacolon*.[60] It has been suggested that the temporary but complete paralysis of the sympathetic supply to the affected parts may bring the two halves of the autonomic nervous system once more into step. To do this, it is necessary to cause paralysis of the anterior roots up to T. 5. The drug and method used are probably of little importance. It has been the writer's experience that while the immediate relief may be spectacular the ultimate results are usually disappointing. On the other hand, one case resulted in an apparently permanent cure. Another series of twelve cases resulted in " cure " (for from 2 to 9 years) in eight instances.

Post-partum hæmorrhage has been successfully treated by spinal block (see Chapter XXIV) as has reactionary *bleeding from the prostatic bed* after suprapubic prostatectomy. In the latter case a very low block is necessary.[61]

Spinal analgesia has also been used in the treatment of peripheral arterial *embolism* of the lower limbs. The subsequent vaso-dilatation may allow the embolus to move on far enough to render operation unnecessary. If not, embolectomy can be performed under the existing analgesia.[62]

An intrathecal injection of 2 to 4 c.cm. of 25 per cent. magnesium sulphate has been used to mitigate intolerable root pains such as occur in *tabes*. The injection may have to be repeated at weekly intervals.[63]

Intrathecal absolute alcohol has also been used for the relief of pain in *inoperable carcinoma* and is said to be safer than the alternatives of chordotomy, excision of the pre-sacral nerve or sacral nerve block with alcohol. The injection is, of course, a hypobaric one and the patient lies with his head low, his affected side uppermost and the spine flexed laterally by sandbags so that the nerve roots aimed at lie at the highest level. The body is also tilted forwards so that the posterior roots will be affected rather than the anterior ones. Various techniques for injection have been recommended[64, 65] but the writer has found the following procedure safer and more reliable than any described. A small bore tuberculin syringe is used and the solution is injected extremely slowly until pain relief is obtained or until 0·5 c.cm. has been used, whichever occurs first. Fifteen minutes is the average time taken, the needle is then removed and after another quarter of an hour the patient is turned on to his back. If the pain has not been relieved or returns later, the injection is repeated using 0·25 cm. more solution. Occasionally a third session is necessary in which 0·5 c.cm. more than the original volume is injected.

Similar doses of intrathecal absolute alcohol have also been used for intractable *sciatica*, 148 " cures " having been reported in 178 cases.[66] In view of the possibility of subsequent degenerative changes, however, it seems unwise to employ the technique except in cases of inoperable neoplasm.[67] Paralysis of the bladder is an occasional complication.[68] It should be noted that the alcohol must be sterilized in an autoclave in order to avoid the risk of introducing living spores.

It has been observed in America that the distillate from the " pitcher plant " (*Sarracenia purpurea*) has a beneficial effect on certain types of neuralgia and the active principle appeared to be the NH_4 ion. A technique has been worked out for giving ammonium salts intrathecally for intractable pain.[70] The lumbar puncture is performed with the patient tilted slightly head downwards. 50 c.cm. of C.S.F. are removed and to this fluid are added 3 c.cm. of ammonium sulphate or chloride, each c.cm. containing 60 to 65 mg. (6 to 6·5 per cent.). The mixture is re-injected and the patient is rolled on to his back and kept flat with a head-down tilt for an hour. A preliminary procaine analgesia can be used to render the procedure painless but this increases the incidence of complications. Some success in malignant cases has been reported but the risk of permanent paraplegia is a real one.[71]

Diagnostic Spinal Analgesia

It has been shown that normal patients show a rise in temperature in the feet of about 8° C. following a spinal block up to T.4. This can be recorded by an electrical surface thermometer and is due to vaso-dilatation. Use has been made of this observation to determine whether sympathectomy is likely to be of value in the treatment of such conditions as *thrombo-angiitis obliterans, Raynaud's disease*, etc. A very small rise in temperature after spinal block shows that the thrombotic element predominates and that operation will be useless. A comparatively large rise, on the other hand, indicates a high degree of vaso-spasm. Operation will therefore be indicated and can be performed under the existing spinal analgesia.[72] It has recently been pointed out that no sedative or analeptic should be used and that observations may be necessary for as long as two hours.[73]

Contra-indications

The following conditions are usually regarded as contra-indications to spinal analgesia :

(1) Severe shock, advanced myocardial degeneration and an abnormally low blood pressure. (The latter is generally taken to mean a systolic pressure which cannot be raised to 100 mg. Hg

with ephedrine.)[74]   A *high* blood pressure is only regarded as a contra-indication if accompanied by marked arterio-sclerosis[74] (see also under total spinal block).

(2) All diseases of the central nervous system, including mental abnormalities.   There is no doubt that latent neurological diseases can be precipitated by spinal analgesia.   These include disseminated sclerosis,[76] progressive muscular atrophy and spinal syphilis.[77]   If possible, a Wassermann reaction should be obtained, as a positive result is a definite contra-indication (unless the analgesia is to be used in the treatment of tabes).

(3) Respiratory obstruction from any cause is a contra-indication to a *high* spinal block.   The pressure of a large abdominal tumour (e.g. a full-term foetus) will cause splinting of the diaphragm and if a spinal block must be used, continuous oxygen should be given.

(4) Extensive vertebral lesions, e.g. curvature or arthritis.

(5) Sepsis in the region of the proposed lumbar puncture.

(6) Blood stream infections.   It is held by some that the lumbar puncture can infect the cerebrospinal fluid in such conditions.[72]

(7) Young children[78] and nervous patients who will not co-operate.[79]

Observations during Operation

Comfort of Patient.   Analgesia is usually perfect and the patient often sleeps throughout the operation.   Several factors, however, may render him uncomfortable.

(i) The " head-down " position in a hot theatre may give rise to a stifling sensation, which can be greatly mitigated by sponging the face with cold water or by allowing a weak air blast from a fan or pump to play on the face.

(ii) The patient may complain of feeling parched or faint.   A small swab soaked in dilute brandy and placed in his mouth to suck will relieve both conditions.

(iii) **Nausea** and even **vomiting** may occur if the surgeon exerts undue traction on the stomach.   This is partly due to impulses passing along the gastric branches of the vagi and can be reduced by injecting some local analgesic solution under the peritoneum in front of and behind the abdominal portion of the oesophagus if the stomach can be brought down sufficiently.[79]   Unless care is taken, it is possible to paralyse the terminal branches of the phrenic nerves with consequent respiratory embarrassment.[80]   Vomiting may occur apart from manipulation of the viscera, and this is now thought to be due to the direct stimulation of the vomiting centre by the drug employed.[81]   Vomiting is not an unmitigated evil, as a distinct improvement in colour, blood pressure and respiration is frequently seen after emesis during a spinal analgesia.[82]

(iv) **Mental discomfort** can often be avoided if the surgeon refrains from discussing the condition of the viscera in a loud voice and does not use the patient's chest as an arm rest or as a convenient repository for heavy instruments.

If, in spite of the above suggestions, the patient remains uncomfortable and miserable, the inhalation of cyclopropane should be started without more ado. This gas should also be used where possible if a **supplementary anæsthesia** is necessary owing to the premature wearing off of the analgesia. The excess of oxygen which is the accompaniment of cyclopropane administration is particularly beneficial in spinal block.[83] A *very light* narcosis can also be obtained by adding at intervals *small* doses of soluble thiopentone to an intravenous drip saline.[84]

Blood Pressure. It is a mistake to take frequent blood-pressure readings, as this disturbs a conscious patient and may give rise to much soreness of the arm. Sufficient information can usually be obtained by observation of his colour and of the characteristics of his pulse. A drop in pressure is inevitable in high blocks probably owing to a vasomotor paralysis. This is suggested by the fact that no such fall occurs in sympathectomized animals.[85] " Low " blocks entail no appreciable fall in pressure since it has been shown that the anterior roots below L. 2 do not contain vaso-constrictor fibres.[86] One modern theory supposes that in high spinal blocks the suprarenal glands are paralysed and that consequently there is a diminution in the output of adrenaline with fall in blood pressure.[87] It is possible that the absorption of the drug into the blood stream may cause a slight drop in pressure from depression of the vasomotor centre. This factor is probably of little importance since 20 c.cm. of 1 in 1,500 nupercaine injected directly into a vein cause only mild symptoms.[34] As a splanchnic block is automatically included in high spinal analgesia, visceral shock is largely eliminated so that sudden drops in blood pressure during rough traction are avoided. The fundamental difference between the low blood pressure in spinal block and true shock is that in the former condition there is no change in the volume of the circulating blood.[88] It is interesting to observe that if a spinal block is given to a patient in acute pain from an abdominal lesion, an immediate fall in blood pressure accompanies the relief from pain. The suggestion has been made that this is due to the cessation of pressor impulses which have been passing via the posterior roots to the vasomotor centre[89] and which are the cause of the high blood pressure often noted in the initial stages of shock (as pointed out by Parsons and Gray in 1912).

The shallow respiration which may occur in high spinal blocks may tend to lower the blood pressure from the diminished " respiratory pump effect ", but this may be offset by the rise in the CO_2 concentration in the blood causing vaso-constriction of those vessels whose nerve supply has not been paralysed.

In total spinal block the blood pressure is allowed to fall intentionally in order to produce an ischæmic field (see above). Apart from this the prophylactic treatment against a fall of blood pressure consists in the intramuscular injection of some such drug as **ephedrine** gr. $1\frac{1}{2}$, *some time before* the lumbar puncture. The synthetic product **ephetonin** is identical in chemical composition, being phenyl-methyl-amino propanol hydrochloride. It is a racemic mixture of the lævo- and dextro-rotatory salts. (It should be mentioned in passing that ephedrine when mixed with spinal analgesic solutions potentiates their effect and this is *not* due to any vaso-pressor action as no rise in blood pressure occurs if the drug is given by the intrathecal route. The explanation is that ephedrine itself is a local analgesic and quite a marked spinal analgesia can be obtained by injecting the drug alone.[90]) An even more effective analeptic is a **mixture** of 5 units of **pitressin** (pressor principle of posterior part of pituitary) **and** gr. $\frac{3}{8}$ or 25 mg. of **ephedrine**.[91] All the pressor drugs mentioned in Chapter XVII have been used at one time or another to raise the blood pressure in spinal block, the author having been favourably impressed by the action of **methedrine** (q.v.). If the suprarenal-paralysis theory is accepted, the most rational analeptic would appear to be an intravenous infusion of dilute **adrenaline** solution. A continuous drip infusion of 1 in 250,000 adrenaline has, in practice, been found satisfactory[92] at the time, but, in the writer's experience, severe collapse may occur when it is stopped. Alternatively the same concentration of l-*nor*-**adrenaline** (arterenol, levophed) can be substituted as this drug acts mainly by a generalized vaso-constriction instead of partly by an increased cardiac output.[93] Here, again, great care is necessary, (see also Chapter XVII) particularly as *nor*-adrenaline decreases the blood-flow through the kidneys[153] and the liver and in prolonged infusion irreversible changes in these organs might occur.[152] The infusion solution should be slightly acid as *nor*-adrenaline is rapidly oxidized by alkaline saline.

In order to combat a fall in blood pressure which has already occurred, the administration of the above drugs will obviously have less effect. The best treatment is undoubtedly to tilt the patient head downwards unless the collapse has followed the recent injection of a hyperbaric solution. The administration of CO_2 usually causes a slight rise in blood pressure but should be used with great care in spinal analgesia. Quite frequently there is already a high CO_2 content in the blood, and since some of the sympathetic fibres are paralysed, the normal vaso-constriction caused by CO_2 is lessened.[94, 95]

Respiration is usually shallow and regular, but must always be watched for impending failure. This is less likely to occur from phrenic paralysis than from fatigue of the respiratory centre caused by the anoxia resulting from imperfect lung ventilation due to the temporary paralysis of most of the intercostal muscles. If the centre has already been depressed by large doses of morphine, bromethol or barbiturates, respiratory failure is naturally more likely to occur.

The administration of pure oxygen appears to be the most satisfactory treatment. The addition of CO_2 should be made (if at all) with great care for reasons already explained. If the respiratory distress is due to an abnormally high level of motor paralysis, a helium-oxygen mixture is useful (see Chapter IV). The administration of the analeptics mentioned above may be temporarily beneficial.

After-effects

Many of the after-effects which occur after general anæsthesia may also be seen after spinal analgesia, and in particular there are :

Headache. In an observed series of 500 consecutive spinal analgesias, just over 30 per cent. of patients complained of headache and in 13·4 per cent. it was severe.[96] In another consecutive series of 400 cases, headache was complained of in 22·5 per cent.[97] In reviewing the enormous total of 50,000 spinal analgesias it was estimated that the frequency of headache was about 18 per cent.[98] From these figures it is clear that headache is a real bugbear. The condition is said to be more frequent in women than in men and in persons under the age of forty.[99] Curiously enough, the incidence of headache is greater after a low than after a high block. This may possibly be due to the more frequent use of concentrated solutions in the former case.[55] Unlike most other types of headache, the pain is nearly always increased by sitting up and diminished by the adoption of the Trendelenburg position. Headache may occur after the intrathecal injection of any drug or even after simple lumbar puncture. In the latter case it has been shown to be less common if a fine needle is used, so that seepage of cerebrospinal fluid into the epidural space seems to be a contributing factor[100] with " coning " of the brain through the foramen magnum (see later). This is confirmed by the demonstration that an orifice in the dura can persist for at least 14 days after puncture.[101] It is possible that seepage can also be reduced by directing the needle bevel laterally when entering the subarachnoid space. The longitudinal fibres are thus merely displaced instead of being severed as is the case when the bevel is transverse (Labat). It has also been shown that the spinal pressure is usually lower during the period of headache than at the conclusion of the original puncture,[102] and that the intrathecal[103] or peridural[104] injection of warm saline restores the pressure and abolishes the headache temporarily. In very severe and intractable cases, a catheter can be left in the peridural space and saline injected from time to time as necessary. On the supposition that the hypotension is due to inhibition of the choroid plexus, Zappala recommends the intrathecal injection of 1 per cent. glucose.[105] Another view is that the analgesic solution irritates the pia mater slightly, causing excessive absorption of cerebrospinal fluid, i.e. a " chemical meningitis ". In order to produce hydræmia to check this absorption, Harrison has given 4 oz. of 5 per cent. glucose in saline intravenously immediately after operation.[106] Contrary to previous opinion, it has been shown that contamination of the solution with tincture of iodine and slight hyper- and hypo-tonicity have no demonstrable effect on the incidence of " spinal headache ".[107] It has been stated that the intravenous injection of a short-acting barbiturate such as thiopentone immediately before the lumbar puncture diminishes the incidence of headache.[108] If a severe headache has already started, an intravenous injection of 20 c.cm. of 30 per cent. saline may be effective, but 50 per cent. glucose in saline[109] or 2 c.cm. of 50 per cent. magnesium sulphate[110] may be necessary to give relief. Six oz. of 50 per cent. magnesium sulphate given as a four-hourly enema has been recommended by Koster.[111] Mild cases may yield to ordinary treatment or to the application of shortwave diathermy[112] or X-ray therapy to the head.[113] 4 to 6 drops of a 0·5 per cent. alcoholic solution of nitro-glycerin has also proved effective.[114] Prophylactic measures include the rigid adherence to a head-down position for some hours after injection, a semi-darkened room and the prohibition of reading for at least twenty-four hours. The transport of the patient from theatre to bed should be effected on a modified trolley so that tilting can be maintained.[115] It is said that the substitution of the prone for the supine position diminishes seepage of C.S.F. and thus reduces the incidence of headache.[116]   Early ambulation undoubtedly increases the incidence of spinal headache.   In one series of 400 analgesias headache occurred in 42·7 per cent. of patients allowed up on the first post-operative day, in 30 per cent. of patients up on the second day, 14·2 per cent. the third day, and only 4·3 per cent. the fourth day.[97]   There is no doubt that a psychic element is often present and in hospital practice " suggestion " by other patients may play a part in the incidence of headache.

Nausea and Vomiting following spinal analgesia are commoner than are often supposed.   In one series of 500 consecutive cases the incidence was 34·6 per cent.[96]   Intravenous morphine given immediately after the lumbar puncture is said to reduce this distressing complication.[117]   The causation of vomiting *during* the analgesic period has already been discussed.

Hyperpyrexia.   A transient rise in temperature up to 104° F. with shivering is sometimes observed after spinal analgesia.   It is possible that boiling syringes and needles in alkaline or tap water may be the cause.[118]

Trophic Changes.   A diffuse redness of the skin over the sacrum, followed by more or less extensive gangrene, has been noted as a rare sequel to spinal analgesia.   One writer had recorded no less than 7 cases in 365 nupercaine blocks.[119]

Retention of Urine.   This is usually slight and transient, yielding to drugs of the acetylcholine series, e.g. doryl or carbachol (carbamyl choline chloride).   On the other hand, urinary retention may be severe and permanent leaving the patient with a serious risk of ascending infection.   The cause appears to be damage to the sacral nerve roots with consequent spasticity of the internal sphincter.[120]

Other Transient Palsies.   Transient lesions of the cauda equina are not very rare and are characterized by the absence on one or more of the leg tendon reflexes, retention of urine (considered above), incontinence of fæces, sensory loss in the sacral region and loss of sexual function.   In one series of 1,000 spinal analgesias with " heavy duracaine " there were thirteen such complications, whereas in 1,000 stovaine administrations there were none.[121] Palsies of all the cranial nerves except the olfactory, glosso-pharyngeal and vagus have been reported after spinal block, but the sixth (abducens) is by far the commonest (over 90 per cent.).[122] This lesion can also follow a simple lumbar puncture.[123]   The incidence of the condition after all types of spinal block has been

variously estimated as between 1 in 100 and 1 in 250. The squint
generally develops about the third day, practically always dis-
appearing within a few weeks. Permanent diplopia has, however,
been recorded.[124] The causation of this condition is obscure
although the sixth nerve is notoriously vulnerable in all types of
cerebral lesions. It has been suggested that this is so because of
the relative instability of the binocular vision function—phylo-
genetically a recently acquired attribute in man.[125] This somewhat
vague explanation is not very satisfying but the alternative theories
of toxicity from the analgesic solution and inflammation from
low-grade meningitis[126] are also unlikely because bilateral lesions
are uncommon, the nerve is not exposed to a concentrated solution,
and pyrexia does not occur. A more probable explanation is the
mechanical one that a rise in intracranial pressure causes a " coning "
of the brain through the foramen magnum which stretches the sixth
nerve over the apex of the petrous part of the temporal bone. This
is supported by the fact that the paralysis is often preceded by
headache.[127] Complete deafness lasting for some weeks is a very
rare complication.[128]

Permanent Paralysis. This disaster is rare but unfortunately not
so rare as was formerly supposed. In a recent Swedish investigation,[133] six cases of permanent spinal cord lesions occurred after
23,000 spinal blocks, an incidence of 1 in 3,800. Direct trauma to the
spinal cord is very unlikely to occur if a puncture higher than the
space between L.2 and L.3 is avoided.[129] It must be remembered
that regeneration of nerve fibres does not take place within the spinal
cord owing to the absence of the neurilemmal sheath,[130] so that
the prognosis of these cases is always grave. A fatal case has been
reported following spinocaine injection where the whole substance
of the cord in the lumbar region was found to be necrotic. These
post-mortem findings were particularly instructive, as there was
no evidence of direct trauma to the cord, nor of old hæmorrhage
nor of the introduction of infection at the time of puncture.[131]
Cases of ascending myelitis have also been described,[132] one of
which did not begin until four weeks after a spinal block for
appendicectomy.[133] There is some evidence to show that concentrated and grossly hypertonic solutions can cause permanent
damage to nerve tissue.[19] Ampoules of spinal analgesia solution
should never be kept in spirit or antiseptic liquids as an unnoticed
flaw in the glass may cause contamination of the contents with
disastrous results. It seems likely that some of the cases of
permanent paralysis are due to this cause.[134]

Spinal Meningitis. It is imperative to use absolute asepsis for the technique of inducing spinal analgesia or meningitis may follow. For example, syringes and needles should be sterilized by an hour's stay in an electric oven at 160° C. or autoclaved after having been packed through loops in a strip of lint and rolled up like a motor tool-roll. Under wartime conditions there was a considerable increase in this grave complication. Investigations of various series of such cases indicate that organisms can be introduced by such diverse means as unsterilized nail brushes, used for washing hands,[135] a defective filter on a hospital water supply,[136] by contaminated labels gummed to ampoules,[137] rinsing syringes with " sterile water ", or by infected analgesic solution used for the preliminary subcuticular wheal.[138] On the other hand, cases of meningitis have occurred where the most exhaustive search has failed to reveal the source of infection.[139] It is possible that the irritation produced by some injected drugs may enable organisms to gain a foothold. The low-grade meningitis produced is often not susceptible to the sulphonamides or to penicillin, and non-fatal cases show a tendency to relapse. There is evidence that this may be due to the formation of adhesions containing infected C.S.F. which is liberated from time to time.[140] A useful memorandum pointing out some of the more obvious pitfalls in an aseptic spinal technique has been published by the Public Health Laboratory Service and the London Sector Pathologists Committee.[141]

Vertebral Arthritis. Several cases have been reported of persistent pain in the back following spinal analgesia. On X-ray examination changes

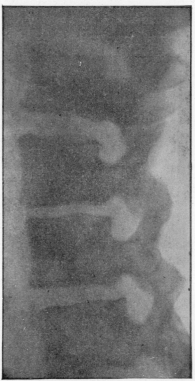

Fig. 94. Skiagram showing diminution of intervertebral joint space due to collapse of disc following spinal analgesia.   (A. D. Everett, *Proc. Roy. Soc. Med.*)

in one intervertebral disc and arthritis limited to one inter-vertebral joint have been demonstrated. It is thought that these changes are caused by the needle striking against the intervertebral disc[142] and giving rise to seepage of the nucleus

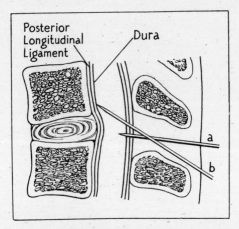

Fig. 95. Flexed spine showing bulging of discs into neural canal. *a.* Spinal needle inserted too far at right angles will hit disc. *b.* Needle inclined towards head will hit next higher vertebral body. (After Dowding, F. H. *U. S. Naval Med. Bull.*)

pulposus through the annulus fibrosus.[143] It seems probable that the acute flexion of the spine assumed prior to lumbar puncture increases the pressure inside the discs and causes them to bulge slightly into the neural canal. A needle pushed too far at right angles to the back is more likely to penetrate the disc than one with a slight inclination towards the head[144] (see Fig. 95).

Mortality and Morbidity

The results obtained with spinal analgesia are extremely difficult to assess, since the most divergent views are expressed. Series of many thousands of administrations are published with no fatalities, whilst other observers give a mortality due to the method as high as 1 in 200.[145] In a survey of spinal analgesias administered in the State of New Jersey there were 14 deaths in 4,360 cases (1 in 311).[146] In the large series of 15,652 administrations in eighteen American hospitals, the immediate mortality (on the table) was 40, or about

1 in 400.[147] In a single American hospital 33,811 spinal blocks were administered during eleven and a half years and the fatalities which were judged to be directly due to the method numbered 30 or 1 in 1,127.[148] A recent statistical study of 3,500 spinal blocks in an Australian General Hospital gives the immediate mortality of 3·1 per thousand (1 in 323).[149] Statistics are, of course, unreliable owing to the impossibility of discovering accurately in which cases the analgesia caused or contributed to the patient's death. Prior to the introduction of the muscle relaxants the general feeling among anæsthetists was that while spinal block had a greater immediate mortality than general anæsthesia in suitable cases, the total morbidity was not increased owing to the added protection from operative shock. It is doubtful if this is now true. Furthermore, it used to be thought that there is little difference in the pulmonary complications whether spinal, general, or combined anæsthesia is used, provided that the patient had no chronic infection before operation,[150] but a statistical investigation suggests that comparable cases anæsthetized with cyclopropane had less sequelæ.[151]

References

1. BIER, A. *Deut. Zeitschr. f. Chir.*, 1899, **51**, p. 361.
2. NEEDLES, J. H. *Anat. Record*, 1935, Nov. 25.
3. KAFKA, Y. *Die Zerebüssrospinalfligkeit*, Leipsig, 1930.
   HASLAR, J. K. *Brit. Med. Jour.*, 1942, April 4, p. 453.
4. HEWER, C. L. *Brit. Med. Jour.*, 1943, Aug. 21, p. 245.
   EPSTEIN, S. H., and MARVIN, F. W. *New Eng. Jour. Med.*, 1933, **207**, p. 259, and WOLMAN, I. J., *et al. Amer. Jour. Clin: Path.*, 1946, Mar. (Technical Sec.), p. 32.
5. HORSLEY, J. S. *Lancet*, 1937, Jan. 16, p. 141.
6. LEVINSON. "Cerebro-spinal Fluid in Health and Disease," 3rd. edit., 1929.
   GREENFIELD and CARMICHAEL. "Cerebro-spinal Fluid in Clinical Diagnosis." 1925.
7. EMMETT, J. L. *Pro. Staff. Mtgs. Mayo Clin.*, 1933, July 19.
8. ARROWOOD, J. *Pro. Roy. Soc. Med.* (An. Sec.), 1950, May 5.
9. SEBRECHTS. *Rapports et Discussions IXe Congrès. Soc. intern. Chir.*, 3, p. 838.
10. BLACK, W. R., and WALTERS, G. A. B. *Brit. Med. Jour.*, 1937, Jan. 20, p. 218.
11. LAKE, N. C. *Brit. Med. Jour.*, 1937, Feb. 6, p. 297.
    HEWER, C. L. *Brit. Med. Jour.*, 1937, Feb. 13, p. 360.
12. GILLIES, J. *Anæsthesia in Casualty Service*, H.M. Stat. Off., 1940.
13. COHEN, E., and KNIGHT, R. *Anesthesiology*, 1947, **8**, p. 594.
14. HOWARTH, F., and COOPER, E. R. A. *Lancet*, 1949, Nov. 17, p. 937.
15. *Lancet* (Annotation), 1950, Feb. 11, p. 268.
16. LIENHOOF, F. *Schmerz, Narkose, Anesthesie*, 1936, Dec., p. 145.
17. PITKIN, C. P. *Brit. Jour. Anæsth.*, 1930, **7**, p. 2.
    FALKNER HILL. *Lancet*, 1930, *i*, p. 124.
18. ROMBERGER, F. T. *Anesth. & Anal.*, 1943, Sept.-Oct., p. 252.
19. DINSDALE, T. *Anæsthesia*, 1947, Jan., p. 17.

20. BROCKMAYER, M. L., *et al.*   *Surg. Gyn. & Obst.*, 1949, **88**, p. 528.
21. { LEMMON.   *Ann. Surg.*, 1940, Jan., p. 141.
     { NICHOLSON, M. J., *et al.*   *Amer. Jour. Surg.*, 1941, Sept., p. 403.
22. LEE, J. A.   *Lancet*, 1943, Aug. 7, p. 156.
23. FRASER, R. J.   *Anesth. & Anal.*, 1943, Jan.-Feb., p. 38.
24. MAXSON, L.   " Spinal Anesthesia," 1938.
25. LEMMON, W. T., and PASCHAL, C. W.   *Surg. Gyn. & Obst.*, 1942, May, p. 948.
26. MARTIN, R. C., *et al.*   *Arch. Surg.*, 1945, Mar., p. 130.
27. TUOHY, E. B.   *Jour. Amer. Med. Ass.*, 1945, May 26, p. 262.
28. ARROWOOD, J. G., and FOLDES, F. F.   *Arch. Surg.*, 1944, Oct., p. 241.
29. { JONESCO, J.   *Brit. Med. Jour.*, 1909, **2**, p. 1395.
     { TAIT, D., and CAGLIERI.   *Abst. Jour. Amer. Med. Ass.*, 1900, **35**, p. 6.
     { LE FILLIÂTRE.   *Precis de Rachianesthésie Générale.* 1921. Paris.
30. GRIFFITHS, H. W. C., and GILLIES, J.   *Anæsthesia*, 1948, Oct., p. 134.
31. BULL, D. C., and ESSELTYN, C. B.   *Amer. Jour. Surg.*, 1936, Jan.
32. LUNDY, J. S.   *Pro. Staff. Mtgs. Mayo Clin.*, 1931, vol. 6, p. 378.
33. { DONALD, C.   *Pro. Roy. Soc. Med.* (An. Sec.), 1930, March 7.
     { FINSTERER, H.   *Brit. Med. Jour.*, 1932, Aug. 27, p. 400.
34. HARRIS, T. A. B., and RINK, E. H.   *Guy's Hosp. Rep.*, 1937, Jan.
35. { HOWARD JONES.   *Pro. Roy. Soc. Med.* (An. Sec.), 1930, May, p. 919.
     { HOWARD JONES.   *Brit. Jour. Anæsth.*, 1930, **7**, p. 99.
     { HOWARD JONES.   *Lancet*, 1930, Jan. 25.
36. WILSON, W. E.   *Brit. Jour. Anæsth.*, 1934, Jan., p. 43.
37. KOSTER, *et al.*   *Arch. Surg.*, 1938, Oct., p. 601.
38. HEWER, C. L.   *Brit. Jour. Anæsth.*, 1939, April, p. 17.
39. HEARD, K. M.   *Anesth. & Anal.*, 1938, May-June, p. 124.
40. { VAN DER POST, C. W. H.   *Brit. Jour. Anæsth.*, 1938, April, p. 117.
     { GURD, F. B., *et al.*   *Ann. Surg.*, 1939, Nov., p. 872.
41. HUGHES, J.   *Brit. Med. Jour.*, 1939, June 17, p. 1124.
42. WILSON, W. E.   *Pro. Roy. Soc. Med.* (An. Sec.), 1944, Nov. 3.
43. SEBRECHTS.   *Brit. Jour. Anæsth.*, 1934, Oct., p. 4.
44. LAKE, N. C.   *Lancet*, 1938, July 30, p. 241.
45. MACINTOSH, R. R.   *Lancet*, 1948, Oct. 16, p. 612.
46. GRAHAM, H. F.   *Amer. Jour. Surg.*, 1931, March, p. 557.
47. Technique as practised at the Lahey Clinic.
48. EVERSOLE, U. H.   *New Eng. Jour. Med.*, 1936, March 5, p. 468.
49. DESSLOCH, J. C.   *Anesth. & Anal.*, 1939, Nov.-Dec., p. 353.
50. CAVE, J. H.   *Brit. Jour. Anæsth.*, 1938, July, p. 158.
51. { THOMSON-WALKER, Sir J.   *Brit. Med. Jour.*, 1923, *i*, p. 137.
     { CAMPBELL, M. F.   *Jour. Urol.*, 1930, Sept.
52. STOWERS, J. E.   *Jour. Missouri Med. Ass.*, 1931, May.
53. RUSSELL, A. S. D., and SWORN, B. R.   *Brit. Med. Jour.*, 1932, May 14, p. 882.
54. LAKE, N. C.   *Brit. Med. Jour.*, 1933, Jan. 14, p. 77.
55. CRANKSHAW, T. B., and KAYE, G.   *Anæsthesia*, 1947, Oct., p. 127.
56. HASLER, J. K.   *Lancet*, 1932, Jan. 9, p. 80.
57. SHORYON, H. J., and L. M.   *Jour. Mental Sci.*, 1943, Jan., p. 69.
58. PARAMORE, R. H.   *Brit. Med. Jour.*, 1930, Jan, 4, p. 15.
59. { COOPER, V. H., and LANG, P.   *Brit. Med. Jour.*, 1951, Feb. 17, p. 338.
     { WILLIAMS, M. H. C.   *Lancet*, 1947, Jan. 18, p. 100.
60. TELFORD, E. D., and SIMMONS, H. T.   *Brit. Med. Jour.*, 1939, Dec. 23, p. 1224.
61. ROWBOTHAM, S.   *Anæsthesia*, 1947, April.
62. { AGAR, H.   *Brit. Med. Jour.*, 1943, July 24, p. 179.
     { DALEY, R.   *Brit. Med. Jour.*, 1943, Aug. 7, p. 101.
63. GORDON, A.   *Med. Jour. & Rec.*, 1931, April 15, p. 399.
64. OTTLEY, C.   *Brit. Med. Jour.*, 1938, March 5, p. 510.

65. MILLS, G. P.   *Brit. Med. Jour.*, 1935, Jan. 26, p. 153.
66. DOGLIOTTI, A. M.   *Anesth. & Anal.*, 1935, July-Aug., p. 150.
67. RUSSELL, W. R.   *Lancet*, 1936, March 14, p. 595.
68. HUDSON, O. C.   *New York Med. Times*, 1936, Feb., p. 44.
69. ADSON, A.   *Minnesota Med.*, 1937, March, 135.
70. JUDOYICH, B. D., *et al.*   *Anesthesiology*, 1944, July, p. 341.
71. GUTTMAN, S. A., and PARDEE, I.   *Anesthesiology*, 1944, July, p. 347.
72. TELFORD, E. D., and STOPFORD, J. S. B.   *Brit. Med. Jour.*, 1932, June 18, p. 1116, and 1933, Feb. 4, p. 173.
73. WADDY, F. F.   *Anæsthesia*, 1947, July, p. 93.
74. DOYLE, J. C.   *Anesth. & Anal.*, 1934, May-June, p. 116.
75. SISE, L. F.   *Amer. Jour. Surg.*, 1936, Dec., p. 424.
76. FLEISS, A.   *New York State Jour.*, 1949, May 1, p. 1076.
77. CRITCHLEY, M.   *Pro. Roy. Soc. Med.* (Neur. Sec.), 1937, Mar. 18.
78. VEAL, J. R., *et al.*   *Amer. Jour. Surg.*, 1936, Dec., p. 600.
79. HOWARD JONES, W.   *Med. Press and Circ.*, 1934, Oct. 3.
80. ASHWORTH, H. K.   *Pro. Roy. Soc. Med.* (An. Sec.), 1938, Feb. 4.
81. COTUI, F. W.   *Anesth. & Anal.*, 1934, July-Aug., p. 144.
82. ABELSON, L.   *Anesth. & Anal.*, 1935, March-April, p. 24.
83. SAKLAD, M.   *Amer. Jour. Surg.*, 1936, Dec., p. 527.
84. HAND, L. V., and SISE, L. F.   *Lahey Clin. Bull.*, 1939, March, p. 18.
85. BRADSHAW.   *Ann. Surg.*, 1936, July, p. 41.
86. HARRIS, T. A. B.   *Brit. Jour. Anæsth.*, 1939, July, p. 131.
87. PITKIN, G.   *Anesth. & Anal.*, 1940, Sept.-Oct., p. 241.
88. SCHUBERTH, O. O.   *Acta Chir. Scand.*, 1936, 78.
89. FALKNER-HILL.   *Brit. Jour. Anæsth.*, 1937, Jan., p. 446.
90. RUBEN, J. E., *et al.*   *Science*, 1948, **107,** p. 223.
91. RAGINSKY, B. B.   *Trans. Internat. Coll. Surg.*, 1938, **1,** p. 66.
92. EVANS, F. T.   *Lancet*, 1944, Jan. 1, p. 15.
93. CHURCHILL-DAVIDSON, H. C.   *Brit. Med. Jour.*, 1951, Dec. 29, p. 1551.
94. BOSTON, F. K.   *Brit. Jour. Anæsth.*, 1939, Jan., p. 77.
95. LEWIS, D. L., and PALSER, E. G. M.   *Brit. Med. Jour.*, 1938, June 4, p. 1202.
96. JENNINGS, W. K., and KARABIN, J. E.   *Amer. Jour. Surg.*, 1939, Nov., p. 317.
97. YULIN, H., and CHIA-ERM, C.   *China Med. Jour.*, 1951, May-June, p. 251.
98. THORSEN, G.   *Acta Chir. Scand.*, 1947, **95,** suppl., p. 121.
99. GRÖNDAHL, N. B.   *Acta Chir. Scand.*, 1932, Dec., p. 51.
100. ALLEN, H. W.   *Brit. Med. Jour.*, 1934, Aug. 25, p. 349.
101. FRANKSSON, C., and GORDH, T.   *Acta Chir. Scand.*, 1946, Sept. 10, p. 443.
102. SHEPPE, *Amer. Jour. Med. Sci.*, 1934, Aug., p. 247.
103. PICKERING, G. W.   *Brit. Med. Jour.*, 1939, May 6, p. 907.
104. RICE, G., and DABBS, C.   *Anesthesiology*, 1950, Jan., p. 17.
105. ZAPPALA, G.   *Policlinico*, 1934, June 18.
106. HARRISON, P. W.   *Arch. Surg.*, 1936, Jan., p. 99.
107. KOSTER, H., *et al.*   *Arch. Surg.*, 1937, July, p. 148.
108. JARMAN, R.   *Brit. Jour. Anæsth.*, 1937, Oct., p. 20.
109. SHAW, R. W.   *Irish Jour. of Med. Science*, 6th Series, No. 73, 1932, Jan.
110. KOSTER, H.   *Amer. Jour. Surg.*, 1930, June, p. 1165.
111. KOSTER, H.   *Surg. Gyn. & Obst.*, 1929, Nov. 29, p. 617.
112. FRANKEN, H.   *Brit. Jour. Anæsth.*, 1935, Jan., p. 85.
113. SCHUBERT, E. Y.   *Schmerz, Narkose, Anesthesie*, 1939, April, p. 11.
114. BACKER, G.   *Schmerz, Narkose, Anesthesie*, 1936, No. 9.
115. MOUAT, T. B.   *Brit. Med. Jour.*, 1944, April 15, p. 532.
116. BENDIT, M.   *Lancet*, 1944, Oct.. 14, p. 517.
117. ROCHFORD, J. D.   *Jour. R.A.M.C.*, 1944, Nov., p. 250.

118. Jost, T. A.   *Anesth. & Anal.*, 1935, July-Aug., p. 191.
119. Contempre, J.   *Le Scalpel*, 1934, June 16, p. 859.
120. Rieser, C.   *Jour. Med. Ass.*, 1941, July 12, p. 98.
121. Ferguson, F. R.   *Pro. Roy. Soc. Med.*(Neur. Sec.), 1937, March 18.
122. Hayman, I. R., and Wood, P. M.   *Ann. Surg.*, 1942, **115,** p. 864.
123. Dattner, B., and Thomas, E. W.   *New York State Jour. Med.*, 1941,
        41, p. 1660.
124. Heard, K. M.   *Anesth. & Anal.*, 1938, May-June, p. 124.
125. Fairclough, W. A.   *Brit. Med. Jour.*, 1945, Dec. 8, p. 801.
126. Babcock, W. W.   *New York State Jour. Med.*, 1913, **98,** p. 897.
127. Bryce-Smith, R., and Macintosh, R. R.   *Brit. Med. Jour.*, 1951,
        Feb. 10, p. 275.
128. Adams, A. W.   *Bristol Med. Clin. Jour.*, 1937, Summer, p. 143.
129. Hewer, C. L.   *Pro. Roy. Soc. Med.* (An. Sec.), 1933, Jan. 25.
130. Hinds-Howell, C. M.   *Lancet,* 1932, Jan, 16.
131. Brain, W. R., and Russell, D.   *Pro. Roy. Soc. Med.* (Neur. Sec.),
        March 18.
132. Martin, J. P.   *Pro. Roy. Soc. Med.* (Neur. Sec.), 1937, March 18.
133. Elstad, D.   *Norsk. Mag. f. Large.*, 1936, Sept. p. 959.
134. Macintosh, R. R.   " Lumbar Puncture and Spinal Analgesia," 1951.
        Livingstone.
135. Yuylsteke, C. A.   *Brit. Med. Jour.*, 1947, Feb. 1, p. 179.
136. Barrie, H. J.   *Lancet*, 1941, Feb. 22, p. 242.
137. Hewer, C. L., and Garrod, L. P.   *Brit. Med. Jour.*, 1942, Feb. 28,
        p. 306.
138. Evans, F. T.   *Lancet*, 1945, Jan. 27, p. 115.
139. Davidson, I. A.   *Lancet*, 1947, Dec. 13, p. 883.
140. Kremer, M.   *Brit. Med. Jour.*, 1945, Sept. 8, p. 309.
141. *Lancet*, 1947, Dec. 13, p. 883.
142. Milward, F. J., and Crout, J. L. A.   *Lancet*, 1936, July 25, p. **133.**
143. Everett, A. D.   *Pro. Roy. Soc. Med.* (Orthop. Sec.), 1941, Oct. 11.
144. Dowding, F. H.   *U.S. Naval Med. Bull.*, 1944, Oct., p. 666.
145. Saunders, E. W.   *Ann. Surg.*, 1931, Nov., p. 931.
146. Bortone, E.   *Anesth. & Anal.*, 1932, *xi*, p. 256.
147. Babcock, M. E.   *Anesth. & Anal.*, 1932, July, p. 187.
148. Veal, J. R., *et al.*   *Amer. Jour. Surg.*, 1936, Dec., p. 606.
149. Crankshaw, T. B., and Kaye, G.   *Anæsthesia,* 1947, Oct., p. 127.
150. { Fairley, H. P.   *Brit. Jour. Anæsth.*, 1932, July, p. 162.
        { Walters, G. A. B.   *Brit. Jour. Anæsth.*, 1932, Oct., p. 33.
151. Campbell, S. M., and Gordon, R. A.   *Canad. Med. Ass. Jour.*, 1942,
        April, p. 347.
152. Grayson, J., and Johnson, D. H.   *Brit. Med. Jour.*, 1952, Mar. 8,
        p. 547.
153. Davidson, H. C., *et al.*   *Lancet*, 1951, **2,** p. 803.

CHAPTER XVI

REDUCTION OF HÆMORRHAGE DURING OPERATION

Local methods—Controlled hypotension—Spinal Block—Arteriotomy— Methonium compounds—Negative Pressure to Limbs

Loss of blood during operation is not only a source of danger to the patient but is a major inconvenience to the surgeon. It will therefore be agreed that a bloodless field is most desirable if this can be obtained without added risk.

Local methods of attaining ischæmia have been employed for many years and include the use of rubber bandages and tourniquets to limbs, and the infiltration of the operative field with vaso-constrictive solutions.

CONTROLLED HYPOTENSION

In pre-anæsthetic days, the excessive psychic and traumatic shock frequently caused fainting at the beginning of an operation. This was welcomed not only by the patient whose agony ceased, but also by the surgeon as bleeding was greatly reduced.

The idea of purposely producing a low blood pressure with a view to reducing bleeding from wounds has been developed intensively during the past few years. It has been found that a systolic blood pressure of about 60 mm. Hg will assure a practically bloodless field and usually appears to maintain a capillary circulation sufficient for the tissues provided that the blood is fully oxygenated and that vaso-dilatation is ensured. So far, three methods have been employed.

Spinal Block

Total spinal block (intrathecal) is considered in Chapter XV. As most of the sympathetic system is paralysed the blood pressure is largely dependent on the patient's position and this constitutes the basis of control.[1]

High epidural block. If a block is carried up to the level of T. 3 the systolic pressure usually falls to between 60 and 80 mm. Hg whatever was the initial pressure.[2] This effect is again caused by sympathetic paralysis and is accompanied by vaso-dilatation. See also Chapter XIV.

Arteriotomy

This technique is founded on experimental work in animals in which the effects of bleeding through an arterial cannula were studied.[3] It was found that it was possible to maintain a state of extreme hypotension for 135 minutes and if at the end of this time the blood was returned through the same cannula, recovery was

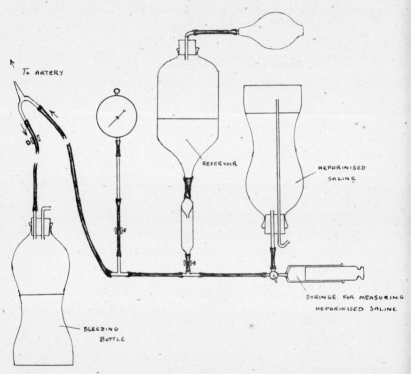

FIG. 96.   Diagram of apparatus for arteriotomy.   (Bilsland, by permission of *Anæsthesia*.)

quicker than if an intravenous re-transfusion was given.   The method was first used in man to control blood loss in cerebral surgery.[4]   The apparatus (Hales')[5] consists of a Y-shaped glass cannula which is introduced into the patient's radial artery.   One limb of the Y goes to a standard blood bottle containing 50 c.cm. of 3·8 per cent. sodium citrate solution into which the blood is withdrawn.   When 500 c.cm. have been collected it is transferred to the reservoir which is connected to the second limb of the Y from which it can be re-transferred through a safety drip-feed by raising the pressure by means of a hand bellows. Clotting is avoided by a 3-way tap and syringe controlling a supply of 500 c.cm. saline to which 5,000 units of heparin have been added.[6] This method is indistinguishable from hæmorrhagic shock and is presumably accompanied by vaso-constriction which would seem to constitute a theoretical disadvantage. Indeed in one technique a brachial plexus block is included in order to inhibit the arteriospasm which otherwise makes both the withdrawal and return of blood difficult.[10]

Drugs which block autonomic ganglia

The autonomic ganglia can be blocked by various drugs, those which have been investigated most fully being tetraethyl ammonium chloride and the methonium compounds. Since these drugs have an unselective action the effect produced is that of sympathetic and parasympathetic paralysis unlike the mainly sympathetic paralysis produced by spinal blocks. The chief side-actions on conscious patients are dryness of the mouth, paralysis of accommodation, gut distension (occasionally progressing to paralytic ileus) and difficulty in micturition. Since the blood pressure can be controlled to an appreciable extent by posture, it is practically certain that the hypotension is caused by loss of vasomotor tone.[9] Although the hypotensive effect of tetraethylammonium chloride was first described in 1914,[7] it has never been popular owing to its transient effects and various side-actions.

Pentamethonium (C.5) $\begin{cases} \text{bromide (lytensium)} \\ \text{iodide (antilusin)} \end{cases}$ was originally introduced as an antidote to the muscle relaxant decamethonium (q.v.) but was soon found to cause a marked fall in blood pressure. It is put up in 2·5 c.cm. ampoules containing 50 mg. of the drug.

Hexamethonium (C.6) $\begin{cases} \text{bromide (vegalysen)} \\ \text{iodide (hexathide)} \end{cases}$ has a very similar action to pentamethonium but is thought by some observers to have a more constant effect.[8] The methonium compounds are quaternery ammonium substances with very low lipoid solubility so that they probably become attached to the surface of the cells upon which they act but do not actually enter them.

Various techniques have been used, an initial intravenous dose of 20 mg. of either drug being common, subsequent injections, after a wait of at least three minutes, being given to maintain the systolic pressure at about 60 mm. Hg. If possible, a head-up tilt is maintained. It has been pointed out that young healthy adults tend to develop tachycardia with little hypotension and thus require a larger dose and steeper Trendelenburg tilt than older ones, especially those with arteriosclerosis who show little change in pulse rate but marked hypotension.[11]   Some workers believe in giving the comparatively large initial dose of 50 mg. to healthy adults but the technique cannot be regarded as safe.   A Gordh needle or one of its many modifications is useful for these multiple injections.

The excretion of penta- and hexa-methonium halides seems to be almost entirely through the kidneys, the actual mechanism being mainly glomerular filtration with minimal tubular excretion.[12] While a moderate degree of induced hypotension with the methonium drugs does not appear to impair renal function to an appreciable extent[17] yet in volunteers the glomerular filtration rate and urine flow dropped sharply and this prolongs the action of the drugs.[18] In patients with diseased kidneys, methonium hypotension may accelerate the rise in blood urea and precipitate uræmia.[19]   Even if this does not occur, the renal function may be further impaired.[20]

Effects on the liver have not yet been fully worked out but it has been observed that if the blood pressure drops below 60 mm. Hg., this organ becomes cyanosed, turgid and rubbery, indicating some degree of anoxia.   It seems certain that occult liver damage can result[21] and a fatal case of necrosis has been reported.[24]

Negative Pressure to Limbs

An ingenious adjunct to any method of controlled hypotension has recently been evolved.   It is well known that compression of the

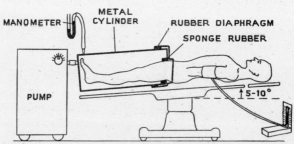

Fig. 97.   Negative-pressure device, showing application of cylinders to patient's leg.   (J. W. Saunders, *Lancet.*)

legs and thighs, e.g. by tight bandaging, raises the systolic blood pressure and conversely the application of negative pressure lowers it.   A metal cylinder encloses each of the patient's legs, a seal at the top of each thigh being made with a rubber diaphragm.   After a *moderate* fall of pressure has been induced, a vacuum of from 30 to 40 mm. Hg. is applied to the legs by means of a powerful suction pump, and this usually ensures a further pressure drop of about 30 mm. Hg. independent of posture. As the air pressure can be varied at will between wide limits, this technique probably reduces some of the risks of controlled hypotension.[22]

Anæsthetic Technique

When using controlled hypotension, the anæsthetist must remember that he has converted a comparatively fit patient into a temporarily shocked one and he will consequently require a greatly reduced dosage of narcotic drugs. Furthermore the reduced blood supply to vital organs makes it imperative that full oxygenation be ensured or some degree of anoxia will occur.

Post-operative Care

At the end of operation with the patient flat, the systolic pressure should be about 100 mg. Hg. If much below this figure a head-down slope must be adopted and if necessary 10 mg. of methedrine should be injected. It is most important that the head should not be raised in transit to the ward and constant supervision is essential until the blood pressure becomes stable.

Complications

Sudden death has occurred during controlled hypotension and is almost certainly due to coronary insufficiency. It is unfortunate that coronary disease occurs with increasing frequency in young patients who are apparently quite healthy and show normal ECGs. The condition may therefore be quite undiagnosable[13] and it is in patients suffering from it that the chief danger lies. The coronary blood flow is determined mainly by the aortic pressure[14] so that severe hypotension may reduce the flow to the point at which cardiac failure occurs.[15]

Embolism and thrombosis may take place in the brain as is shown when the patient recovers consciousness to find himself paralysed in one or more limbs. In conscious hypertensives, a 26 per cent. reduction of mean artificial pressure resulted in a 12 per cent. reduction of cerebral blood flow while the oxygen consumption remained unaltered. This resulted in symptoms of anoxia.[16] Under general anæsthesia, however, there is diminished cerebral oxygen consumption so that there is less risk of anoxia with mild degrees of hypotension. Blindness has occurred but the exact cause is obscure.[25]

Reactionary hæmorrhage is almost certainly increased in incidence as might be expected.

From a consideration of these facts it must be inferred that at the present time controlled hypotension should be reserved for patients suffering from a fatal disease or gross disability for the relief of which an operation is necessary which cannot be undertaken unless a bloodless field is provided.[15]

Contra-indications

It is obvious that to reduce the blood pressure seriously for a considerable time must be fraught with danger in many conditions amongst which would be placed the following :

angina and any state suggestive of coronary insufficiency ;

late stages of pregnancy in which fœtal death from anoxia might occur ;

cachectic and shocked patients ;

Addison's disease ;

chronic hypertension associated with pulmonary or renal disease;

tendency to cerebral thrombosis.

References
1. GRIFFITHS, H. W. C., and GILLIES, J.   Anæsthesia, 1948, Oct., p. 134.
2. BROMAGE, P. R.   Anæsthesia, 1951, Jan., p. 26.
3. KOHLSTAEDT, K. G., and PAGE, I. H.   Arch. Surg., 1943, 47, p. 178.
4. GARDNER, W. J.   Jour. Amer. Med. Ass., 1946, 132, p. 572.
5. HALE, D. E.   Anesthesiology, 1948, 9, p. 498.
6. BILSLAND, W. L.   Anæsthesia, 1951, Jan., p. 20.
7. MARSHALL, C. R.   Trans. Roy. Soc. Edin., 1914, 50, p. 379.
8. SHACKLETON, R. P. W.   Brit. Med. Jour., 1951, May 12, p. 1054.
9. { PATON, W. D. M.   Brit. Med. Jour., 1951, i, p. 773.
     McMICHAEL, J.   Pro. Roy. Soc. Med. (Sec. Med.), 1952, Feb. 26 (discussion).
10. MORTIMER, P. L. F.   Anæsthesia, 1951, July, p. 128.
11. { ENDERBY, G. E. H., and PELMORE, J. F.   Lancet, 1951, Mar. 24, p. 663.
      HUGHES, S.   Lancet, 1951, Mar. 24, p. 666.
12. YOUNG, I. M., et al.   Brit. Med. Jour., 1951, Dec. 22, p. 1500.
13. BLUMGART, H. L., et al.   Amer. Heart Jour., 1940, 19, p. 1.
14. ECKENHOFF, J. E., et al.   Amer. Jour. Physiol., 1947, 148, p. 582.
15. HAYWARD, G.   Anæsthesia, 1952, April.
16. KETY, S. S., et al.   Jour. clin. Invest., 1950, 29, p. 402.
17. EVANS, B., and ENDERBY, G. E. H.   Lancet, 1952, May 24, p. 1045.
18. { McQUEEN, E. G.   Med. Jour. Austral., 1952, i, p. 769.
      MACKINNON, J.   Lancet, 1952, July 5, p. 12.
19. ROSENHEIM, M. L.   Pro. Roy. Soc. Med. (Sec. Med.), 1952, Feb. 26.
20. BLAINEY, J. D.   Lancet, 1952, May 17, p. 990.
21. BROMAGE, P. R.   Lancet, 1952. July 5, p. 10.
22. SAUNDERS, J. W.   Lancet, 1952, June 28, p. 1286.
23. MILNE, G. E., and OLESKY, S.   Lancet, 1951, i, p. 889.
24. SHACKMAN, R., et. al.   Anæsthesia, 1952, Oct. p. 217.
25. GOLDSMITH, A. J. B., and HEWER, A. J. H.   Brit. Med. Jour., 1952, Oct. 4, p. 759.

CHAPTER XVII

COLLAPSE AND RESUSCITATION

Primary Cardiac Failure—" Status Lymphaticus "—Shock

THE anæsthetist may be confronted with two main types of collapse : firstly, sudden primary cardiac failure, and, secondly, the more gradual deterioration in a patient's condition conveniently described as shock, and which may, if severe and untreated, lead to secondary cardiac failure.

PRIMARY CARDIAC FAILURE

The *signs* of this rare catastrophe are obvious. The colour suddenly changes to a grey pallor, the pupils dilate widely and become inactive, the pulse is imperceptible and respiration becomes sighing in character and finally ceases.

The *causes* of primary cardiac failure are not so clearly defined. It is often associated with a light anæsthesia, usually maintained by chloroform or a mixture containing this drug. A severe surgical stimulus, the introduction of adrenaline into the circulation and status lymphaticus (q.v.) may be factors. The inadvertent injection of local analgesics into veins has also led to the condition, as has spinal analgesia.[1]

Without going into the exact mechanism of the cardiac failure, it is probable that in the early stages the heart is either : (i) beating very feebly ; (ii) in ventricular fibrillation ; or (iii) quiescent. This subject is considered further under " Chloroform ".

The *treatment* of primary cardiac failure is now fairly well standardized and can be summarized as follows :—

(i) Whatever may be the stage of the operation, it must be suspended at once and the patient tilted into a steep Trendelenburg position. There is no doubt that immediate **inversion** alone has frequently led to recovery.[2] The head-down tilt must not be allowed to persist for long or congestion will ensue. If the type of operating table permits, a head-down and head-up tilt can be alternated as it is said that " *rocking* " alone can produce an artificial circulation as well as an efficient respiratory exchange.[3] Too much faith should not be placed in this manœuvre.

(ii) The lungs should be slowly and rhythmically inflated with

pure oxygen (e.g. with the emergency tap on an intermittent
flow gas-oxygen apparatus (q.v.)). If no pressure is available,
efficient **artificial respiration** must be instituted, the Silvester
technique being shown by comparative tests to be the best in the
supine position.[4] The "respiratory pump" effect of the forced
breathing will aid a feeble circulation provided that such is in
existence. At the end of two to three minutes the situation must
be reviewed. If there is no improvement in colour or contraction
of the pupils, and if no pulse or heart beat can be detected it is
obvious that no efficient circulation is present and immediate steps
must be taken to restore it.

(iii) **Cardiac Puncture, Injection** and **Infusion.** The injection of
many different drugs into the heart has been followed by the restora-
tion of its normal rhythm. For instance, success has been reported
with adrenaline,[5] strophan-
thus, digitalis, camphor,
nikethamide, procaine,
strychnine and dextrose.[6]
Since these drugs act in
the most diverse ways,
the opinion is gaining
ground that it may be
the stimulation of the
needle which brings about
recovery.[7] As long ago

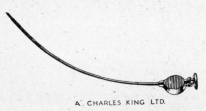

A. CHARLES KING LTD.

Fig. 98. Cardiac puncture and injection
needle. Hewer's modification of
Shipway's.

as 1887 it was shown that in twenty-two out of sixty dogs killed
with chloroform cardiac puncture alone restarted the heart.[8]
Furthermore, it has been proved that the intra-cardiac injection of
such drugs as adrenaline is not devoid of danger, as serious damage
may be done to the musculature. For example, abscesses in the
heart wall have been observed post-mortem.[9] A good deal of
recent research has been done upon cardiac puncture, and it is now
known that the auricles are more sensitive to stimulation than the
ventricles.[10] Auricular puncture is performed with a slightly
curved 5-inch needle inserted through the third right intercostal
space close to the sternum and directed downwards and towards
the middle line. In children the auricle lies within about 2 inches
of the anterior border of the sternum, whilst in adults the depth
varies from $3\frac{1}{2}$ to $4\frac{1}{2}$ inches.[6] It seems reasonable, therefore, to
perform auricular puncture with the special needle illustrated, and
if no response follows to inject from 50 to 100 mg. procaine in a
1 per cent. solution if there is reason to suppose that the ventricles

are fibrillating (see also cardiac surgery), adrenaline (up to 0·5 c.cm. of a 1 in 1,000 solution) should be reserved for those cases which show complete cessation of the heart's action either by vision or by palpation when cardiac massage is being performed. Owing to the difficulty of deciding at once whether fibrillation or arrest has occurred, it has been suggested that a mixture containing 9·5 c.cm. 1 per cent. procaine and 0·5 c.cm. 1 in 1,000 adrenaline should be at hand for immediate injection in primary cardiac failure.[11]

The first beats produced by cardiac puncture are usually extrasystoles followed by normal rhythm, but if the preceding period of anoxia has been prolonged, arrhythmia may develop into ventricular fibrillation. A more certain way of stimulating a stopped heart is by means of rhythmic electrical impulses. A special needle electrode has been devised in America which acts as an artificial pace-maker and imitates the normal sinus impulse. The complete apparatus weighs 16 lb. and is said to be very efficient.[12]

Intra-ventricular infusion of blood or saline has been suggested and one case of temporary resuscitation after this procedure has been reported.[13] The writer has had success in restarting an infant's heart by the rapid injection of 2 c.cm. saline into the left ventricle. It would seem wise to try distending the heart with an innocuous solution before injecting drugs whose action is largely unpredictable. Another way of temporarily filling an empty heart is to bandage the limbs rapidly with a rubber bandage from the periphery to the trunk.[14]

(iv) **Cardiac Massage.** If cardiac puncture has failed to elicit a response, massage of the heart must be attempted without delay. The first successful case was reported in 1902.[15] In 76 cases of primary heart failure collected from the literature, 20 were successfully revived by cardiac massage (Pieri). In children with flexible chest walls, subdiaphragmatic massage is usually effective, but in adults it may be necessary to detach the diaphragm from the left costal margin.[16] Definite squeezing movements of compression at the rate of from 60 to 80 per minute are carried out, an efficient circulation being indicated by a return of a pink colour to mucous membranes and by contraction of the pupils. If the aorta can be compressed distal to the origin of the left subclavian artery, the blood flow to the cerebral and coronary arteries will be increased.[124] Massage should not be abandoned for a considerable time,[17] one case being reported in which the heart responded after twenty-nine minutes.[18] When this event has occurred, an appreciable interval should elapse before closing the abdomen in order to make certain that the cardiac action is permanent. During the whole process, rhythmic infiltration of the lungs with oxygen should be maintained, and procaine or procaine amide given intravenously if this drug has not already been injected into the heart.[19] When a natural circulation has been re-established, spontaneous respiration as a rule soon returns, but if it is delayed for long it may be desirable to employ some form of mechanical artificial respiration. The somewhat elaborate " Drinker " apparatus is admirable for such cases.[20] The patient, with the exception of his head, is placed in an airtight chamber with a rubber diaphragm round his neck and intermittent negative pressure is applied to his body. His lungs thus expand, drawing in air from the outside as in normal respiration. An additional advantage of the " Drinker " machine is the maintenance of any desired temperature. Largely owing to the generosity of Lord Nuffield, a modification of this apparatus is available in most large hospitals in Great Britain.

(v) **Intra-arterial Perfusion.** In 1906 it was shown that the perfusion of Ringer's solution with adrenaline and hirudin into the central end of the carotid arteries of dogs killed by deliberate overdosage of chloroform and ether restarted the heart uniformly in five minutes although cardiac massage frequently failed. After ten minutes' cessation of circulation, consciousness was rarely restored, while after twenty-three minutes in adults and thirty-five minutes in puppies complete return of the circulation could not be accomplished by this method.[21] Later work has suggested that, as a last resort, the perfusion of 0·023 per cent. of calcium chloride in normal saline (0·25 c.cm. of saturated solution to 1 litre saline) into the brachial or carotid artery might be tried in man. A pressure of 150 mm. Hg. is desirable and can be obtained by keeping the funnel 6½ feet above heart level. The solution should be at body temperature and 1 c.cm. of 1 in 1,000 adrenaline chloride may be added, whilst oxygen can be kept bubbling through the liquid.[22] The chief aim of this proceeding is to maintain a suitable intra-coronary pressure, which is now recognized as being essential to the maintenance of the heart beat.[23] In the dog, it has been demonstrated that the blood flow through the coronary arteries varies with the mean aortic pressure.[24]

In Russia, several cases of resuscitation in battle casualties were described by injecting blood into an artery at a pressure of from 160 to 200 mm. Hg. It is said that under these circumstances the aortic valves close and that the blood is forced into the coronary arteries and the peripheral arterial tree. The lungs should be inflated rhythmically at the same time.[25] More recently several successful cases of resuscitation of patients moribund from severe traumatic shock during operation have been recorded in this country.[26] In an emergency, an arterial transfusion can be carried out with a standard intravenous set, the pressure being obtained by double bellows. It is preferable, however, to have the cork secured in the bottle, to use pressure tubing and minimize the risk of air embolus by a float in the drip chamber as in the Macintosh-Pask device (Fig. 67). (See also under arteriotomy.)

The chances of recovery after primary cardiac failure seem to depend almost entirely upon the length of time that the circulation has failed. The first cells in the body to be affected by anoxia are those of the cerebral cortex, and it has been shown in animals that irreparable damage occurs after about eight minutes of oxygen lack (see Chapter I). It would therefore appear probable that permanent recovery is unlikely if more than five minutes have elapsed between cardiac arrest and the establishment of an efficient circulation.[4] This is borne out in practice, and four different results may follow efforts at resuscitation :

(i) If an efficient circulation is re-established rapidly recovery may be complete.[27]

(ii) Slight damage to the cortical cells may be indicated by prolonged coma,[28] by convulsions or by mental deterioration after recovery.[29]

(iii) The heart may regain its normal rhythm and respiration may be restored, but the cerebral cortex has been so badly damaged that consciousness will not be regained. The patient is, in fact, in a similar condition to that of a " decerebrate " animal and will eventually die.[30] A case illustrating this condition has been fully reported recently. Death occurred on the 26th day of unconsciousness following cardiac massage for primary failure which supervened after the induction of spinal analgesia.[31]

(iv) In rare instances the heart will not respond at all, and cessation of the massage results in death.

From the above considerations it will be seen that time is the all-important factor in treating primary cardiac failure, and the measures which have been described carried out *at once* offer the only hope of recovery. They should be done in the order given and time will be saved if a cardiac puncture set is included in the emergency injection outfit normally kept in a sterile condition on the anæsthetic trolley.[32]

A word of warning to the young anæsthetist may not, perhaps, be out of place here. It must be reiterated that, if chloroform has not been used at all, primary cardiac failure during anæsthesia is a very rare condition. Before resorting to drastic measures, it is essential to be convinced that the circulation really has failed and that the condition is not one of excitement on the part of the surgeon !

The subject of resuscitation of the new-born is discussed in Chapter XXIV.

" STATUS LYMPHATICUS "

There is no doubt that " status lymphaticus " or more correctly " status thymico-lymphaticus ", has been unjustifiably used as a label for the cause of deaths occurring under general and local anæsthesia which could be explained in other ways. Several attempts have been made to discredit the existence of the condition[33] but many observers of great eminence such as E. H. Campbell, W. N. Kemp, Alan Moncrieff and Sir Bernard Spilsbury have been convinced that status lymphaticus is a definite entity. It is an undoubted fact that post-mortem examination of many children dying suddenly either during anæsthesia or after some shock or emotion, or even for no apparent reason at all, reveals the presence of definite changes. Occasional cases in adults are reported,[34] especially during labour.[35] It is worth noting that in a recent statistical survey of 142 fatalities associated with anæsthesia, three patients died from primary cardiac failure with no abnormal post-mortem finding, except general hyperplasia of lymphatic tissue and marked thymic enlargement (37, 50 and 50 grammes[125]). E. H. Campbell has summarized the modern view of this condition as " those who have had personal experience with such cases and those who have given the subject careful investigation and study cannot doubt the existence of a pathological condition of such lowered resistance and hyper-susceptibility that the patient so affected is in danger of sudden death from trivial causes ".[36]

History. Status lymphaticus has been recognized as a clinical entity for over 300 years, and a graphic account with accurate post-mortem observations was made by Felix Platter, Professor of Medicine at Basle in 1641.[37] The condition was named status lymphaticus by Paltauf in 1889.

Diagnosis. It is extremely difficult to recognize status lymphaticus during life, but the following characteristics are suggestive : Fat, flabby children with pale, smooth skin, scanty hair and adenoid facies. Adrenal insufficiency may be shown by leucocytosis, low blood pressure, hypoglycæmia, increased coagulation time and lowered alkaline reserve. Allergic symptoms may also be present.[38] In an analysis of 249 cases of status lymphaticus at autopsy the condition was found to be six times as common in males as in females.[39]

Moncrieff considers that the following features in infants are very suggestive of this condition. (1) Intermittent head retraction and stridor. (2) Attacks of syncope sometimes accompanied by dyspnœa and cyanosis. (3) An enlarged thymus shown by X-ray examination.

The three " classical " signs are usually given as :

"Sergent's Sign." Delay or failure in reddening when the skin of the chest or abdomen is lightly scratched.

"Orroya's Sign." Delay in the contraction of the pupil to light. More useful eye signs, however, appear to be follicular conjunctivitis and bilateral trachoma.[40]

"Schridde's Sign." Prominence of lymphoid follicles on the pharyngeal wall between the tonsils.

These signs must be regarded as inconstant and unreliable.

Post-mortem Changes. Largely owing to the work of Sir Bernard Spilsbury, the post-mortem findings are now well recognized, and comprise (a) a markedly enlarged thymus gland (which might conceivably cause pressure on the trachea,[41] vagus or recurrent laryngeal nerves[42]) ; (b) hyperplasia of lymphoid tissue throughout the body, especially marked in the case of Peyers' patches and solitary follicles ; and (c) fatty degeneration of the heart with narrowing of the aorta.[43]

In anæsthetic deaths occurring in " status lymphaticus ", chloroform or a mixture containing it has generally been used, but a few fatal cases have been recorded under ether, ethyl chloride and nitrous oxide.[44]

The **causes** of the cardiac failure in this condition have recently been the subject of much discussion,[45] as indeed has the mechanism of the disorder as a whole.[46, 47, 48] It is outside the scope of this book to go deeply into the matter, but it appears to the author that the most reasonable theory is that advanced by Kemp, who considers that it is caused by a temporary hypofunction of the adrenal cortex in a child already handicapped by inadequate thyroid function due to insufficiency of dietary iodine. (It should be noted that a condition closely resembling status lymphaticus has been produced experimentally by removing seven eighths of a dog's adrenal cortical tissue.) " The lymphatic glands and the thyro-thymic apparatus attempt to compensate for this lack of adrenal cortical secretion and the subsequent upset in body chemistry that this lack involves.   Hence the enlarged thymus, far from being the cause of status lymphaticus, is a compensatory hyperplasia on the part of the thyroid-thymus defence mechanism."[45]

Treatment. X-ray therapy is said to be beneficial probably by raising the calcium content in the serum and cerebrospinal fluid.[49] The administration of calcium gluconate and parathyroid before anæsthesia has been suggested with the same object in view.[40] Local irradiation of the thymus gland by X-rays or radium appears to cause a diminution in its size and an amelioration of the general condition.[43] If allergic symptoms are present, skin tests should be applied, and, if positive, desensitization carried out. Kemp considers that one minim of a saturated solution of potassium or sodium iodide should be given thrice weekly with 3 grains of adrenal cortical extract three times a day. In practical anæsthetics there is no doubt that the best way to avoid primary cardiac failure from status lymphaticus is to eschew the use of chloroform or any mixture containing it for children.

SHOCK

The term " shock " was introduced by James Latta in 1795. The whole subject is extremely involved and it is only possible to consider here the aspects which concern the anæsthetist. For a more detailed account of the theoretical viewpoint of shock, the reader is referred to the excellent article by E. A. Pask.[50]

Clinical Signs. The clinical signs of shock occurring during an operation are pallor, sweating, coldness of the skin, rising pulse rate, falling blood pressure (systolic more than diastolic), dilated pupils and spaced or sighing type of respiration. The first four signs are indicative of compensatory sympathetic stimulation. Some of these signs may be modified by the anæsthesia or type of operation. Attempts have been made to reduce degrees of shock to actual figures of blood pressure and pulse rates. Thus McKesson recognized three degrees of shock, but these formulæ do not take into consideration the very great variations from normal which a patient may exhibit even before anæsthesia is induced, and too much reliance should not be placed upon them. A persistently rising pulse rate, combined with a falling pulse pressure, gives perhaps the most reliable indication of the onset of shock. (The latest devices for measuring blood pressures are referred to in the next chapter.) The skin temperature of the forehead can be taken by a mercury thermometer and a fall exceeding 3° F. is indicative of considerable shock.[51]

Pathological Changes. The essential pathological change in shock is now thought to be such a diminution in the total volume of circulating blood that compensatory mechanisms (such as arterial contraction and the discharge of blood from the spleen) are insufficient and the vascular system is no longer adequately filled.[52] This leads to such effects as a fall in blood pressure, tissue anoxia, etc. If death occurs, it is thought to be due to secondary cardiac failure from acute coronary insufficiency. This conception distinguishes true shock from depressed conditions of the circulation, such as that seen during spinal analgesia (q.v.).

Apart from actual loss from hæmorrhage, the location of the missing blood is probably in the capillaries of the relaxed muscles. The former view that it was in the splanchnic area is demonstrably false. Simultaneous red corpuscle counts of blood from the veins and capillaries show a much higher count in the latter,[53] which is probably due to increased permeability of the capillary endothelium from dilatation. It is possible that tissue anoxia can cause a further transudation of fluid from the blood, a further decrease in the effecting blood volume and yet more severe tissue anoxia, thus completing a vicious circle.[54] Attempts have been made to estimate the degree of shock by the hæmo-concentration, but various factors must be allowed for, e.g. the effect of any hæmorrhage on the red blood count, etc.[55]

Although it is true that the alkali reserve is often diminished in shock, recent work suggests that the importance of " acidosis " may have been exaggerated.

The basal metabolic rate is diminished.

The shock syndrome can be produced by so many different conditions that other pathological changes must be considered under causes. The artificial division of shock into " primary " and " secondary " (by E. M. Carvell during the 1914-18 war) will be ignored in this chapter.

Causes. The causes of operative shock can be classified as follows :

    I. Severe emotions, e.g. fear in " psychic shock ".

    II. Loss of fluids.
       (1) water — (*a*) visible and invisible sweating.
            (*b*) respiratory loss.
       (2) blood and plasma — (*a*) hæmorrhage.
            (*b*) extravasation.

III. Trauma to $\begin{cases} \text{(1) nerves in "reflex shock".} \\ \text{(2) muscles, etc., in "histamine shock".} \end{cases}$

IV. Loss of heat, e.g. from exposed viscera and from cold inhaled vapours.

V. Overdose of anæsthetic, relative or absolute.

VI. Oxygen deficiency from obstructed airway, etc.

VII. Excessive duration-time of operation.

Prophylactic Measures

The causes of shock are so varied that it will be necessary to deal with them separately when discussing preventive measures.

Psychic Shock can be practically abolished by making use of preliminary hypnotics, basal narcosis or suggestion (q.v.). Crile recognized the importance of psychic shock many years ago when elaborating his "anoci-association" technique[56] (see also Chapter I).

Dehydration is by no means a negligible factor in shock, since it has been calculated that during an operation of moderate severity no less than 1 litre of fluid is lost.[57] If the surgical condition permits, the patient should be encouraged to drink up to three hours before operation and pre-operative purging reduced to a minimum. Sweating accounts for about three-quarters of the fluid lost, and can be much reduced by avoiding rubber sheeting as far as possible and by the pre-operative administration of an adequate dose of atropine. Respiratory loss can be almost abolished by total rebreathing (q.v.).

If pre-operative dehydration has occurred, it should be established whether this is mainly due to loss of water only, e.g. from inadequate fluid intake, or from salt as well, e.g. from loss of secretions, diarrhœa, vomiting, etc., and appropriate measures should be taken to correct the deficiency.

Hæmorrhage. In the 1914-18 war it was estimated that 25 per cent. of the blood volume could be lost before the blood pressure fell noticeably and that a further loss of 25 per cent. usually proved fatal.[58]

The reduction of blood loss during operation has been given great attention by anæsthetists in recent years and is discussed in Chapter XVI.

It has been shown by microscopic inspection of the peripheral vessels in dogs that the administration of ether causes great diminution of the peripheral compensatory mechanism in hæmorrhage. Cyclopropane does not produce this effect while soluble thiopentone gave variable results. This work confirms the clinical observation that ether should preferably be avoided if hæmorrhage has occurred or is anticipated.[59]

" **Reflex** " **Shock** was at one time thought to be due to exhaustion of the vaso-motor centre from excessive stimulation. The modern view, however, is that there is a definite inhibition of the centre by " nocioceptive " afferent stimuli. This type of shock can be minimized by deep general anæsthesia,[60] and practically prevented by suitable nerve blocking or by curare (q.v.).

" **Histamine** " **Shock** supposes that some histamine-like toxin is produced from lacerated tissues and absorbed.[61] It has been shown that chloroform and ether (but not nitrous oxide) sensitize the capillaries to the action of histamine so that its effects are increased.[62] It would therefore appear desirable to use pure nitrous oxide-oxygen anæsthesia on patients suffering from this type of shock. There is no doubt that the adoption of this practice saved many lives during the 1914-18 war. Some recent workers, however, have cast doubt upon the above theory,[63] and the presence of a depressor substance in the blood of a shocked animal cannot be said to have been definitely proved.[64] Many physiologists, therefore, now hold the view that shock following muscle injury is accounted for by the mere extravasation of blood and plasma.[65] On the other hand, it has been shown that an injection of histamine into some patients produces a temporary fall in blood pressure followed by a considerable rise, and that these patients are the most likely to suffer from operative shock. It has also been shown that this predisposition can be overcome by prophylactic injections of 0·5 mg. to 1 mg. of histamine for eight to ten days before operation. It is thought possible that toxic substances released into the circulation may be the cause of the grave impairment of renal function due to an arterial by-pass or shunt, seen in the " **crush syndrome** ".[66] Some workers, on the other hand, regard the cause as mere anoxia of the kidney cells. If the condition is evident or seems to be impending, an intravenous infusion of up to 1 litre of a 4·28 per cent. solution of sodium sulphate at the rate of 100 drops per minute is said to aid the secretion of urine.[67]

Loss of Heat can to some extent be limited by an adequately heated theatre and an efficient insulating pad (e.g. sorbo rubber) between the patient and the table. The anæsthetist can prevent appreciable heat loss from respiration by avoiding open methods of administration and employing complete rebreathing (q.v.),

Anæsthesia must be maintained at as light a level as is possible for existing conditions, since in very deep narcosis the heat-regulating centre is depressed and metabolism is greatly reduced, thus tending towards further lowering of body temperature.[68] The question of applying external heat to a shocked patient is considered at the end of this chapter.

Overdose of Anæsthetic. An overdose must be carefully avoided, and it is well to bear in mind the **" law of diminishing resistance "**, which was propounded many years ago by Gill. This states that " the amount of a drug required to produce a given depth of anæsthesia diminishes with the time of its administration ".[69] Shock, due mainly to anæsthetic overdose, can be distinguished from that due to other factors by means of the **" depression test "**. A large volume of oxygen is suddenly added to the anæsthetic mixture and the blood pressure is noted. A sudden rise indicates overdosage (especially with nitrous oxide and ethylene). If no appreciable change occurs, the shock is due to other causes.[70] Overdosage of local analgesics, and particularly their introduction into a vein, can produce signs similar to those of shock. If shock develops during the course of an operation, the plane of narcosis can nearly always be lightened with advantage.

Oxygen Deficiency. As mentioned above, if shock has already started, the tissues become short of oxygen and acidosis may occur (Haldane). It therefore seems reasonable to suppose that any further oxygen deficiency will increase the shock. It is fortunate that shock so increases the susceptibility to anæsthetics that even with a weak agent such as nitrous oxide, the oxygen content of the mixed gases can frequently exceed that of normal air. The effects of anoxia on the liver have been discussed in Chapter I.

Time Factor. Modern anæsthesia has made possible operations of a severity and duration unthought of thirty years ago. There is a regrettable tendency, however, to prolong operations unnecessarily, and this must increase shock. The factors already considered become cumulative after a certain length of time.[71] In the past it has been said that a patient must not be left for more than twenty minutes with a systolic pressure below 80 mm. Hg. or a diastolic pressure of less than 60 mm. Hg. If this time be appreciably exceeded death is extremely probable within forty-eight hours.[72] This is a palpable exaggeration as pressures below these are deliberately maintained for considerable periods in the techniques for producing controlled hypotension (q.v.).

Treatment

The treatment of shock occurring during or immediately after operation can be summarized as follows :

(1) LOWERING THE HEAD and, if possible, tilting the whole body into a steep Trendelenburg position. This results in increased venous return ensuring adequate filling of the heart which results in accordance with Starling's law, in a rise of blood pressure and slowing of the pulse rate. On the other hand a change of position every fifteen minutes is desirable or the cephalic congestion will become predominantly venous resulting in cardiac and respiratory embarrassment.[73] See also under " gynæcological operations ".

(2) ENSURING ADEQUATE OXYGENATION OF THE BLOOD by seeing that the airway is perfectly clear and, if necessary, by increasing the oxygen percentage in the inspired mixture. In certain cases only, the addition of 5 per cent. carbon dioxide may be desirable, as it has been shown that acapnia can increase shock.[60] On the other hand, the theory advanced by Henderson[74] that the symptoms of shock were due to a deficiency of CO_2 in the blood is no longer generally accepted.[75]

(3) FLUID REPLACEMENT. *Intravenous* normal **saline** appears at first sight the obvious method. It has been shown (McKesson) that the optimum effect is obtained when the systolic pressure has been restored to within 10 per cent. of the patient's normal figure. A smaller volume of fluid is inefficient while a larger one introduces the risk of cardiac dilatation. The comparatively sudden increase in blood volume almost certainly accounts for the deaths which have occasionally occurred immediately after the transfusion of compatible blood.[76] In practice two signs can be sought for if there is reason to believe that the circulation is being overloaded. The pulse rate shows a second rise and crepitations at the bases of the lungs may indicate the onset of pulmonary œdema. It should be noted that saline for intravenous use must not only be absolutely sterile but free from dead bacteria and other extraneous matter or " reactions " may occur. If fresh triple-distilled water is not available, sterile normal saline should be obtained from the makers in sealed bottles.[77]

In severe shock, venous spasm may slow down the rate of drip to a serious extent and this can often be overcome by injecting 5 c.cm. of 1 per cent. **procaine** into the tubing.[78] This also applies to a blood transfusion.

As an alternative to normal saline, if salt depletion is not present,

4 per cent. **dextrose** in 0·18 per cent. saline (" Bart's " solution) is commonly used.

During the 1914-18 war, Bayliss introduced the 6 per cent. solution of **gum-acacia** in normal saline on the supposition that the vessels were unduly permeable in shock and that a viscous solution would have a more permanent effect than pure saline.[79] Later investigation showed, however, that gum-saline may have a toxic effect on the liver and other organs and may interfere with the gaseous interchanges in the red blood corpuscles.[80] Several deaths have been caused by its employment, the preceding syndrome being characterized by dyspnœa, tachycardia, cyanosis and pulmonary œdema.[81]

Solutions of **isinglass, pectin**[82] and **gelatin**[83] have been tried in America but have not proved very satisfactory.

During the late war, the German army used a plasma substitute called "**periston** " in which a plastic known as polyvinylpyrrolidon (P.V.P.) provided viscosity.[84] This product has since been improved and is now known as **plasmosan** in the United Kingdom and as **subtosan** in France.[85] It is a sterile 3·5 per cent. aqueous solution of P.V.P. with electrolytes, i.e. sodium, potassium, calcium, magnesium and chloride ions. Its pH. is 5·7-7, its S.G. 1·012 and its viscosity about twice that of water. It is supplied in standard 540 c.cm. British transfusion bottles.

Since the end of the war, **dextran (intradex)** has also proved satisfactory. It is a polysaccharide produced by the effects of an enzyme upon sucrose. The large molecule maintains the osmotic tension of the blood and the solution stays in the vessels. It is used in a concentration of 6 per cent. in 0·9 per cent. saline.[86]

Serum and **plasma** have both given much satisfaction in shock unaccompanied by gross hæmorrhage, i.e. in cases where marked hæmo-concentration is present. There are no important differences in action of these two fluids and as they have a high colloidal osmotic pressure they show little tendency to transude through the capillary walls. Both serum and plasma can be dried for storage or transport and reconstituted by the addition of sterile distilled water.[87] Unfortunately, however, they both suffer from the serious drawback that they can transmit the virus of homologous serum jaundice. This risk may be as high as 10 per cent. in those transfused. It is possible that irradiation with ultra violet light may diminish the hazard.[88]

The very slow drip intravenous saline technique introduced by Friedmann in 1913[89] still has its advocates and may be combined with 1 in 250,000 **adrenaline** or *nor*-**adrenaline** (**arterenol levophed**) (see also later and under spinal analgesia). A very careful watch must be kept on the blood pressure when using the latter drug and the danger of embolism following prolonged infusions is not

OH	OH

Adrenaline   CHOH   ĊHOH   *nor*-adrenaline
              CH₂   CH₂
              N   N
            H   CH₃   H   H

negligible.[90]   Suprarenal cortical extract, e.g. " **eschatin** ", has also been used in doses of from 10 to 20 c.cm. in 250 c.cm. saline with the object of restoring capillary tone.[91]   In really desperate cases of shock, fluids can be given intravenously under positive pressure. It is even possible to give 1,500 c.cm. in ten minutes, but very great care must be taken for such heroic measures.[87]   An alternative technique much used in battle casualties is to give fluids into two or three veins simultaneously.[92]

If much hæmorrhage has occurred during operation, or if the patient is known to be anæmic, **whole blood transfusion** may be of great benefit.   It is now recognized that a fairly fast drip transfusion is an excellent prophylactic against shock during severe operations where considerable hæmorrhage is inevitable.   A rate of 40 drops per minute is equivalent to a pint of blood in four hours or a rise of 10 per cent. hæmoglobin in an adult.   This should be regarded as the basic rate and increased in proportion to the amount of bleeding which is occurring[93].   The blood must be of the same ABO group as that of the patient and should always be cross-matched.   Rh-negative blood should be used for (*a*) young women who are Rh-negative, (*b*) all Rh-negative patients who are likely to require further transfusions or who have previously had them ; (*c*) mothers of babies who have had hæmolytic disease ; (*d*) babies suffering from hæmolytic disease.

Really severe anæmia can be treated by using **concentrated erythrocytes** (" packed red cells ").   The fluid is prepared by taking two bottles of blood after maximum sedimentation has occurred, i.e. five to six days, siphoning off the supernatant plasma and adding the red cell deposit from one bottle to the other.

Several cases of fatal air embolism during intravenous infusions have recently been reported. There are two common causes of this disaster. In the first place, if the regulating clip is placed just below the bottle and above the drip-chamber, the pressure of the fluid just below the drip will be less than that of the atmosphere and a slight leak at the rubber-glass junction will result in air being sucked into the infusion.[94] Secondly if the " gas mantle " type of filter is used, it may become choked with sludge during a blood transfusion. An attempt to speed up the rate of drip by applying pressure from a Higginson's syringe can then force air into the infusion.[95] The glass float type of drip chamber (see p. 154) eliminates this risk.

Intra-arterial transfusion (see earlier) is well worth trying in very severe cases of surgical shock.

Intramedullary infusions can be used if for any reason a vein is impracticable. In adults, sternal puncture is the most convenient method, using a winged needle.[96] In infants, infusions can be made into the marrow of the tibia by means of Tocantin's needle[97] (see also under " intramedullary anæsthesia ").

Fluid administered *per rectum* is absorbed slowly, at first into the tissue spaces and lymph, and by the time it actually reaches the blood other substances, such as proteins, are drawn into it from the tissues. In this way the lowering of viscosity and osmotic pressure of the blood (which always occurs after intravenous saline infusion) are negligible, and the fluid having reached the blood stream will stay in it and not transude out again into the capillaries. Consequently, unless an immediate effect is imperative, there is a good deal to be said for using the rectal route, especially after operation. Plain tap water at body temperature is most commonly used, but if salt or glucose are considered necessary they should be given in slightly hypotonic concentrations. Some authorities maintain that glucose is not absorbed below the ileo-cæcal valve[98] but the writer considers this to be unlikely. Wesley Bourne dislikes glucose on account of the hyperglycæmia present during shock and uses a hypotonic alkaline solution containing potassium, which is said to be most stimulating in depressed states (Nothmann *et al.*). The concentrated stock solution is potassium bicarbonate ($KHCO_4$) 100 g., disodium phosphate crystals ($Na_2HPO_4 : 12H_2O$) 358 g. dissolved in 2 litres of distilled water ; 1 oz. of this mixture is added to 1 pint of warm distilled water and 1 pint of this diluted fluid to 50 lb. of the patient's body weight is given *per rectum*.[99]

Subcutaneous saline is not efficient by itself and has been known to cause extensive sloughing of tissues in debilitated patients. The discovery of the " spreading factor " has, however, revived interest in the method.[100] Very briefly the theory is that hyaluronic acid, a viscous polysaccharide, forms the ground substance or cement of tissue spaces. The enzyme **hyaluronidase** depolymerizes this acid and reduces its viscosity to that of water.[101] This enzyme can be isolated from testicular extract and a purified form is now on the market under the names **hyalase, hydase** and **rondase**. Each ampoule contains 1,000 " Benger units " (1 mg.) of sterile powder and this should be freshly dissolved in 1 c.cm. of sterile water. This is sufficient to add to from 500 to 1,000 c.cm. of saline, dextrose or plasma which can then be injected subcutaneously at a greatly accelerated speed. If desired the hyaluronidase can be added to the injection by puncturing the drip tubing with the needle of a hypodermic syringe. This technique can be of outstanding value in shocked patients with collapsed veins and in young children where intravenous therapy presents technical difficulties.

The *intra-peritoneal* route is discussed under abdominal surgery.

(4) INSULIN AND HYPERTONIC GLUCOSE. It has been shown that the blood sugar is high during shock and that the administration of **insulin** will reduce this and simultaneously raise the blood pressure.[102] In the light of these findings it is curious that the intravenous injection of **hypertonic glucose** has also been found to be beneficial. A dose of 50 to 100 c.cm. of 50 per cent. glucose causes a considerable rise in blood pressure within five minutes. This is maintained for about half an hour, when there is a slight drop, followed by a more gradual secondary rise in both systolic and pulse pressures. It is essential to employ chemically pure glucose for these injections or severe reactions may occur.[103] A buffer salt is usually added so that the solution is maintained at the neutral point, but even so venous thrombosis is not uncommon. It seems possible that glucose causes these effects in a similar way to gum-saline by altering the viscosity of the blood.

(5) PRESSOR or " ANALEPTIC " DRUGS may be administered to tide over an emergency, but too much reliance should not be placed upon them, nor should they be used if the cardiac muscle is known to be degenerated. The drugs most commonly used in (alphabetical order) are :

Adrenaline and *nor*-**adrenaline** have already been mentioned. It is now considered practically certain that *nor*-adrenaline is the transmitter at sympathetic nerve endings, and that the enzyme amine-oxidase destroys it, just as acetylcholine is the transmitter at cholinergic nerve endings and that cholinesterase destroys it.[123]

Cycliton (3-5 dimethyl isoxazol-4-carboxylic acid diethylamide) which is put up in a 25 per cent. solution.

Ephedrine (discussed in Chapters XIII and XV).

Icoral, a combination of m-hydroxy-N-ethyldiethyl-amino-ethyl-amino benzol which has a similar action to lobeline, and hydroxy-phenyl-propanolamine which acts in the same way as ephedrine.[104]

Leptazol (azoman, cardiazol, hexazol, phrenazol, triazol) is pentamethylene tetrazol. The B.P. injection is a 10 per cent. solution with a dose of from 3 to 5 c.cm.

Methedrine (desoxyephedrine, pervitin) is N-methyl amphetamine.

$$CH_2CH(NH.CH_3)CH_3$$

This has a very prolonged effect in raising the blood pressure, and the writer has been favourably impressed by it. The intramuscular dose is 15 to 30 mg., but if an immediate effect is required 15 mg. can be given intravenously as well as 15 mg. intramuscularly.[105]

Neosynephrine (meta-sympatol) is α-hydroxy-β-methyl-amino-3-hydroxy-ethyl benzene.

$$CHOH.CH_2NH.CH_3$$
$$OH$$

This drug is closely allied to adrenaline and should not be used in cases of thyrotoxicosis[106] (q.v.). The adult intravenous dose is from 4 to 5 mg.

Nikethamide (anacardone, coramine, corvotone, nikamide) is pyridine-β-carbonic acid diethylamide.

$$CO.N \begin{cases} C_2H_5 \\ C_2H_5 \end{cases}$$

Five c.cm. of the 25 per cent. solution injected intravenously usually causes an immediate rise in blood pressure and respiratory stimulation. An intramuscular injection gives a more prolonged effect.

Paradrine is p-hydroxy-α-methyl phenyl ethylamine hydrochloride.

$$CH_2CH.NH_2CH_3$$

HO

It has had some vogue in America to raise the blood pressure during spinal analgesia. The adult intramuscular dose is from 10 to 20 mg., or it can be given intravenously in about half these quantities.[107]

Phedracine (**Preparation 2020 Ciba**) is trimethoxybenzyldihydroimidoazol hydrochloride.

$$CH_3O$$
$$CH_3O \quad CH_3O$$

$$CH_2C. \; NH$$
$$N \quad CH_2$$
$$CH_2$$

The usual intramuscular dose is 0·2 g. and the intravenous dose 0·1 g.[108]

Pholedrine (**paredrinol, pholetone, veritol**) is chemically β(p-oxyphenyl) isopropylmethylamine.

$$CH_2CH(NH.CH_3)CH_3$$

HO

The adult intramuscular dose is 1 c.cm. and the intravenous dose 0·2 to 0·25 c.cm. of the 2 per cent. solution. Although animal experiments were not very encouraging,[109] good results have been obtained in man with this drug.[110]

The above drugs are given by the intramuscular, or, preferably, the intravenous route, but **amphetamine** (**benzedrine**) (benzyl-methyl-carbamine)

$$CH_2CH.NH_2CH_3$$

occurs as a vapour at ordinary temperatures and pressures. The drug has been added to the anæsthetic mixture by a special device attached to the gas-oxygen apparatus.[111]

The mode of action of pressor drugs is not entirely clear as the normal mechanism of maintaining blood pressure is still not certain. The current theory[121] is that it depends on three factors : it is high in proportion to the volume of circulating blood, and to the constriction of the arteries by (a) sympathetic impulses depending on the release of nor-adrenaline at the sympathetic nerve endings, and (b) by pressor amines from the adrenal glands ; it is reduced by the activity of the enzyme mono-amine oxidase present in the blood vessels.[122] If this view is correct, it would seem logical to give nor-adrenaline by infusion as this reinforces the normal mechansim of increasing vascular tone. Adrenaline acts in a similar way but has a greater effect on the heart. Both these drugs, however, reduce the renal blood flow when given to anæsthetized patients with hypotension.[113] Ephedrine and methedrine probably act by inhibiting mono-amine oxidase. Neosynephrine, phedracine and pholedrine may act similarly or directly on the heart and blood vessels.[112] Nikethamide and leptazol act mainly as medullary stimulants causing vaso-constriction. This group in greater than analeptic dosage produce convulsions. The pharmacological actions of the three pressor drugs in commonest use can be summarized in the following table.

Drug	Cardiac Output	Peripheral Resistance	B.P.	Pulse Rate	Blood flow to			
					Muscles	Skin	Intestines	Kidney
Adrenaline ..	+ +	−	+	+	+	−	? +	−
nor-adrenaline..	0	+ +	+	−	− −	−	−	−
Methedrine ..	+	−	+	0	+	−	? +	+

It must be confessed that at the present time the choice of drugs is apt to depend less on their specific effects than on the intensity of advertising propaganda of their respective manufacturers.

(6) THE MAINTENANCE OF BODY TEMPERATURE is important both during operation and afterwards. On the other hand, electric cradles and other devices must be used with discretion as excessive peripheral vaso-dilatation may divert much-needed blood away from the vital organs (see below).

(7) VITAMIN ADMINISTRATION. It is thought by some that lipoid-soluble anæsthetics such as chloroform and ether interfere with the proper functioning of the fat-soluble vitamins stored in the liver. If concentrated solutions of vitamins A and D (e.g. " dekadexolin ") are injected just before operation, it is claimed that shock is diminished if chloroform or ether is used as the anæsthetic agent.[114]

It must be realized that hypotension occurring during an operation can be due to causes other than shock. A very rough classification[126] can be based on the pulse rate as under :

(1) Hypotension with raised pulse rate due to reduction of cardiac output as described above under " shock ".

(2) Hypotension with unchanged pulse rate due to reduction of vasomotor tone as in spinal block (q.v.) and best treated by analeptic drugs.

(3) Hypotension with bradycardia possibly due to overaction of the vagal mechanism and sometimes overcome by atropine.

Shock occurring before Operation

In air raid and battle casualties, as well as in industrial and road accidents, the anæsthetist may be called upon to deal with patients already severely shocked. If at all practicable, efficient anti-shock measures must be taken before the administration of an anæsthetic. These have already been described and will include rest, relief of pain, fluid replacement, stimulants and oxygen therapy.

It should not be forgotten that one of the effects of trauma is marked delay in the emptying of the stomach, and the anæsthetist must always be on his guard against regurgitation in shocked patients.[115]

The importance of heat used to be stressed, but recent work by Blalock has modified our previous views. A shocked patient is suffering from a depletion of the circulating blood volume. If external heat is applied, the blood vessels of the skin dilate, and it has been estimated that as much as 500 c.cm. of blood can be diverted from the vital organs. Furthermore, the increased heat creates a greater tissue demand for oxygen which may not be forthcoming. The present view is that coldness of the skin is a protective reflex in shock and that heat should be applied internally (as by hot drinks) rather than externally.

Some divergence of opinion exists as to the choice of anæsthetic technique for shocked patients and it has even been stated that the actual agent used does not matter provided that it is administered properly. This is definitely not the case and certain lessons have been learnt from the last two wars. For example, it is agreed by all that further depression must be avoided and no anoxia allowed. Shocked patients are very sensitive to *all* anæsthetics and require much smaller doses than normal.

It is the writer's view that any inhalation anæsthetic should be given by means of a closed circuit, the method of choice being nitrous oxide with a relatively high percentage of oxygen. It is often possible to use a higher proportion of oxygen than is present in atmospheric air and yet to obtain satisfactory anæsthesia in severely shocked patients. If any adjuvant is necessary, cyclopropane is preferable to ether (as mentioned above) while chloroform should seldom be used. For chest casualties, cyclopropane-oxygen is ideal. The North African campaign has demonstrated that contrary to expectations it is perfectly practicable to use cyclopropane near the front line of rapidly moving armies.[116] A recent investigation into shocked patients whose plasma volume had been reduced by trauma has suggested that cyclopropane-oxygen was preferable to all other anæsthetics.[117] Local blocks can sometimes be used profitably, but large quantities of analgesic solutions and spinal blocks cause further depression of circulation and should be avoided. The intravenous barbiturates have proved extremely useful during the late war, but they should be given in the smallest possible doses and combined with an analeptic in order to minimize further falls in blood pressure and respiratory depression. There is experimental evidence to show that in animals suffering from moderate loss of blood, a smaller dose of thiopentone will cause respiratory failure than in normal animals. Disastrous results can follow the *indiscriminate* use of the intravenous barbiturates in shocked patients as was shown after the Japanese air raid on Pearl Harbour on December 7th, 1941.[118]

The Medical Research Council has recently issued a memorandum on the lessons learned about traumatic shock in the second World War and the reader is referred to this for much detailed information which is impossible to give in this book.[119]

Finally it should be noted that badly shocked patients very readily develop pulmonary complications. It is, in fact, the view of a prominent physiologist that a terminal broncho-pneumonia is often only an expression of delayed shock.[120]

References

1. MILLS, G. P.   *Brit. Med. Jour.*, 1935, Jan. 26, p. 153.
2. { JONES, B. S.   *Brit. Med. Jour.*, 1912, *i*, p. 421.
   { SHIPWAY, F.   *Brit. Jour. Anœsth.*, 1932, Jan., p. 75.
3. EVE, F. C.   *Brit. Med. Jour.*, 1947, Aug. 23, p. 295.
4. { WATERS, R. M., and BENNETT, J. H.   *Anesth. & Anal.*, 1936, May-June.
   { GREENFIELD, J. G.   *Jour. Neurol. & Psychiat.*, 1938, *i*, p. 306.
   { WALLACE, E. J. G.   *Brit. Med. Jour.*, 1952, Aug. 2, p. 278.
5. SCHAFER, E. S., and BAIN, W. A.   *Pro. Roy. Soc. Edin.*, 1932, Jan., p. 139.
6. { SHIPWAY, F.   *Pro. Roy. Soc. Med.*, (An. Sec.), 1931, Dec. 4.
   { BLATCHLEY, D.   *Brit. Med. Jour.*, 1935, May 30, p. 1134.

7. { BODON, C.   *Lancet*, 1923, *i*, p. 586.
{ GLOVER, R. M.   *Brit. Med. Jour.*, 1926, *ii*, p. 342.
8. WATSON, B. A.   *Trans. Amer. Surg. Ass.*, 1887, **5**, p. 275.
JOHNSON, S., and SIEBERT, W. J.   *Amer. Heart. Jour.*, 1928, **3**, p. 279.
9. { SMIRNOW, A. J.   *Zeitschr. f. d. ges. exper. Med.*, 1927, **57**, p. 554.
{ DOOLEY, M. S.   *Anesth. & Anal.*, 1936, Sept.-Oct., p. 246.
10. HYMAN, A. S.   *Arch. Int. Med.*, 1930, **46**, p. 553.
11. ANDERSON, R. M., *et al.*   *New Eng. Jour. Med.*, 1950, **243**, p. 905.
12. { HYMAN, A. S.   *Arch. Int. Med.*, 1932, **50**, p. 284.
{ HEWER, C. L.   *Brit. Med. Jour.*, 1935, Aug. 3.
13. GOVERNALE, S. L., and RINK, A. G.   *Brit. Med. Jour.*, 1944, July 8, p. 43.
14. WOODWARD, W. W.   *Lancet*, 1952, Jan. 12, p. 82.
15. { ROOME, N. W.   *Surg. Gyn. & Obst.*, 1933, **56**, p. 161.
{ BOST, T. C.   *Lancet*, 1918, *ii*, p. 552.
16. { NORBURY, L. E. C.   *Lancet*, 1919, *ii*, p. 601.
{ COLEMAN, R. C.   *Brit. Med. Jour.*, 1921, *i*, p. 47.
17. OGILVIE, W. H.   " Recent Advances in Surgery," 2nd edit., p. 147.
18. BOHN, G. L.   *Brit. Med. Jour.*, 1939, Oct. 7, p. 725.
19. LAMPSON, R. S., *et al.*   *Jour. Amer. Med. Ass.*, 1948, Aug. 28, p. 1575.
20. Described in *Lancet*, 1931, *i*, p. 1186.
21. CRILE and DOLLEY.   *Jour. Exper. Med.*, 1906, **8**, p. 713.
22. KEMP, W. N.   *Brit. Jour. Anæsth.*, 1933, July, p. 156.
23. MACLEOD, J. J. R.   " Physiol. and Biochem. in Modern Med.", 1930, p. 383.
24. WRIGHT, S.   " Applied Physiology," 1947.   Oxford Univ. Press, p. 447.
25. *Soviet War News,*, 1944, **982**, p. 3.
26. { DEVITT, D., and WIDGEROW, C.   *Brit. Med. Jour.*, 1951, Aug. 4, p. 278.
{ BAYLES, O.   *Anæsthesia*, 1951, Oct., p. 233.
{ BINGHAM, D. L. C.   *Lancet*, 1952, July 26, p. 157.
27. { BALL, W. G.   *Brit. Med. Jour.*, 1926, April 24.
{ MILLS, G. P.   *Brit. Med. Jour.*, 1935, Jan. 26, p. 153.
{ COLE, P. P.   *Brit. Med. Jour.*, 1935, March 9, p. 503.
{ GRANT, R. A.   *Brit. Med. Jour.*, 1935, p. 64.
28. PETTY, M. J.   *Lancet*, 1919, *ii*, p. 784.
29. MOLLISON, W. M.   *Pro. Roy. Soc. Med.* (An. Sec.), 1916, **10**, p. 9.
30. LANGLEY, G. F.   *Brit. Med. Jour.*, 1935, March 9, p. 503.
31. HOWKINS, J., *et al.*   *Lancet*, April 6, p. 488.
32. BAILEY, M.   *Brit. Med. Jour.*, 1941, July 19, p. 84.
33. *Joint Com. Med. Res. Counc. & Path. Soc. Gt. Brit. & Ire.*, 1931.
34. PINEY, A.   *Brit. Med. Jour.*, 1941, Sept., 20, p. 423.
35. COOKE, R. G.   *Brit. Med. Jour.,*, 1944, April 1, p. 457.
36. CAMPBELL, E. H.   *Penn. Med. Jour.*, 1937, **41**, p. 907.
37. PLATTER, F.   " Observationes in hominis affectibus pleurisque," 1641.
38. CAMPBELL, E. H.   *Anesth. & Anal.*, 1940, July-Aug., p. 228.
39. SYMMERS.   *Belleview Hospital, New York.*
40. MADAN, K. E.   *Anesth. & Anal.*, 1940, July-Aug., p. 224.
41. RABSON, S. M.   *Jour. Pediat.*, 1949, **34**, p. 166.
42. TAYLOR, J. F.   *Pro. Roy. Soc. Med.* (An. Sec.), 1939, Dec. 1.
43. { *Brit. Jour. Anæsth.*, **8**, No. 3, p. 81.
{ MONCRIEFF, A.   *Pro. Roy. Soc. Med.* (Dis. Chil. Sec.), 1938, Jan.
{ MILLAR, W. G., and ROSS, T. F.   *Jour. Path. and Bact.*, 1942, Oct., p. 455.
44. DAVIES, W.   *Brit. Jour. Anæsth.*, **8**, No. 3, p. 112.
45. KEMP, W. N.   *Anesth. & Anal.*, 1932, **11**, No. 3, p. 128.
46. PRICE, F. W.   " Textbook of Pract. of Med.", 1930.
47. SLOT, G.   *Pro. Roy. Soc. Med.*, 1929, May, p. 901.
48. CHALMERS, R.   *Brit. Med. Jour.*, 1932, Feb. 13, p. 308.

49. HENSON, C. W.　*New York State Jour. Med.*, 1933, Sept. 1, p. 860.
50. PASK, E. A.　*Brit. Jour. Anœsth.*, 1941, July, p. 129.
51. CLUTTON-BROCK, J.　*Pro. Roy. Soc. Med.* (An. Sec.), 1947, May 2.
52. *Rep. Shock Com., Med. Res. Counc.*, 1918.
53. COWELL, E. M.　*Brit. Med. Jour.*, 1939, April 29, p. 883.
54. MOON, V. H.　" Shock and Related Capillary Phenomena," 1938. Oxford.
55. GOULD, R. B.　*Med. Press. & Circ.*, 1943, Sept. 8, p. 151.
56. CRILE and LOWER.　" Surgical Shock," 1920.　Philadelphia.
57. COLLER, F. A., and MADDOCK, W. G.　*Jour. Amer. Med. Ass.*, 1932, **99,** p. 875.
58. *Med. Res. Counc. Special Reports*, 1919, Nos. 25 and 26.　London.
59. HERSHEY, S. C., et al.　*Anesthesiology*, 1945, July, p. 362.
60. McDOWALL, R. J. S.　*Brit. Med. Jour.*, 1933, April 22, p. 690.
61. CANNON, W. B., and BAYLISS, W. B.　*Rep. Shock Com. M.R.C.*, 1919.
62. WRIGHT, S.　" Applied Physiology," 3rd edit., p. 309.
63. O'SHAUGNESSY and SLOME.　*Brit. Jour. Surg.*, 1935, **22,** No. 87.
64. HOLT, R. L.　*Pro. Roy. Soc. Med.* (Surg. Sec.), 1935, April 3.
65. BLALOCK, A.　*Arch. Surg.*, 1930, **20,** p. 959.
66. McMICHAEL, J.　*Brit. Med. Jour.*, 1932, Dec. 5, p. 671.
67. MORGAN, A.　*Med. Jour. Austral.*, 1942, Sept. 5, p. 193.
68. FEATHERSTONE, H. W.　*Brit. Med. Jour.*, 1937, July 31, p. 225.
69. GILL, R.　" The $CHCl_3$ Problem," **2,** p. 81, etc.
70. McKESSON, E. I.　*Canad. Med. Ass. Jour.*, 1927, **17,** p. 1314.
71. GILLIES, J.　*Pro. Roy. Soc. Med.* (An. Sec.), 1943, March 5.
72. KAYE, C.　*Austral. & N.Z. Jour. Surg.*, 1937, April, p. 772.
73. BURSTEIN, C. L.　" Fundamental Considerations in Anesthesia," 1949. New York, p. 53.
74. HENDERSON, Y. ⎰ *Amer. Jour. Physiol.*, 1908, **21,** p. 126.
　　　　　　　⎱ *ibid.*　　　　　1909, **24,** p. 66.
　　　　　　　　 ibid.　　　　　1910, **25,** p. 385.
75. ROOME, N. W.　*Surg. Gyn. & Obst.*, 1933, **56,** p. 161.
76. PYGOTT, F.　*Brit. Med. Jour.*, 1937, Mar. 6, p. 496.
77. BAILEY, H.　*Brit. Med. Jour.*, 1938, Feb. 5, p. 294.
78. ORGANE, G. S. W., and SCURR, C. F.　*Brit. Med. Jour.*, 1948, Oct. 30, p. 787.
79. BAYLISS, W. M.　" Wound Shock and Hæmorrhage," 1919.
80. RAVEN, R. W.　*Brit. Med. Jour.*, 1940, June 8, p. 950.
81. STUDDIFORD, W. E.　*Surg. Gyn. & Obst.*, 1937, April, p. 772.
82. McMICHAEL, J.　*Brit. Med. Jour.*, 1942, Dec. 5, p. 671.
83. EVANS, E. I., and RAFAL, H. S.　*Ann. Surg.*, 1945, April, p. 478.
84. HECHT, G., and WEESE, H.　*Münch. med. Wschr.*, 1943, **90,** p. 11.
85. ⎰ THROWER, W. R., and CAMPBELL, H.　*Lancet*, 1951, May 19, p. 1096.
　　⎱ ARDEN, G. P., et al.　*Lancet*, 1951, May 19, p. 1099.
86. ⎰ BULL, J. P., et al.　*Lancet*, 1949, Jan. 22, p. 134.
　　⎱ MAYCOCK, W. D.　*Lancet*, 1952, May 31, p. 1081.
87. ⎰ BOND, D. D., and WRIGHT, D. C.　*Ann. Surg.*, 1938, Apr., p. 500.
　　⎱ RAVEN, R. W.　" War Wounds and Injuries," 1943.　London.
88. BLANCHARD, M. C., et al.　*Jour. Amer. Med. Ass.*, 1948, **138,** p. 341.
89. FRIEDMANN, M.　*Munch. med. Woch.*, 1913, **60,** p. 1022.
90. WALTER, C. W.　*Jour. Amer. Med. Ass.*, 1935, **104,** p. 1688.
91. MORGAN, A. D.　*Med. Jour. Austral.*, 1942, Sept. 5, p. 193.
92. BINNING, R.　*Lancet*, 1945, April 21, p. 515.
93. WINTERTON, W. R.　*Jour. Obstet. Gyn. Brit. Empire*, 1937, June, p. 510.
94. ⎰ SIMPSON, K.　*Lancet*, 1942, *i*, p. 697.
　　⎨ MACINTOSH, R. R., and MUSHIN, W. W.　" Physics for the Anæsthetist." Oxford, p. 134.
95. DOLTON, E. C., et al.　*Lancet*, 1945, April 28, p. 531.

96. BAILEY, H. *Brit. Med. Jour.*, 1944, Feb. 5, p. 181.
97. ELLISON, J. B. *Brit. Med. Jour.*, 1944, Feb. 19, p. 266.
98. MCNEALY, R. H., and WILLENS, J. P. *Surg. Gyn. & Obst.*, 1929, **49**, p. 794.
99. BOURNE, W. *Yale Jour. Biol. & Med.*, 1938, Dec., p. 155.
100. DURAN-REYNALS, F. *Jour. exp. Med.*, 1929, **50**, p. 327.
101. GAISFORD, W., and EVANS, D. G. *Lancet*, 1949, **2**, p. 505.
102. MINNITT, R. S. *Pro. Roy. Soc. Med.* (An. Sec.), 1932, Dec. 2.
103. POLAK, *et al.* *Amer. Jour. Obst. & Gyn.*, 1931, **22**, p. 817.
104. SCHOEN, R., and LEMMEL, C. *Klin. Woch.*, 1933, No. 21.
105. DODD, H., and PRESCOTT, F. *Brit. Med. Jour.*, 1943, Mar. 20, p. 345.
106. JOHNSON, C. A. *Surg. Gyn. & Obst.*, 1936, July, p. 35.
107. ALTSCHULE, M. D., and GILMAN, S. *New Eng. Jour. Med.*, 1939, Oct. 19, p. 600.
108. JONES, F. A., and WILSON, C. *Lancet*, 1938, Jan. 22, p. 195.
109. SCHOENEWALD, G., *et al.* *Lancet*, 1940, March 23.
110. DODD, H., and MERTON, C. *Brit. Jour. Surg.*, 1939, July.
111. TOVELL, R. M. *Anesth. & Anal.*, 1938, Sept.-Oct., p. 271.
112. ELMES, P. C., and JEFFERSON, A. A. *Brit. Med. Jour.*, 1942, July 18, p. 65.
113. CHURCHILL-DAVIDSON, H. C., *et al.* *Lancet*, 1951, Nov. 3, p. 803.
114. LEAK, W. N. *Brit. Med. Jour.*, 1939, Dec. 9, p. 1163.
115. GREEN, H. N., and HARBORD, R. P. *Pro. Roy. Soc. Med.* (An. Sec.), 1946, Dec. 6.
116. BINNING, R. *Brit. Med. Jour.*, 1944, May 5, p. 620.
117. CROOKE, A. C., *et al.* *Brit. Med. Jour.*, 1944, Nov. 25, p. 683.
118. HALFORD, F. *Anesthesiology*, 1943, Jan., p. 67.
119. " Observations on General Effects of Injury in Man." M.R.C. No. 277. H.M.S.O. 1951.
120. GREEN, H. N. *Pro. Roy. Soc. Med.* (An. Sec.), 1946, Dec. 5.
121. *Brit. Med. Jour.* Annotation. 1951. Dec. 29, p. 1571.
122. THOMPSON and TICKNER. *Jour Physiol.*, 1951, **115**, p. 34.
123. BURN, J. H. *Brit., Med. Jour.* 1952, Apr. 12, p. 784.
124. CARTER, M. G. *Jour. Amer. Med. Ass.*, 1951, **147**, p. 1347.
125. BROWN, G. *Adelaide Hosp. Rep.*, 1950, **30**, p. 45.
126. INGLIS, J. M. *Lancet*, 1952, Aug. 23, p. 362.

CHAPTER XVIII

ANÆSTHESIA AND ANALGESIA FOR NEURO-SURGERY

THE demands made by cranial surgery upon anæsthesia have increased very greatly in the last few years. When the late Sir Victor Horsley first made craniotomy a relatively safe operation in this country, a duration of half an hour was rarely exceeded, and chloroform was a perfectly satisfactory anæsthetic. This " rapid " technique was developed by the late Sir Percy Sargent and others who extended the scope of cranial surgery considerably, and although extensive tumours were removed, the time of operation was usually under one and a half hours. Ether, generally administered by the endotracheal route, gave excellent results in such cases. More recently, however, the " slow " method, in which the late Dr. Harvey Cushing took such a prominent part, has, to a certain extent, come into vogue. In one well-known clinic, the average duration of major cranial operations is five hours, whilst a time of twelve hours has on occasion been exceeded.[1] The vexed question as to whether the end-results justify the immense time taken by surgeons of the " slow " school is of great interest,[2] but cannot with propriety be discussed in a book of this nature. There is no doubt, however, that these excessively long operations have profoundly modified anæsthetic technique, since the continued use of toxic drugs, such as chloroform or ether, is not permissible, as severe toxic symptoms may ensue. The other difficulties which confront the anæsthetist are the frequent use of the diathermic cautery, the necessity to keep the brain volume at its minimum, the impossibility of approaching the face when the operation has started and the patient's position which is often anything but physiological.

Posture

As a rule, subtemporal decompressions, frontal explorations, and gasserectomies are performed with the patient lying on his back or in the sitting position. The latter posture frequently leads to an unstable blood pressure and if the intracranial venous pressure is negative, air embolism is an ever-present danger. Some surgeons like the anæsthetist to compress the jugular veins from time to time in order to raise the venous pressure and demonstrate open

veins.[3] Cerebellar and occipital explorations formerly took place
in the prone position with the head fixed on a special rest and flexed
as far forward as possible. This position frequently raised an
already high intracranial pressure with disquieting effects upon the
respiratory centre. The introduction of the Crutchfield caliper has

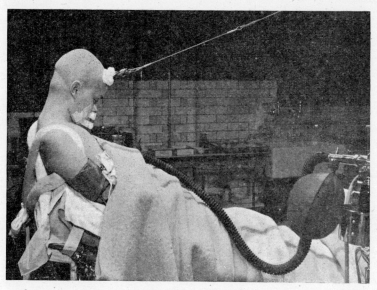

Fig. 99.   The Crutchfield caliper in use for operation upon the posterior
fossa.   The patient is held forward by the wire attached to the caliper
and is also supported by pillows to help maintain him in a semi-sitting
position.   A foot-piece prevents the patient sliding down the table.
(Photo, *Neuro-surgical Department, St. Bartholomew's Hospital.*)

proved a boon to the anæsthetist. This device is fixed into the
frontal bones and a steel wire supports the head in a flexed position
with the patient half sitting up.[10] The intracranial pressure is not
raised and the surgeon enjoys better access than in the prone
position.

Operations for the removal of prolapsed intervertebral discs,
laminectomies, etc., are now usually performed in the lateral position
which causes no special difficulty. Sometimes, however, the surgeon
requires the prone posture which necessitates careful management.
It is imperative that unimpeded movements of the thorax and
abdomen should be permitted and this is usually attained by

arranging for the body weight to be borne on longitudinal sandbags under the shoulders and pelvis. It is important to avoid a rigid transverse support below the abdomen or pressure on the inferior vena cava may cause imperfect filling of the heart and congestion of the veins of the epidural space. Pressure on the stomach can cause regurgitation, and it is wise to pass a stomach tube after tracheal intubation and to leave it in position throughout the operation.

Premedication

Heavy premedication before cranial operations is usually inadvisable, a mild sedative accompanied by reassurance being preferable. If morphine or an allied preparation is used, it must be ascertained that the patient reacts normally to it as a surprising proportion of people are nauseated or may actually vomit. Pethidine can often be used profitably instead of morphine combined with atropine instead of the normal scopolamine in order to stimulate rather than depress respiration. Similarly if full basal narcosis is deemed to be necessary, rectal paraldehyde is preferable to bromethol. Opiates are particularly dangerous in patients with high intracranial pressure and with cerebellar lesions.

Local Analgesia

Local analgesia alone is useful when the patient is comatose, and for comparatively short operations in adults such as repair of scalp lacerations, subtemporal decompression, ventriculography, cisternal encephalography, etc. The method is, however, unsuitable for lumbar encephalography owing to the intense headache produced, and also for prefrontal leucotomy on account of the patient retaining terrifying recollections.[4]

The *technique* of local analgesia for cerebral operations is simple. A polygon is described around the proposed field by means of wheals not more than 5 cm. apart and connected by subcutaneous infiltration. The periosteum is insensitive so that subperiosteal injections are unnecessary. If, however, muscle is included in the area, it must be injected. The process of trephining is always described by a conscious patient as definitely unpleasant.[5] The dura is not sensitive except towards the base of the skull and along the course of the middle meningeal artery, while the brain itself is quite insensitive, except in the region of the Sylvian fissure. Procaine-adrenaline solution is suitable for short procedures, amethocaine being substituted for longer operations.

Basal Narcosis Combined with Local Analgesia

When a prolonged cranial exploration or the removal of an extensive tumour is contemplated, the average patient has not sufficient fortitude to face the ordeal with pure local analgesia. Even assuming that no pain whatever is felt, the strain of keeping in one uncomfortable position for several hours is insupportable. Enthusiasts for local techniques should read the description of a patient's sensations during a prolonged craniotomy in the book entitled " A Journey round my skull " by Frigyes Karinthy.

It might be thought that the ideal method would be to combine a basal narcotic with local analgesia. This is often satisfactory for short craniotomies and many such operations have been performed under the morphine-bromethol-local technique. An advantage of bromethol in cranial surgery is that it lowers the blood pressure and is thought by some to affect the intracranial pressure in the same way.[6] Observers are, however, not agreed upon this point.[7] The dangers of respiratory depression when using these agents has already been mentioned. If very prolonged operations are attempted, the effects of the drug may wear off and the patient may get into a restless, non-coöperative state and become uncontrollable. Repeated injections of hyoscine are sometimes of use in such a condition,[8] but to be absolutely certain of continuous quietude, some form of general anæsthesia is necessary. In many neurosurgical clinics local analgesia has been largely replaced by general techniques.[9]

Local and General Anæsthesia

In chordotomy for the relief of pain due to inoperable neoplasms, the level of analgesia obtained by division of the spino-thalamic tracts in the antero-lateral columns must be accurately known. In consequence, these operations were performed under local analgesia which proved most unpleasant ordeals for both patients and surgeons. A modified method has recently been used with success.[10] After a normal induction, narcosis is maintained by means of nitrous oxide and oxygen given through a naso-pharyngeal tube, the mouth and free nostril being occluded with adhesive strapping. Local infiltration of the tissues is carried out after the patient has been placed in position and the operation is started, and continued until the surgeon is ready to incise the cord. The pharyngeal tube and strapping is then removed and the patient is allowed to regain consciousness. The antero-lateral columns are incised and the resulting level of analgesia is ascertained by response to pinprick.

When satisfactory, intravenous thiopentone is given, the naso-pharyngeal tube is replaced and the operation completed under nitrous oxide and oxygen. It is, of course, essential to have a coöperative patient to whom the whole procedure has been carefully explained beforehand.

Intravenous Anæsthesia

Lumbar encephalography is performed in the sitting position and can be done quite satisfactorily under intravenous thiopentone anæsthesia. After induction, the needle is kept in the vein and just enough of the 5 per cent. solution is injected from time to time to avoid reflex movements. The head is held by an assistant and its position altered as required. Narcosis is usually too light for an artificial airway to be tolerated, but the jaw must be kept forward to avoid the slightest respiratory obstruction.

Endotracheal Anæsthesia

In the writer's opinion, the only satisfactory anæsthetic technique for major craniotomies is the endotracheal one. Several points must be borne in mind.

In the first place it is essential to maintain a perfectly clear airway with no pressure in the respiratory circuit. This is best attained by the passage of the largest orotracheal tube which can be inserted without trauma. An inflatable cuff is not necessary but a plain Magill's tube is liable to kink in certain positions of the head. A flexible metal case slipped over the tube[11] (illustrated) is some

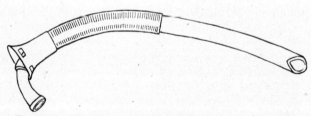

Fig. 100.   Flexible metal case to fit over orotracheal tube.
(J. C. Bournè, *Brit. Med. Jour.*)

protection from kinking, but the writer prefers the armoured tracheal tubes now obtainable with the metal spiral embedded in their walls. Introduction of such a tube is most easily effected under light general anæsthesia followed up by a relaxant such as tubocurarine or gallamine. If difficulty is experienced, the tube can be threaded on to a small blunt-ended gum-elastic catheter which is passed previously and subsequently withdrawn. The tube should be lubricated with a long-acting analgesic jelly[12] such as " Brennan's paste " :—

> Paraff. dur. gr. xv.
> Cera alb. gr. xxx.
> Paraff. moll. alb. $\mathfrak{Z}$i.
> Nupercaine base 10 per cent.

An equally effective lubricant is 5 per cent. xylocaine ointment which has the advantage of a water-soluble base which has no action on rubber. Having inserted the tube, it should be adjusted so that its tip lies approximately half-way between the cords and the bifurcation of the trachea. This gives a certain latitude for alteration of the position of the patient's head. Otherwise extreme flexion may pull the tip of the tube out of the trachea and extreme extension may cause it to impinge on the carina and cause a bout of coughing.[13] When it is certain that the tube is accurately placed, it must be firmly fixed with a harness or strapping so that there is no possibility of it being dislodged during the operation. The anæsthetist must make perfectly certain that the breathing is absolutely free before the sterile towels are fixed in position rendering further access to the face impossible. It is worth noting that slight respiratory obstruction practically never gets less as time proceeds. On the contrary it nearly always becomes worse.[13]

Anæsthesia can be maintained with high flows of nitrous oxide (about 60 per cent.) and oxygen (about 40 per cent.) with minimal trichlorethylene. Ether should seldom be used, even in the absence of the diathermy, as it raises the intracranial pressure. A semi-closed circuit is generally used with the expiratory valve set to blow off at practically no pressure. Alternatively the T-piece technique can be employed with both arms of the T composed of wide-bore corrugated rubber tubing. With a total gas flow of about 8 litres a minute, extremely quiet respiration can be obtained and the open end of the tube is accessible to the hand and ear of the anæsthetist who can thus be certain that respiration is unimpeded.[14] Small doses of thiopentone (which lowers intracranial pressure) can be given from time to time into the intravenous drip tubing.[16]

It is important to maintain a constant level of narcosis and to keep a chart of systolic, diastolic and pulse rate readings so that changes are noted at once and their causes ascertained. A high intracranial pressure is often accompanied by tachycardia. In this condition it is dangerous to open the dura, as the brain may become extruded and strangulate unless the incision is rapidly extended. A small intravenous dose of hexamethonium will rapidly lower the blood pressure and secondarily the intracranial pressure (q.v.). In some clinics the arteriotomy method of controlling pressure is adopted and blood can be withdrawn or re-transfused as required[15] (see Chapter XVI). These methods have largely replaced the intravenous injection of hypertonic saline, glucose[19] or sucrose which

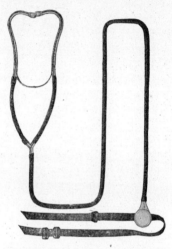

Fig. 101.   Stethoscope connected
to small plastic chest-piece for
slipping under inflating cuff.
B.O.C.

were formerly much used to lower the intracranial pressure.[20] Hypothalamic circulatory failure is usually shown by fall in blood pressure followed by a rise in pulse and respiratory rates. Medullary anoxia, on the other hand, is characterized by bradycardia and a high blood pressure.[3]   If any of these changes occur, they should be reported to the surgeon for appropriate action.

Blood pressure readings are not always easy to take but various devices are available. In one the flat stethoscope end is screwed into a 2 inch square plate which, in turn, is sewn to the lower angle of the fabric containing the inflation cuff. The stethoscope is consequently fixed in position by winding on the cuff and does not tend to slip like the usual separate brachial stethoscope attached to a narrow band. Alternatively small plastic chest pieces are now obtainable which can be slipped under the inflating cuff over the brachial artery (Fig. 101). The tubing for the bellows, gauge and stethoscope should be in lengths of about 7 ft. for neuro-surgical work.[17] A recent development is the cuff inflator illustrated which

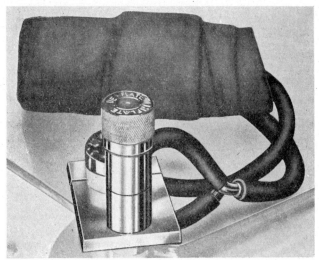

M.I.E LTD.

Fig. 102. Sphygmomanometer cuff inflator. (Williams'.) M.I.E.

is attached to the reduced oxygen pressure pipe-line and avoids the necessity for bellows.[21]

If available, a sphygmoscope can be used which eliminates the stethoscope altogether and affords visual measurement of the systolic and diastolic pressures by means of two cuffs on the arm or leg.[18]

References

1. GILLESPIE, N. A. *Anesth. & Anal.*, 1935, Sept.-Oct., p. 225.
2. MENNELL, Z. *Brit. Jour. Anæsth.*, 1935, Oct., p. 3.
3. HUNTER, A. R. *Pro. Roy. Soc. Med.* (An. Sec.), 1952, Mar. 7.
4. FLEMING, G., and MCKISSOCK, W. *Lancet*, 1943, March 20.
5. KAYE, G. *Austral. & N.Z. Jour. Surg.*, 1937, Oct., p. 141.
6. WOOD, D. A. *Anesth. & Anal.*, 1933, **12**, p. 38.
7. BEECHER, H. K. V. " The Physiology of Anæsthesia," London, 1938.
8. DOTT, N. M. *Pro. Roy. Soc. Med.* (An. Sec.), 1933, March 3.
9. RENTON, D. G. *Austral. & N.Z. Jour. Surg.*, 1938, July, p. 37.
10. Technique used by neuro-surgical unit, St. Bartholomew's Hospital.

11. BOURNE, J. C.　*Brit. Med. Jour.*, 1947, Oct. 25, p. 654.
12. BRENNAN, H. J.　*Lancet*, 1938, Feb. 5, p. 315.
13. HEWER, A. J. H.　*Pro. Roy. Soc. Med.* (An. Sec.), 1952, Mar. 7.
14. BULLOUGH, J.　*Brit. Med. Jour.*, 1952, Jan. 5, p. 28.
15. { GARDNER, W. J.　*Jour. Amer. Med. Ass.*, 1946, **132,** p. 572.
       HALE, D. E.　*Anesthesiology*, 1948, **9,** p. 498.
       BILSLAND, W. L.　*Anæsthesia*, 1951, Jan., p. 20.
16. LEE, J. A.　*Brit. Jour. Anæsth.*, 1945, Jan., p. 101.
17. FLOOD, A. D.　*Brit. Med. Jour.*, 1944, Nov. 25, p. 696.
18. EVANS, D. S., and MENDELSSOHN, K.　*Brit. Med. Bull.*, 1946, vol. 4,
       No. 2, p. 99.
19. MENNELL, Z.　*Pro. Roy. Soc. Med.* (An. Sec.), 1933, Mar. 3.
20. HAHN, E. V., *et al.*　*Amer. Med. Ass.*, 1937, **108,** p. 773.
21. WILLIAMS, T. M.　*Brit. Med. Jour.*, 1951, Nov. 3, p. 1087.

CHAPTER XIX

ANÆSTHESIA AND ANALGESIA FOR DENTAL SURGERY
Local Analgesia—General Anæsthesia—General Analgesia

LOCAL ANALGESIA

AT the present time local analgesia is usually employed for dental extractions in adults who dislike nitrous oxide and when the injections can be made into normal tissues. In certain cases also an immediate extraction may be necessary when the services of an anæsthetist are not available. Local analgesia is inadvisable in young children and where the needle point would have to penetrate inflamed or septic tissues.[1] The indiscriminate employment of the method has led to severe complications and even death, and dentists generally are realizing the very real dangers of disseminating infection.[2]

The **syringes** used for dental work are sometimes constructed of metal with large finger grips so that considerable pressure can be

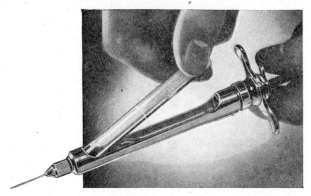

Fig. 103. Dental cartridge syringe ejector type.

exerted. The needles must be sharp, a fresh one being preferable for each case. Owing to the difficulty of rapid sterilization, cartridge syringes are tending to displace the metal ones. The glass cartridges are filled with 2 c.cm. sterile procaine and adrenaline and are sealed at each end with rubber corks. One of these is fixed

295

by a flange and when inserted into the holder is pierced by one end of a double pointed stainless steel needle. The other rubber cork acts as a plunger and slides down the cartridge which becomes the

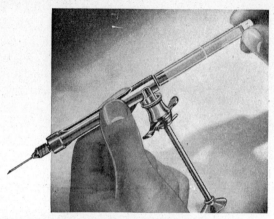

FIG. 104. Dental cartridge syringe breech-loading type.
(Amalgamated Dental Trade Distributors, Ltd.)

barrel of the syringe. The method of inserting the cartridge into the holder varies with different makes and two common types are illustrated.

Cocaine is still used to some extent in spite of its obvious disadvantages. It has, however, been largely displaced by 2 per cent. *procaine* and 1 in 100,000 *adrenaline*, and latterly by *nupercaine* (0·1 per cent. with adrenaline).

Infiltration Analgesia. Two injections are usually made at an angle of 45° to the long axis of the tooth to be extracted, the mucous membrane being pierced near the free margins of the inter-dental tags in front of and behind the tooth. A single injection is then made into the lingual side of the gum towards the apex of the tooth. This method is generally employed when one or two teeth are to be extracted. Many observers think, however, that an appreciable delay in healing is usual.[3]

Nerve Block Analgesia is mainly used for multiple extractions, the chief nerves concerned being the anterior, middle and posterior superior dental nerves from the maxillary division of the trigeminal, the inferior dental and lingual nerves from the mandibular division of the trigeminal, and the nasopalatine and anterior palatine nerves from Meckel's ganglion. The successful blocking of the required nerves in the various fossæ and foramina demands an exact anatomical knowledge and considerable practice. It is worth noting that the addition of hyaluronidase to the analgesic solution increases the chance of a successful block from a greater spread of fluid.[30]

So-called " **Pressure Analgesia** " is sometimes used for the removal of dental pulp. A strong solution of cocaine on a small piece of absorbent material or solid cocaine is forced under pressure into the pulp. The latter can then be removed relatively painlessly.[4]

GENERAL ANÆSTHESIA

Before the induction of general anæsthesia for short dental operations, a prop should usually be inserted. If the central

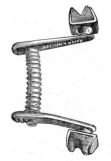

FIG. 105. Wingrave's swivel prop.

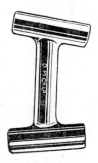

FIG. 106. Lateral prop (Mushin's).

incisor teeth are not affected, a swivel prop enables both sides of the mouth to be reached without changing and gives considerably more room than do the clumsier metal, wood and rubber varieties. If, however, a side prop is needed, the one designed by Mushin is useful. It is made of chromium-plated German silver with rubber biting plates having a fine canvas impression. These plates are set at an equal angle to the central rod and subtend an angle of 20°.[5]

Young children are generally anæsthetized with the single-dose open **ethyl chloride** technique, which gives ample time for six or eight extractions. This method is extremely rapid and safe, as evidenced by the fact that at large children's hospitals many thousands of cases are done yearly without ill-effects.[6] One series of no less than 123,000 consecutive administrations has been reported without accident[7] and another of 125,000.[8] The disadvantages of ethyl chloride are the unpleasant smell (greatly masked in the scented product) and a slight tendency to cause nausea and vomiting after administration. The majority of children, however, are fit to go home within half an hour of operation.

Various attempts have been made to give continuous ethyl chloride for prolonged dental operations, and an ingenious apparatus

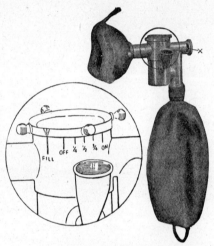

Fig. 107. " Oxford " closed inhaler for divinyl ether (modified from Goldman's). X=inlet valve to allow inspiration of air should bag inadvertently become empty. Enlargement in circle shows wheel control for vapour concentration. (*Lancet*).

called a " somnator " had some vogue in Germany. By this means ethyl chloride can be inhaled by the nose, mouth or both from small masks. A special liquid containing 15 per cent. of mixed additions (valerian, camomile, alcohol, etc.) is used, as the higher boiling point prevents unnecessary freezing.[9]

Di-vinyl ether can be substituted for ethyl chloride and given in a simple closed inhaler as illustrated[10] ; 3 c.cm. from an ampoule is the average amount for a " single-dose " technique. The outstanding advantage of this method is the absence of nausea and vomiting. In a series of 364 administrations to patients from seven

weeks to fifty years old there was no nausea or vomiting. It is
therefore considered by some to be permissible to give a single-dose
di-vinyl ether anæsthesia to out-patients unprepared for operation.[11]
This, however, hardly seems a sound practice.

Trichlorethylene in doses of about 1·5 c.cm. can be used instead
of di-vinyl ether in the same inhaler.[12]

If the necessary apparatus is available and the anæsthetist is
one of experience, children can be dealt with quite satisfactorily
for short dental extractions by **nasal nitrous oxide and oxygen** as
described later. It has been estimated that the average cost per
case of the actual drugs used in these alternative methods is[13] :

> 3·3d. for ethyl chloride.
> 8·6d. for di-vinyl ether.
> 1·87d. for nitrous oxide and oxygen.

In *adult patients*, **nitrous oxide** is the anæsthetic *par excellence*
for dental extractions. The single-dose method will only suffice
for one or two teeth and the nasal administration of **nitrous oxide
and air** is necessary for longer procedures. It is, however, not
always easy to maintain an even level of anæsthesia indefinitely
by such means, and nasal **nitrous oxide-oxygen** is undoubtedly
preferable if the operation is likely to exceed five or ten minutes.
An intermittent-flow apparatus (see Chapter V) is ideal for this
work as the pressure of the gases can be increased to avoid air
dilution from the mouth without altering their proportions. If the
anæsthetist has to take his own apparatus to a dental surgery, the
Walton and McKesson machines are heavy and take some time to
set up. The simpler and lighter type of two-bag apparatus
originated by Hewitt in 1892 and modified by Macintosh is quite
suitable for this purpose.[14]

Composition nose-pieces, which can be moulded to fit any type
of nose, are preferable to the older metal pattern. The provision
of thin rubber flaps is an advance on pneumatic pads, as any increase
in gas pressure tends to apply them more tightly to the nose and air
leaks are thus avoided. A drop or two of scent such as eau de Cologne
placed inside the nose-piece immediately before starting the
anæsthesia avoids the objectionable smell of rubber.

Most patients will breathe through the nose if this is suggested
tactfully, but occasionally mouth breathing occurs just before
consciousness is lost. In this event, the mouthpiece should be
applied until anæsthesia is established.

For " difficult " patients, a Marrett's bottle (see Chapter VII) containing trichlorethylene can be plugged into the exit tube. A surprisingly small quantity of the vapour of this drug added to the gas-oxygen mixture will convert an uneven and stormy anæsthesia into a smooth and tranquil one.

In order to prevent the possibility of inhaling fragments of teeth, fillings, etc., a pack should be placed behind the site of extraction. This usually consists of a bleached honeycomb marine sponge attached to a stout thread.

The degree of safety afforded by nitrous oxide either alone or mixed with air oxygen for dental extractions is of a very high

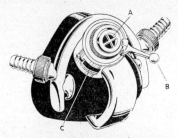

Fig. 108. Nasal inhaler for gas-air anæsthesia (Karn's). A. Adjustable spring-loaded expiratory valve. B. Lever which simultaneously opens C. Air aperture and shuts off the gas supply.[15]

order. As the result of a questionnaire sent out in America, it was reported that a total of 1,161,820 dental cases were anæsthetized by these methods with two fatalities, a mortality rate of only 0·00017 per cent. Another series of 300,000 has been reported with no fatality.[16]

If no facilities exist for the administration of nitrous oxide and oxygen, **intravenous narcosis** can be used for operations of medium duration.[17] There have, however, been disquieting fatalities following such injection,[18] and on the whole it seems wise not to use the sitting position in the dental chair with this technique, at any rate when dealing with patients who are cachectic, or who have low blood pressures.[19] The airway tends to become obstructed during dental surgery and if this is allowed to occur with the respiratory depression produced by the barbiturates, a serious situation may arise. The rate of recovery is slower than after gas, and the patient should never be allowed to go home unaccompanied.[20] The technique for hexobarbitone and thio-pentone administrations has been discussed in Chapter X. A small initial dose of barbiturate such as 0·2 g. of thiopentone can be given and followed up by nasal gas and oxygen. This combined technique gives a pleasant induction and a rapid recovery.[21]

For somewhat longer dental operations, **naso-pharyngeal inhalation** of nitrous oxide and oxygen can be carried out by means of two rubber tubes. These are ordinary endotracheal tubes cut short so that their distal ends lie just above the glottis. Their average length is $6\frac{1}{2}$ inches in men and $5\frac{3}{4}$ inches in women. They should be of the largest size that will pass easily through each nostril and should have a short bevel of 45 degrees. They are connected via metal angle-pieces and short lengths of rubber tubing to a Y-piece fitted with an expiratory valve and a rubber covered forehead plate. When in position, a light gauze pack is inserted. With the aid of adequate premedication and an efficient intermittent flow apparatus, the whole procedure can often be carried out under pure N_2O—O_2. It does not afford quite the same freedom from respiratory obstruction as does naso-tracheal anæsthesia, but on the other hand it is followed by fewer unpleasant sequelæ. The method is unsuitable in cases of nasal obstruction, and for muscular men and young children.[22]

If a really long dental operation is contemplated, such as the removal of unerupted or impacted teeth, dentigerous cysts, etc., it is wise to have the patient admitted for a night to a hospital or nursing home and to employ the **nasal endotracheal** method of anæsthesia[23] (see Chapter VIII). The dental surgeon can then proceed deliberately with the operation, knowing that a perfect airway is assured and that no septic material can be inspired into the air passages. The use of suction will ensure a dry field and may greatly facilitate the operative procedure (see Chapter XX).

The whole subject of anæsthesia in dental surgery is dealt with admirably in " Essentials of General Anæsthesia ", by R. R. Macintosh and F. B. Bannister, to which book the reader is referred for further particulars.

GENERAL ANALGESIA

The preparation of teeth for filling is frequently an extremely painful process, and various methods have been tried to produce insensitivity of the pulp. For example, the introduction of pure phenol into the cavity, the application of cold by means of an ethyl chloride spray or an oxygen jet, and the submucous injection

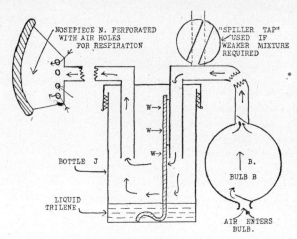

FIG. 109. Diagrammatic sketch of apparatus for the production of analgesia by self-administered trichlorethylene. (Hill, *Pro. Roy. Soc. Med.*)

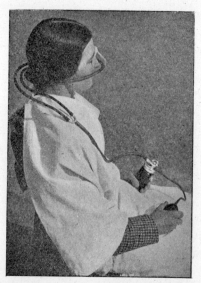

FIG. 110. The apparatus shown in position for dental analgesia. (Hill, *Pro. Roy. Soc. Med.*)

of local analgesics have all been tried with varying success. The induction of analgesia with **nitrous oxide and oxygen or air** is, however, much more certain, and can usually be prolonged indefinitely. It is, at first, surprising to see a patient in an apparently normal condition and fully conscious, but quite insensitive to pain. The proportion of oxygen or air will naturally be considerably higher than that obtaining with anæsthesia. The late S. R. Wilson pointed out that the analgesic state is more readily attained when using air than oxygen with the nitrous oxide. An adaptation of Minnitt's obstetric apparatus (q.v.) is eminently

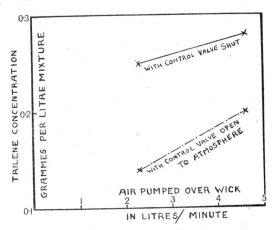

FIG. 111. Graph showing output of trilene by apparatus.
(Hill, *Pro. Roy. Soc. Med.*)

suitable for dental work, and a public demonstration of this technique was given at Guy's Hospital by Kemshole in March, 1935. Since that date several varieties of apparatus have been specially designed for producing analgesia for dentistry and the method has attained much popularity in America.[24]

The *sensations* experienced by the patient are usually (*a*) a feeling of warmth, (*b*) tingling or numbness starting in the extremities, (*c*) tinnitus, and (*d*) a feeling of well-being, resignation and occasionally dizziness or floating in space.

The *signs* observable are few. The patient should have a normal colour and an apathetic appearance and should carry out instructions. He will probably have a somewhat guttural speech.

If the patient's eyes become fixed, staring or closed, or if he becomes unco-operative or unruly, he is entering the second (or excitement) stage of anæsthesia and the nitrous oxide percentage must be reduced.[25]

It now seems certain that **trichlorethylene and air** provides a more simple and efficient type of general analgesia for dentistry (see Chapter VII). The patient squeezes a rubber hand bulb which supplies a weak vapour to a nose piece[26] (see Figs. 109, 110 and 111).

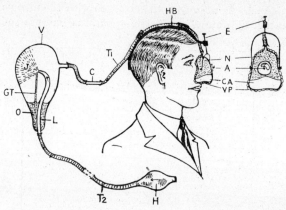

Fig. 112.   Vaporizer for trichlorethylene analgesia in dentistry. Diagrammatic lay-out of apparatus illustrated in Fig. 113.

(Scher : *Dental Record*.)

VP=Vinyl portex rim.   CA=Clear acrylic area.   A=Steel pin pivot for revolving aperture.   N=Nose hood.   E=Adjustable earphone clamp.   H.B.=Headband. T_1 and T_2=Rubber tubing.   C=Glass connector.   V=Vaporizer.   J=Trilene spray.   GT=Capillary bore glass tube.   O=Aperture of conduit for ascending liquid.   L=Liquid.   H—Higginson-type bulb.

A slightly different type of nasal inhaler[27] is shown in diagrammatic form in Fig. 112 and is photographed in action in Fig. 113.

Ethyl chloride has also been used recently for analgesia. For short cases, no apparatus at all is necessary. The lips are smeared with vaseline, a dental prop is inserted and a 2 inches by 6 inches oblong of gauze is crumpled up and placed between the teeth. The patient is told to breathe through his mouth and ethyl chloride is sprayed on to the gauze at intervals for about forty-five seconds. A total of 6 c.cm. is usually sufficient. The gauze is then pushed aside and the dental procedure effected. Complete analgesia usually lasts from one to two minutes and after-effects are rare.[28]

For longer dental operations such as painful drilling, nasal administration can be used. A special nose fitting is strapped to the forehead and enables the patient to inhale a weak ethyl chloride vapour by squeezing a rubber hand-bulb.[29] This method is probably not so efficient as that described with trichlorethylene.

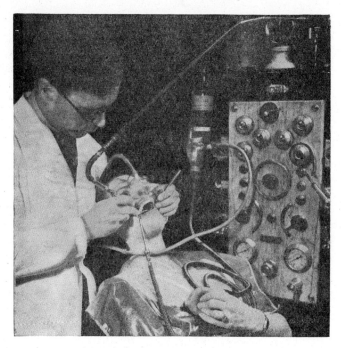

Fig. 113. Dental drilling in progress under trichlorethylene analgesia with Scher's vaporizer (*Dental Record*).

References

1. ROUNDS, F. W.   *Anesth. & Anal.*, 1937, Sept.-Oct., p. 276.
2. { MILLER, H. C.   *Jour. Amer. Dent. Ass.*, 1932, Jan.
   { FRIEDMAN, R.   "Modern Dentistry," 1932, Feb.
3. { BOYLE, H. E. G.   *Pro. Roy. Soc. Med.* (An. Sec.), 1927, March 4.
   { SEYBOLD, J. W.   *Jour. Amer. Dent. Ass.*, 1931, Sept.
   { HARMS, B. H.   *Anesth. & Anal.*, 1932, Jan.-Feb., p. 43.
4. { Technique of Funk, of Chicago.
   { COLEMAN, F.   *Pro. Roy. Soc. Med.* (Spec. Discus.), 1924, March 12.
5. MUSHIN, W. W.   *Lancet*, 1936, May 8, p. 1062.
6. { SHIPWAY, F.   *Pro. Roy. Soc. Med.* (An. Sec.), 1927, March 4.
   { SANDIFORD and CLAYTON.   *Brit. Med. Jour.*, 1928, July 28.
   { SINGTON, H.   *Brit. Med. Jour.*, 1930, Feb. 1, p. 217.
   { HEWER, C. L.   *Brit. Med. Jour.*, 1930, Feb. 8, p. 262.

7. SISE, L. F., and WOODBRIDGE, P. D. *New Eng. Jour. of Med.*, 1930, Aug. 7, p. 273.
8. KNIBERG, B. " Dental Cosmos," 1933, Jan.
9. GOULD, R. B. *Brit. Med. Jour.*, 1934, June 16, p. 1073.
10. BOSTON, F. K., and SALT, R. *Lancet*, 1940, Nov. 16, p. 623.
11. GOLDMAN, V. *Brit. Med. Jour.*, 1936, July 18, p. 122.
12. GALLEY, A. H. *Pro. Roy. Soc. Med.* (An. Sec.), 1943, May 7.
13. ORD, J. W. E. *Brit. Med. Jour.*, 1940, April 13, p. 638.
14. MACINTOSH, R. R., and BANNISTER, F. B. " Essentials of General Anæsthesia," 3rd edit., p. 190.
15. KARN, R. *Brit. Dent. Jour.*, 1933, April 13.
16. McCARDIE, W. J. *Pro. Roy. Soc. Med.* (An. Sec.), 1923, March 2.
17. GOLDMAN, V. *Dent. Mag. & Oral Topics*, 1933, Nov., p. 1153.
18. *Brit. Dent. Jour.*, 1934, Feb. 15, p. 218.
19. JARMAN, R. *Brit. Dent. Jour.*, 1934, March 15.
20. TREWICK, J. A. *Dent. Gaz.*, 1936, Feb., p. 331.
21. PRATT, F. B. *Brit. Med. Jour.*, 1939, Sept. 9, p. 555.
22. MUSHIN, W. W. *Brit. Med. Jour.*, 1941, Jan. 11, p. 46.
23. MAGILL, I. W. *Pro. Roy. Soc. Med.* (An. Sec.), 1923, March 2.
24. AMBROSE, J. *Dental Record*, 1940, June, p. 266.
25. RUBINSTEIN, M. N. *Anesth. & Anal.*, 1938, Nov.-Dec., p. 345.
26. HILL, B. *Pro. Roy. Soc. Med.* (Odont. Sec.), 1944, March 27.
27. SCHER, E. A. *Dental Record*, 1946, Sept., p. 217.
28. ROCHFORD, J. D., and BROADBENT, B. T. *Brit. Med. Jour.*, 1943, May 29, p. 664.
29. FORMAN, S. A. *Anesth. & Anal.*, 1942, Nov.-Dec., p. 318.
30. LOOBY, J. P., and KIRBY, C. K., *Jour. Amer. Dent. Ass.*, 1949, **38,** p. 1.

CHAPTER XX

ANÆSTHESIA AND ANALGESIA FOR ENDOSCOPY, BRONCHOGRAPHY, FOR NASAL, ORAL AND MAXILLO-FACIAL SURGERY, AND FOR OPERATIONS UPON THE PHARYNX AND LARYNX. USE OF SUCTION

THE gradual perfecting of the technique of endotracheal anæsthesia has reduced the necessity for the employment of local analgesia in nasal and oral surgery, but it is still preferable in certain cases. In bronchoscopy, for example, the same tube must be used for anæsthesia, for vision, for suction and for any necessary surgical manipulations. The technical difficulties of general anæsthesia are, of course, much less in œsophagoscopy and gastroscopy, but some surgeons also prefer the use of local analgesia for these proceedings, although they are more upsetting to the average patient than is bronchoscopy.[1] Those who have themselves endured an œsophagoscopy under local analgesia will not need convincing of its unpleasantness. Examinations and operations carried out through a direct-vision laryngoscope should, as a rule, be performed under local analgesia although contact of the instrument with the tongue may set up undesirable movements.[2] The old view that excessive hæmorrhage was inevitable in intra-nasal operations performed under general anæsthesia has been shown to be erroneous provided that a perfectly free airway is maintained and that the preliminary preparation is carried out efficiently. There is, however, undoubtedly more bleeding than with local analgesia unless some type of controlled hypotension is employed. Techniques for some of the commoner operations will now be considered in some detail.

Local Analgesia for Bronchoscopy, Œsophagoscopy and Gastroscopy[3]

One hour and a half before operation the patient is given an adequate dose of morphine or omnopon and scopolamine. Half an hour before examination of an adult, the morphine or omnopon is repeated. The mouth and pharynx are then swabbed with equal parts of cocaine 10 per cent. and adrenaline 1 : 1,000, 60 minims of each, mixed in a glass container. The solution is applied by means of a swab of long fibre wool firmly rolled on to a long-curved applicator. After painting the lips, gums and dorsum of the tongue, the swab is held just below the arches of the pillars of the fauces, first to one side, and then to the other side of the uvula ; the posterior pharyngeal wall is thus anæsthetized sufficiently. No retching is produced if the applicator be kept firmly applied to one spot without any general brushing or swabbing action.

After two or three minutes devoted to this region, the swab is next caused to slide gently into each pyriform sinus in turn, the handle of the applicator being raised and turned slightly outwards ; here again the production of nausea can be eliminated, if unnecessary or rapid movements are avoided. When bronchoscopy is to be performed it is advisable, in addition, to introduce the swab into the larynx, allowing it to lie for half a minute between the cords, particular care being taken to see that the wool is securely fastened.

If complete analgesia of the tracheo-bronchial tree is required, as in bronchoscopy, 15 minims of the cocaine-adrenaline solution may be injected through the glottis into the trachea by means of a laryngeal syringe.

When cocainizing the mouth and pharynx it is important to squeeze excess of the solution out of the swab, because cocaine poisoning may be produced if any is swallowed.

When the swab is introduced into the larynx, however, it is advisable to leave the wool saturated, so that a few drops of the solution may trickle down the trachea.

The whole procedure should take about ten minutes ; a further pause of ten to twenty minutes is desirable before the actual examination. After the introduction of a bronchoscope the cough reflex may still be present even after the full preparation described above, and this is, in suppurative cases, desirable. If, however, it is desired to abolish it, as in the removal of foreign bodies, or the introduction of lipiodol, a few more minims of the mixture already used may be injected into the mouth of the bronchoscope from a syringe without a needle, the solution trickling down the tube into the bronchus under inspection. Alternatively, the cocaine and adrenaline may be applied directly to the lower bronchi by means of a swab carried on a bronchoscopic holder.

In the case of children it is wise to avoid the application of cocaine, because of their susceptibility to the drug. Chevalier Jackson's work leaves no doubt on this point. For them, pre-medication with rectal paraldehyde (q.v.) followed by nitrous oxide-oxygen with possibly a trace of trichlorethylene is a suitable method. Even in adults, the use of cocaine is not entirely devoid of risk.[4] Some authorities consider that it is safer to substitute 1 in 1,000 nupercaine for cocaine[5]. 2 per cent. amethocaine is also efficient but is probably as toxic as the cocaine solution described, several fatalities before and during bronchoscopy having been recorded.[6] A simple but effective technique for bronchoscopy is (1) to give the patient an amethocaine lozenge (gr. 1) to suck fifteen minutes before examination and (2) to inject 2 c.cm. 2 per cent. amethocaine solution by a hypodermic syringe through the crico-thyroid membrane in the sitting position.[7] Some anæsthetists, however, dislike injecting solution through a puncture hole when it can be sprayed through the glottic opening. A short-acting barbiturate such as soluble thiopentone can be injected intravenously to produce unconsciousness during the actual examination. It is imperative, however, for the local analgesia technique to be efficient, as if the unprepared glottis is touched during quite deep intravenous anæsthesia alone a severe spasm usually occurs.

When the patient is returned to his bed, it is a wise precaution to pin a card to the front of his pyjama jacket reading :—

> AS THIS PATIENT'S THROAT
> IS INSENSITIVE, NO FOOD
> OR DRINK MUST BE GIVEN
> BEFORE . . . M.

the time being filled in for three hours after the topical application.

General Anæsthesia for Bronchoscopy and Œsophagoscopy

Intravenous thiopentone combined with curare has been tried for bronchoscopy[8] but in the author's opinion this technique is not uniformly satisfactory, the chief objection being prolonged respiratory depression afterwards. This can be partly overcome by using a more evanescent relaxant such as gallamine, deca-methonium or succinylcholine (q.v.). An amethocaine spray of the glottis can be incorporated in the technique.[9] Alternatively, after cocainization of the glottis a deep plane of general narcosis can be induced and maintenance carried out with a mixture of nitrous oxide-oxygen-trichlorethylene passed into the tube of the bronchoscope. Ether should not be used owing to the risk of ignition.

With the ordinary open ended bronchoscope, the anæsthetist has little control over the patient's respiration while anæsthetic vapour may prove an annoyance to the bronchoscopist. Both difficulties can be overcome by using the fitting illustrated. A metal sleeve

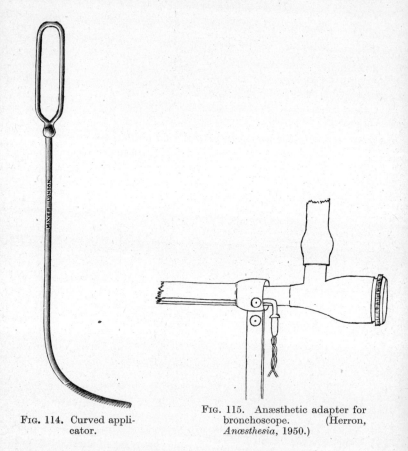

FIG. 114. Curved appli-
cator.

FIG. 115. Anæsthetic adapter for
bronchoscope. (Herron,
Anæsthesia, 1950.)

welded on to a Magill's T-piece is used as a push-on fit to the proximal end of the bronchoscope. An unbreakable watch-glass window is fitted for vision. This arrangement converts the system into a practically closed one with adequate control over respiration. When suction is required or if biopsy forceps must be passed, the attachment is temporarily disconnected.[10]

Œsophagoscopy is best carried out under nasotracheal anæsthesia.

This obviates the respiratory obstruction which is otherwise caused by the displacement forwards of the larynx and trachea by the passage of the œsophagoscope. This may be either mechanical or spasmodic.

Anæsthesia for Bronchography in Children

The work now being done in the detection and localization of early bronchiectasis in children has necessitated a special anæsthetic technique such as that worked out by A. H. L. Baker.[11] Forty-five minutes before operation a hypodermic injection of hyoscine is given : children aged two to four years receiving gr. 1/600, four to twelve years gr. 1/450, and those aged twelve to

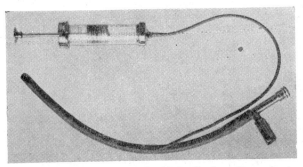

Fig. 116. Special endotracheal tube for bronchography in children. (Way & James, *Lancet*, 1950.)

sixteen years gr. 1/300. Twenty-five minutes later bromethol is given per rectum in doses of $0 \cdot 1$ g. per kilo. body weight. After complete anæsthesia has been obtained by nitrous oxide-oxygen-divinyl ether, an oral endotracheal tube is passed and a saline gauze pack inserted ; 10 to 20 c.cm. lipiodol is then slowly introduced through a fine catheter inserted down the Magill's tube and projecting about $\frac{1}{4}$ inch beyond its distal end. By suitable posturing the lipiodol can be dropped into either bronchus at will and the upper and lower zones of the bronchial tree filled. If desired the same apparatus as that used for tracheal suction can be used (see Fig. 128).

Alternatively the special endotracheal tube illustrated can be used. Anæsthesia is maintained with nitrous oxide-oxygen-trilene and the radiopaque fluid introduced by a syringe into the side tube.[12] In an emergency the bronchial tree can be quickly emptied by a suction catheter passed through the Cobb's adapter.

Local Analgesia for Intra-nasal Surgery

One hour before operation, omnopon- or morphine-scopolamine is given as before.[3]

Half an hour before the operation the induction of analgesia is begun. The nostrils are first purified with 2 per cent. mercurochrome. The mucous surfaces of the nasal fossæ are then painted over with a paste recommended by Albert Gray ; it consists of :

> Cocaine hydrochloride, ℥ 2.
> Desiccated adrenal gland, gr. 24.
> Chloretone, min. 5.
> Liquid paraffin, min. 220.
> " Vaseline," ad 1 oz.

This is applied by means of a wool swab carried on a flat-ended probe ; it is painted on to all parts of the nose except the roof, in the region of the cribriform plate; the lateral walls of the nose under cover of the inferior turbinals are included if antrostomy is to be performed. No pain or bleeding should be caused by its application.

About five or ten minutes are spent in covering the whole surface of the nasal mucous membrane, care being taken that no lumps of paste adhere to the probe for fear of cocaine dropping into the pharynx. All excess is wiped away.

At the end of the surface application Sluder's method of nerve blocking is employed. Two long and two short silver wire probes are employed. They are tipped with wool, which is then smeared with cocaine paste.

The two short ones are slipped up as far towards and as high up as possible to lie at the roof of the nose near the point of entrance of the nasal branch of the naso-ciliary nerve. The long ones are slipped backwards and obliquely upwards at an angle of about 30° to lie just behind the posterior ends of the middle turbinal bodies ; they will be felt to impinge on the anterior wall of the sphenoidal sinus.

After a lapse of twenty minutes from the termination of the preparation, the patient is ready for operation. Such proceedings as submucous resection of the septum, turbinectomy, ethmoidectomy, intra-nasal antrostomy, or opening of the sphenoidal sinuses can then be carried out. This technique avoids to some extent the great discomfort and reactionary hyperæmia which follow preliminary packing of the nose with gauze soaked in cocaine-adrenaline solution.

An alternative technique is known as **postural instillation.**[13]   The analgesic solution is a mixture of 2 c.cm. 8 per cent. cocaine hydro-chloride, 2 c.cm. 1 per cent. sodium bicarbonate and 1 c.cm. 1 in 1,000 adrenaline hydrochloride. A 2 c.cm. syringe is fitted with a solid ended needle 2 inches long bent in the middle to an angle of 45° and perforated with three lateral holes near its end. The patient first lies on his left side with a pillow under his left shoulder so that his head is in the lateral position at an angle of 45° to the vertical. One-third of the total volume of solution (1·7 c.cm.) is drawn into the syringe and a few drops are massaged into the anterior part of the septum. The remainder is injected equally along the floor of each nasal cavity. At the end of ten minutes, a further 1·7 c.cm. are introduced into the two sides, the patient then pinches his nose and rolls on to his face with the head flexed. Finally he rolls on to his right side and relaxes his grip on his nostrils. The remainder of the solution is now inserted and in ten minutes' time the patient is ready for operation. If a septum resection is to be performed it may be necessary to inject 1 or 2 c.cm. of 1 per cent. procaine into the columella.

Local Analgesia for Tonsillectomy

Owing to advances in general anæsthesia for oral surgery, there now seems small reason for subjecting patients to a proceeding which at best can only be described as unpleasant. Local analgesia for tonsillectomy is, however, still widely used on the Continent, where the standard of general anæsthesia is often unsatisfactory, and a short description of the technique will now be given.[14]

The fauces are first sprayed with 10 per cent. cocaine or 2 per cent. nupercaine, after warning the patient not to swallow any of the solution. After five minutes an injection of 0·75 per cent. procaine with adrenaline is made into the upper and lower poles of the tonsils and just outside the margin of the anterior and posterior pillars. A long needle, the point of which is curved almost to a right angle, is helpful.[15] By the time that the second tonsil is injected the first will be ready for dissection. Discomfort can be minimized by using no gag and by giving the patient frequent rests, during which he can relax his jaw muscles. Greater gentleness in manipulation must be exercised, and a longer time allowed than if general anæsthesia is employed.

This method is occasionally followed by collapse and even death, which is apparently due to primary cardiac failure.[16] The writer knows of two such disasters.

Local analgesia is unsuitable for the removal of tonsillar remains and for fibrotic tonsils where adhesions obliterate the retrotonsillar space. The most serious objection to the use of local analgesia for tonsillectomy is the increased risk of sepsis. Thirty cases of deep cervical infection following tonsillectomy (three fatal) were investigated, and it was found that over 90 per cent. had a local infiltration.[17] Pulmonary complications are also commoner with local than with general anæsthesia, presumably owing to the aspiration of blood, etc.[18]

General Anæsthesia for Oral Surgery

Guillotine enucleation of tonsils in children is generally carried out under the single-dose ethyl chloride or di-vinyl ether methods. The use of chloroform or C.E. mixtures for this purpose cannot be too strongly condemned.

Premedication with rectal paraldehyde is extremely useful in nervous children (see Chapter II).

Dissection enucleation demands quiet anæsthesia with relaxed muscles for an indefinite period. Although the actual technique of dissection tonsillectomy varies with different surgeons, the use of the Davis gag, introduced into this country by Boyle in 1921, has become almost universal. The position of the patient may be (i) sitting in a dental chair, as is frequently the case in America, where the whole proceeding may be carried out under nasal nitrous oxide-oxygen anæsthesia. In this position it is impossible to be sure that the patient will inhale no blood. In the writer's opinion the technique is dangerous and has nothing to recommend it. (ii) The " Butlin " position with the head slightly lower than the body and rotated to the right by a sandbag placed behind the left shoulder. (iii) The " thyroid " position, with the head in the mid-line but hyperextended. The gag may be held in position by an assistant or fixed with an adjustable " jack ", which either rests on the patient's chest direct or transfers some of the strain to the shoulders through the medium of a strap. Various attempts have been made to support the end of the gag by outside objects such as the edge of an instrument table or a hook in the ceiling via an adjustable cord. In the author's opinion a better means of support is a simple bipod whose arms rest on the sterile towel under the patient's head.[19] Anæsthesia may be maintained by endopharyngeal nitrous oxide-oxygen-ether through the metal pipe on the tongue depressor of the gag or preferably by the single-tube nasal endotracheal method (see Chapter VIII). The latter technique enables a gauze pack to be used and avoids any possibility of blood finding its way into the trachea. The tracheal tube should *not* be lubricated with an analgesic preparation.

If adenoids are present, blind nasal intubation is not without risk, but if it is used the tube should be left in until the operation

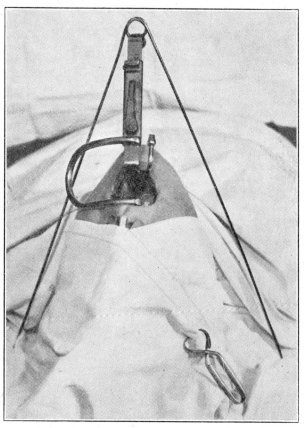

Fig. 117. Davis gag in position supported by bipod. (Draffin, *Brit. Med. Jour.*)

is completed. After the tonsils have been enucleated, the writer has found that the most convenient technique is to grip the tube in the pharynx with forceps and to withdraw the proximal end through the nose and bring it out through the mouth. The angle-piece is then reconnected and anæsthesia maintained for as long as is necessary.

The repair of hare-lip and cleft-palate in infants can be carried out with the open endotracheal technique using an armoured tube to avoid kinking (Fig. 118).

Partial or complete rebreathing with a bag is not, as a rule, suitable for babies owing to their small tidal capacity.[29]

Suitable sizes of tube are as follows :

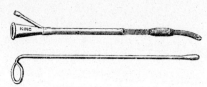

Fig. 118. Armoured tracheal tube for infants with soft rubber end. Gases are fed into the side tube thus providing an open circuit. (Magill.)

For babies aged less than three months, size OO (external diameter 4 mm.).

For babies aged from three to nine months, size OA (external diameter 5 mm.).

For babies aged from nine to fifteen months, size O (external diameter 6 mm.).

For babies aged from fifteen to twenty-one months, size I (external diameter 7 mm.).

Alternatively the device shown in Fig. 119 can be used. A short rubber endotracheal tube fits on to a curved metal tube which is in turn connected by a bayonet joint to the metal chin-piece provided with a large gas inlet and a rubber expiratory valve.

Two curved metal wings can be strapped to the patient's chin to prevent rotation. The whole attachment can be made to fit into the tongue depressor of a Davis' gag if a slot is cut in its upper surface.[21]

Prior to these operations on infants a culture should be made from the throat in order to exclude the presence of the Klebs-Loeffler bacillus and hæmolytic streptococcus. Apart from surgical considerations, it has been shown that even slight trauma can cause post-operative œdema of the glottis in the presence of these organisms.[22]

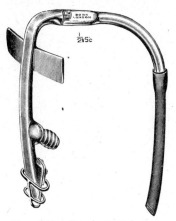

Fig. 119. Orotracheal attachment
for repair of cleft-palate and hare-
lip. (Humby and Hawksley, *Brit.
Med. Jour.*)

Maxillo-facial Surgery

A very large number of operative procedures are included under
this heading but the guiding principles for anæsthesia can be
simplified quite easily. An endotracheal tube should practically
always be passed either through the nose or throat as dictated by
the site of operation. A water-tight seal is essential owing to the
brisk hæmorrhage which so often occurs. This can be effected
either by a cuffed endotracheal tube (q.v.) or by careful gauze
packing. In " cold " plastic surgery of the face, controlled hypotension with one of the methonium drugs is now sometimes used to
minimize bleeding.

The late war has emphasized difficulties in connection with
gunshot and bomb wounds involving fractures of the maxilla and
mandible accompanied by profuse hæmorrhage into the mouth.
The writer has found the following anæsthetic technique useful
for splinting or wiring the fractures. The patient is placed in a
Trendelenburg position with his head extended. The pharynx is
cleared of blood and debris by means of a small suction catheter
passed through a nostril. If no suction pump is available, an
aural or bladder syringe can be used. The other nostril and glottis
are then cocainized, intravenous thiopentone is given to the point of
unconsciousness and followed up by nitrous oxide-oxygen-ether by
means of a face-piece. A naso-tracheal tube is then passed and

a lubricated gauze pack carefully inserted. If foreign matter has passed down the trachea, it is essential to perform a thorough tracheo-bronchial toilet by suction. It has been shown that the longer debris is left in the upper respiratory passages, the more likely is pulmonary infection to occur.[23]

After some fractures of the maxilla and mandible (e.g. those due to road accidents) partial or complete loss of consciousness may occur often accompanied by paralysis of the palatal muscles and much œdema of the pharyngeal tissues. These factors may result in a dangerous degree of respiratory obstruction which can often be relieved by the gentle insertion of a half-length Magill tube through the least damaged nostril. The tube should be lubricated with an analgesic preparation and when its tip reaches the posterior pharyngeal wall, the obstruction is frequently relieved. If the patient is unconscious, blood and debris can then be aspirated from the trachea and bronchi by passing a small gum-elastic catheter through the naso-pharyngeal tube.[24]

General Anæsthesia for Nasal Surgery

Plastic operations on the nose and such intra-nasal procedures as submucous resection of the septum, drainage of sinuses, removal of growths, etc., are now usually performed under orotracheal

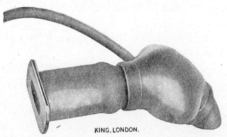

KING, LONDON.

Fig. 120.   Shipway's ballooned airway for
intra-nasal surgery.

anæsthesia with a cuffed tube (q.v.). If the preliminary cocainization of the nose has been carried out with as much care as if local analgesia only was to be used, there should be very little hæmorrhage and in the writer's opinion controlled hypotension is rarely necessary.

If it is impossible to administer an endotracheal anæsthesia for an intranasal operation, a fairly efficient substitute is an airway fitted with an inflatable balloon combined with a gauze pack.[25]

The rotating adapter illustrated fits most types of airway and enables gas mixtures to be administered. A rubber flap tucked *inside* the lips minimizes air leakage. The telescopic airway also illustrated permits accurate fitting for any patient.[26]

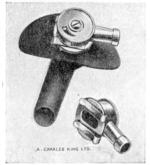
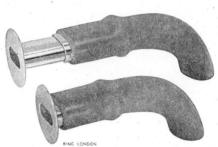

FIG. 121. Rotating adapter, rubber flap and telescopic airway (Charles's).

Whatever method of general or local anæsthesia is used for nasal and oral surgery, too much attention cannot be paid to the exclusion of fluids from the larynx and trachea. The ease with which fluids can enter the air passages is well illustrated by Singer's technique of introducing lipiodol into the lungs by simply dropping the oil on to the base of the protruded tongue of a conscious patient.[27] General and local anæsthesia enable liquids to enter the trachea even more readily, as is demonstrable by bronchoscopy after tonsillectomy. Blood can frequently be seen in the trachea and bronchi if no efficient precautions have been observed, especially if the operation has been performed in the sitting position.[28]

There is no doubt that the routine use of suction and of endo-tracheal anæsthesia with adequate packing for nasal and oral operations has diminished the incidence of post-operative pulmonary complications. The author investigated the after-effects of 500 such cases without finding a single patient who developed lung trouble sufficiently severe to prolong his stay in hospital beyond the normal limit.

After operation the patient should be placed on his side with the foot of the bed raised.

Operations upon the Larynx and Pharynx

The excision of extensive malignant growths involving the larynx and pharynx (e.g. laryngectomy and lateral pharyngotomy) may necessitate preliminary laryngotomy or tracheotomy (see Chapter VIII).

If laryngo-fissure is to be performed for a moderate sized laryngeal growth, however, it may be possible to maintain anæsthesia by a small stiff tracheal catheter passed through the mouth under vision. If the anæsthetic agents used are N_2O—O_2—chloroform or trilene and air, diathermy can be used at any stage of the operation. When the larynx has been opened, the trachea can be packed off with a gauze strip leaving the catheter lying in the posterior commissure of the larynx. Should this impede the surgeon's work it can be temporarily retracted out of the way. If complete hæmostasis cannot be secured at the end of the operation, the catheter and gauze pack are withdrawn and a ballooned Magill's tube passed through the nose so that the cuff lies in the larynx. This manœuvre may be impossible, but it can frequently be done if the nostril is wide and preliminary cocainization of the nose has been performed. A new unwrinkled cuff is also helpful. Inflation will now cause the cuff to exert pressure on the bleeding area and the laryngo-fissure can be closed. The tube is left in place for eight hours, retention being helped by morphine injections and 2 per cent. amethocaine sprayed down the tube. The cuff is then allowed to deflate and after a few minutes the patient is asked to cough. If any blood appears the cuff is reinflated for a further two hours and the same test applied. When no blood is coughed up the tube is gently withdrawn.[29]

The Use of Suction

The employment of suction is now almost universal in nasal and oral surgery. The main advantages are a dry field, less interference with vision when clearing away fluids, and less trauma to tissues than with swabbing.

The desirable features of an electric suction pump are :

(i) It must be efficient[30] (a vacuum of 25 inches Hg is usual).

(ii) It should be almost noiseless.

(iii) If the electric motor is of the brush type, the commutator must be enclosed to avoid sparking and the switch should be of the safety type.

(iv) If the pump is enclosed, the exhaust vapour must not pass into the case (see Chapter IX), but after being filtered should be available for providing an air-ether mixture in case of emergency.

(v) A trap or other device should be incorporated to prevent the suction bottle being overfilled and clogging the pump.

If the pump is to be *portable*, provision will also have to be made for variations in voltage and for continuous and alternating electric supplies. *Transportable* pumps, on the other hand, need not have this provision and can be heavier in build.

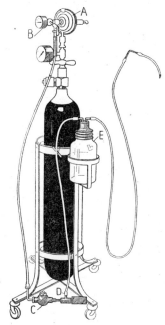

Fɪɢ. 122. Injector-type suction apparatus working from oxygen cylinder. (M.I.E. Co.)
A. Reducing valve.
B. Reduced pressure gauge.
C. Foot control button.
D. Suction tube nozzle.
E. Suction bottle.

It should be noted that if A.C. current is available, electric motors of the induction type can be used and are inherently safer from the ignition risk point of view than the brush type necessary for D.C. supplies.

In hospital work it is most desirable to have a large pump working at a low speed in some distant room, connected with the operating theatres through permanent piping.[31] All noise and danger are thus eliminated.

If an electric supply is not available, an extractor which works from a water main can be used or an injector deriving its power from a steam pipe or from an oxygen or compressed air cylinder.[32] (Fig. 122.)   Finally, it is possible to use a pedal-operated pump.

References.

1.   NEGUS, V. E.   *Brit. Med. Jour.*, 1939, Dec. 23, p. 1223.
2.   LAYTON, T. B.   *Pro. Roy. Soc. Med.* (Laryng. Sec.), 1937, Feb. 5.
3.   Technique of Mr. V. E. Negus, M.S., King's College Hospital.
4.   DAVIDSON, M.   *Brit. Med. Jour.*, 1932, Oct. 1, p. 619.
5.   ABEL, A. L.   *Practitioner*, 1936, April, p. 509.
6.   DOANE, J. C., and COHN, E. M.   *Anesthesiology*, 1945, July, p. 421.
7.   ORGANE, C.   *Pro. Roy. Soc. Med.* (An. Sec.), 1946, May 3.
8.   BOURNE, J.   *Brit. Med. Jour.*, 1947, **2**, p. 654.
9.   SCURR, C. F.   *Brit. Med. Jour.*, 1950, Dec. 9, p. 1311.
10.   HERRON, R. A. C.   *Anæsthesia*, 1950, Jan., p. 40.
11.   BAKER, A. H. L.   *Brit. Jour. Anæsth.*, 1941, Jan., p. 112.
12.   WAY, C. L., and JAMES, G. C. W.   *Lancet*, 1950, June 10, p. 1073.
13.   MOFFETT, A. J.   *Anæsthesia*, 1947, Jan., p. 31.
14.   COSTELLO, J. W.   *Brit. Med. Jour.*, 1932, May 7, p. 839.
15.   MOREY, G.   *Brit. Med. Jour.*, 1934, Dec. 1, p. 990.
16. { " Medico-legal."   *Jour. Amer. Med. Ass.*, 1933, Feb. 11.
     { *Rep. Austral. Soc. Anæsth.*, 1937, May 3.
17.   SHAPIRO, S. L.   *Arch. of Oto-laryngology*, **11**, No. 6.
18.   *St. Bart's. Hosp. Jour.*, 1935, Feb., p. 107.
19.   DRAFFIN, D. A.   *Brit. Med. Jour.*, 1951, July 7, p. 53.
20.   AYRE, P.   *Anesth. & Anal.*, 1937, Nov.-Dec., p. 330.
21.   HUMBY, C., and HAWKSLEY, M.   *Brit. Med. Jour.*, 1943, March 13, p. 317.
22.   GILLESPIE, N. A.   *Brit. Jour. Anæsth.*, 1939, Dec., p. 3.
23.   SHACKLETON, R. P. W.   *Lancet*, 1944, March 25, p. 396.
24.   RICHARDS, H. J.   *Brit. Med. Jour.*, 1950, May 13, p. 1113.
25.   SHIPWAY, F.   *Brit. Med. Jour.*, 1935, April 13, p. 767.
26.   CHARLES, H.   *Brit. Med. Jour.*, 1937, Feb. 27, p. 449.
27.   NEGUS, V. E.   *Pro. Roy. Soc. Med.* (An. Sec.), 1933, May 5.
28.   MYERSON, M. C.   *Laryngoscope*, 1924, **34**, p. 63.
29.   LEWIS, C. R.   *Brit. Med. Jour.*, 1943, Feb. 6, p. 162.
30.   SCOTT-PINCHIN, A. J., and MORLOCK, H. V.   *Brit. Med. Jour.*, 1932, Jan. 23, p. 154.
31. { CLAUSEN, R. J.   *Brit. Med. Jour.*, 1932, Jan. 30.
     { HEWER, C. L.   *Brit. Med. Jour.*, 1932, Feb. 6.
32. { LAKE, N.   *Lancet*, 1924, *ii*, p. 1166.
     { SAHER, N. F., and SALT, R.   *Brit. Med. Jour.*, 1943, June 26, p. 790.

CHAPTER XXI

ANÆSTHESIA AND ANALGESIA FOR THYROID AND THYMIC SURGERY

Simple Goitres—Toxic Goitres—Obstructive Goitres—Total Thyroidectomy for Congestive Heart Failure—Estimation of Basal Metabolic Rate—Thymectomy.

FROM the anæsthetic point of view, thyroid operations can be divided into four groups :

(a) For the partial removal of simple goitres.
(b) For the relief of toxic goitres.
(c) For the relief of obstructive goitres.
(d) Total thyroidectomy for congestive heart failure.

Simple Goitres are those causing no toxic or obstructive symptoms. They are usually removed for cosmetic reasons, and the anæsthesia presents no special difficulty. A good technique is : preliminary hypodermic injection of pethidine-scopolamine, local infiltration of neck with adrenaline-saline (described in detail later) and inhalation of nitrous oxide-oxygen with minimal trilene.

Toxic Goitres are usually divided into primary and secondary types. As a general rule primary toxic goitre occurs in young patients and causes mainly nervous symptoms while the secondary variety is commoner in an older age group and the brunt of the disorder falls upon the cardiovascular system.

Patients suffering from toxic goitre exhibit various signs and symptoms which are of particular importance to the anæsthetist and are described in detail in the monograph published by S. Rowbotham entitled "Anæsthesia in Operations for Goitre" (1945).

(1) *Mentality.* The great majority of such patients are abnormally apprehensive of an operation and may be in the extreme of terror. It is therefore obvious that a pure local analgesia is unsuitable and that some form of basal narcosis is strongly indicated.

(2) *Circulatory Disturbances.* The commonest forms of such disturbances are tachycardia and auricular fibrillation. In older patients with secondary toxic goitre, the condition may be complicated by a high blood pressure and arteriosclerosis. It is a recognized principle that in the treatment of this condition the

pulse rate should be reduced as far as possible before operation by rest, iodine medication, etc.   If the resting pulse rate is above 150 the risk of operation is fairly high, although, in the author's practice, several patients exceeded the rate of 180 and subsequently recovered. The highest pulse rate recorded was 190 at the beginning of the operation, rising to 210.   These figures were noted in two instances, in each of which the patients ultimately recovered.

The actual pulse rate is, of course, only one indication of the cardiac defect and must be taken in conjunction with œdema of the legs, ascites, size of the liver, position of the apex beat, etc.

Auricular fibrillation appears to increase the operative risk considerably and renders any estimation of a patient's condition during operation extremely difficult, as the pulse rate does not usually vary greatly and, in any case, is extremely difficult to note. It is a common observation that even a trace of cyanosis coincides with an increased frequency of pulse rate, so that adequate oxygen should always be present in the inspired mixture.   If nitrous oxide-oxygen is employed, the basal narcotic will greatly facilitate this procedure, as will the addition of very small quantities of cyclopropane.

(3) *Exophthalmos* is often present and, if marked, predisposes to conjunctivitis and corneal ulcer after operation.   A drop of liquid paraffin should always be instilled into each conjunctival sac, and an oblong piece of oil-silk or gutta-percha laid over the eyes to prevent towels or face-piece from touching the eyeballs. In extreme cases the lids may have to be strapped or sutured together.

(4) Persistent *loss of weight* in spite of absolute rest, *vomiting* and *diarrhoea* all increase the gravity of the prognosis.

(5) The *basal metabolic rate* does not, in the author's opinion, give much additional help in estimating the operative risk, but may be of assistance in gauging the dose of bromethol necessary and the approximate oxygen consumption during anæsthesia.   It should not be forgotten that a B.M.R. estimation may badly upset the critically ill patient, so that care should be taken in its use.   Various formulæ (e.g. Read's and Gale's) have been devised in order to deduce the B.M.R. from blood pressure and pulse rate figures, but, in the writer's opinion, they are too inaccurate to be of much value.   The estimation of the B.M.R. is considered later in this chapter.

It now seems to be agreed that *the angle of impedance* is of little value in estimating the severity of toxic goitre.

Choice of Anæsthetic Technique

In deciding upon the actual technique, it is obvious that basal narcosis is essential. In desperately nervous patients it is often best to " steal the thyroid ", to use Crile's expression. Permission for operation having been obtained, the date is left vague and the patient is sent to sleep with a basal narcotic before she realizes that the operation is imminent. Although in mild cases the barbiturates,[1] or large doses of morphine and scopolamine, are fairly satisfactory, there is no doubt that as a general rule bromethol or paraldehyde should be employed.[2]

The rectal method of administration is most convenient and there is some evidence to show that bromethol and thyroxin have to a certain extent antagonistic actions.[3]

Local infiltration is also an advantage, since it renders the operation easier by separating tissue planes, and if adrenaline is incorporated in the solution, capillary oozing is minimized. Unfortunately, however, thyrotoxic patients may react badly to adrenaline,[4] and some anæsthetists perform a preliminary test by injecting 0·5 c.cm. of 1 in 1,000 adrenaline subcutaneously and noting the rise in blood-pressure, pulse and respiration rates over a period of one hour (Goetsch's test). For some time past the writer has omitted the procaine from the solution and since no vaso-dilator is then present, 1 in 500,000 adrenaline in normal saline produces an almost ischæmic field in from ten to fifteen minutes. Increased tachycardia is practically unknown with this dilute solution,[5] It is said that the synthetic product known as cobefrin is not so toxic as adrenaline (see Chapter XIII).

Pure nitrous oxide-oxygen is given usually by means of a facepiece. Owing to the basal narcosis, a quiet anæsthesia can usually be obtained with a fairly high proportion of oxygen. If any adjuvant is required, cyclopropane or trilene can be used.

Tracheitis is frequently present after operation from the inevitable baring of the trachea, and this tends to be aggravated by the inhalation of ether and by the passage of tracheal tubes. Ether also adds to the toxicity of an already ill patient and predisposes to vomiting. It should therefore be avoided.[6] It is arguable that the greater smoothness of narcosis obtainable by the endotracheal technique due to the virtual elimination of reflex laryngeal spasm outweighs the possibility of increased tracheitis. If the anæsthetist is unfamiliar with the surgeon's technique or if it is known that the latter individual tends to be heavy-handed, intubation is wise.

Preparation of Patient

This will naturally depend mainly upon the surgeon's wishes, but all are agreed that the pulse should be slowed and steadied, as far as possible, by rest in bed and such drugs as digitalis or strophanthin if auricular fibrillation is present. Iodine, in the form of Lugol's solution, is given until the maximum effect is obtained. In the few days preceding operation, every endeavour should be made to increase the patient's store of carbohydrate by the administration of glucose.[7] If thiouracil has been given previously for the treatment of the thyrotoxicosis, it should be discontinued for at least two weeks before operation and iodine substituted. In the author's experience, difficulties from hæmorrhage may be very great if this advice be ignored.

If the patient's nervousness is extreme, it may be deemed necessary to avoid all mention of operation and a simple saline retention enema is given for three days beforehand. On the day of operation, and about fifty minutes before the time arranged, a bromethol enema is given in exactly the same way as the previous salines. The patient is turned on to her left side and a freshly-prepared 2·5 per cent. solution of bromethol in distilled water is run in slowly at blood heat. The usual dosage for patients with a moderate degree of thyrotoxicosis is 0·1 gm. per kilogramme body weight. Patients whose B.M.R.'s are extremely high may not be sufficiently affected by the standard dose, and the writer's practice was to increase this to 0·11 gm. per kilogramme. Paraldehyde is cheaper than bromethol and appears to act equally well. The author has been well satisfied with 1,000 recent administrations for thyroid operations. The usual rectal dosage of 1 drachm per stone body weight up to 8 drachms is employed (see Chapter II). There is no doubt that paraldehyde causes less respiratory depression than bromethol for a given plane of narcosis. Directly the patient has lost consciousness a drop of liquid paraffin is instilled into each conjunctival sac. The eyes are lightly bandaged over with a piece of oil-silk and the ears are blocked with cotton wool. A hypodermic injection of scopolamine 1/200 gr. combined with not more than ⅛ gr. of morphine is then given and the patient gently transferred to the trolley and thence to the operating table. The pre-operative use of atropine is unwise in patients having a high B.M.R.[8] If the patient is aware that an operation is about to be performed it is preferable to give the morphine-scopolamine about half an hour before the bromethol or paraldehyde.

Anæsthesia During Operation

The patient's position is of the greatest importance. The special adjustable thyroid rest is of much help, since the anæsthetist can obtain the exact degree of head extension quite smoothly. The insertion and withdrawal of sandbags under the shoulders may upset a patient considerably and cause coughing. The head should not be extended too far as this may actually impede the surgeon's

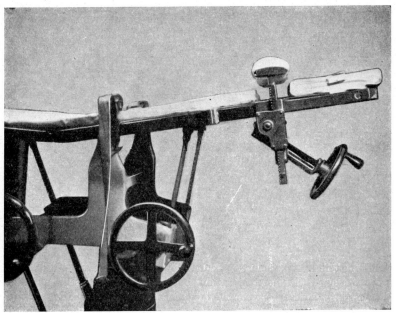

FIG. 123. Operation table with shoulder-rest raised (Kny-Scherer).
Photo by C. Langton Hewer.

task by tightening the anterior muscles of the neck especially in male patients. The correct position of the head having been obtained, the wrists are securely fixed. The table shown in the photograph has padded rests to which the wrists are strapped. It is not sufficient to have the hands tucked under the buttocks as the patient may move before general anæsthesia is induced. This is, in any case, an unsatisfactory proceeding, as cases have been known of gangrene of the fingers occurring from loss of circulation from pressure. The whole table is given a slight foot-down tilt to decrease vascularity in the neck. In order to facilitate heat-loss, patients with thyrotoxicosis should as a rule be left with their legs bare (i.e. without bedsocks) and mackintoshes near the wound should be avoided.

The face-piece of a gas-oxygen machine is next fixed in position by a harness, such as Clausen's face-piece retainer.[9] Incidentally the rubber should *not* be interleaved with a layer of canvas which destroys the elasticity. The face-piece is of special design, with the adapter for the flexible hose inserted just above the nose instead of on the top, as is usual. This arrangement gives the surgeon considerably more room. Pure nitrous oxide-oxgyen is then

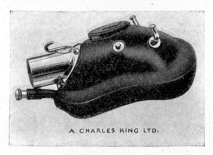

A. CHARLES KING LTD.

Fig. 124.   Goitre face-piece with hooks
for retainer (McKesson, modified by
Hewer).

administered. The closed-circuit technique gives an admirable anæsthesia with quiet respiration, but the " circle " system should be used as an absorber near the face-piece is difficult to manage.

If paraldehyde has been used as the basal narcotic, it is possible for a " build-up " of the vapour concentration of the drug to occur with a closed-circuit (as mentioned in Chapter II) with consequent laryngeal spasm or coughing.   In these circumstances it is therefore better to use a semi-closed circuit.

If intubation is decided upon, it should be carried out at this stage, the nasal tube being lubricated with nupercaine ointment.

The skin of the neck is sterilized either with ether and spirit or Harrington's solution or with C.T.A.B. Iodine and picric acid should be avoided, as severe rashes and toxic symptoms may occur. The greatest care is necessary to avoid intravenous injection, as there is little doubt that most of the fatalities which have occurred during infiltration have been due to this cause.   A continuous-flow syringe is convenient and the point of the needle should be kept moving, the infiltration being made as a collar in the line of the proposed incision. The mid-point is usually half-way between the lower border of the cricoid cartilage and the supra-sternal notch. Sufficient extension both upwards and downwards must be made to ensure that both flaps will be thoroughly infiltrated when they are dissected up by the surgeon.

Observations During Operation

It is the anæsthetist's duty to make careful and continuous observation of the patient's state during operation and to be in a position to advise the surgeon of her condition at any time.

Cyanosis must not be permitted, as except in plethoric patients it is a sign of anoxia (see Chapter III). The detection of minor grades of cyanosis is not always easy. In the first place the face is covered, and, secondly, the green towels which are now fashionable throw a blue-green shadow and tend to exaggerate cyanosis. The lighting system must also be taken into consideration. Plain daylight, of course, gives natural colouring, but the shadowless lamps, commonly used, do not. Some give an intense yellow beam which tends to mask cyanosis, while others throw a greenish light which exaggerates it. It is best to disregard the face and to judge of the colour entirely by the capillary oozing from the wound. If endotracheal anæsthesia is not being used, some respiratory obstruction may occur temporarily from laryngeal spasm while the lobes of the thyroid gland are being dislocated. This may require a higher percentage of oxygen in the inspired gases and in extreme cases an emergency intubation may be necessary, but this is very rare if the surgeon is reasonably gentle.

The best artery in which to feel the pulse is the superficial temporal just in front of the ear, and the rate should be recorded at least every five minutes, some attempt also being made to estimate its volume. It sometimes happens that during the operative manipulation the pulse on one or both sides may become imperceptible from pressure. In this event the pulsation of the common carotids can usually be seen and can be counted for rate. As a general rule the pulse slows on beginning the administration of nitrous oxide-oxygen. The tendency of the pulse rate is of more importance than its actual value, and this should be taken into consideration when advising the surgeon of the desirability of terminating the operation after one lobe has been removed, or, in extreme cases, after tying one artery. Auricular fibrillation often ceases after the administration of bromethol. If it does not, there may be extreme difficulty in gauging the patient's condition as the exact pulse rate is impossible to determine. Many operating theatres are now equipped with mains-operated electric clocks, fitted with centre-second hands, and these are a great help in taking rapid pulse rates in thyroid cases. Failing these, a stop-watch fitted on the anæsthetic apparatus should be used as shown in Fig. 29. An ordinary wrist-watch is almost useless.

Some surgeons require the patient to cough just before the final suturing in order to make certain that hæmostasis is complete. The simplest way to effect this is to interpose one inspiration of strong ether vapour in the nitrous oxide and oxygen mixture. This usually results in three or four coughs and some straining for about fifteen seconds. The alternative method of altering the gas percentages is much less certain and renders the rapid resumption of smooth anæsthesia more difficult.

Immediate After-treatment. This will naturally depend, to some extent, upon the individual surgeon, but the following points are useful. A rectal saline containing $\frac{1}{2}$ drachm of Lugol's solution should be given immediately on the patient returning to bed. In very toxic cases it is an advantage to give the same during the last part of the operation, since it has been shown that an anæsthetized person will retain practically twice as much as a conscious one. If the rectal tube has been left in place from the paraldehyde or bromethol injection, the clip is removed, any remaining solution allowed to flow out and the Lugol's solution run in. If vomiting is excessive an intravenous infusion of 4 per cent. glucose in 0·18 per cent. saline is useful. Lugol's solution may be added if desired.

It is most important for highly toxic patients to be kept cool, and the nursing staff must be dissuaded from heaping blankets upon them. It is, in fact, undesirable to operate upon desperately ill thyroid patients in very hot weather.

The post-operative thyroid crisis, accompanied by extreme restlessness and tachycardia, can frequently be averted by the inhalation of oxygen. The oxygen tent is undoubtedly ideal for this purpose, but, unfortunately, patients with toxic goitre may be very disinclined to use it and some even appear to suffer from definite claustrophobia.[11] This psychic factor can be diminished in hospital by keeping the tent constantly in the ward so as to accustom the patients to the sight of it, and by explaining its use before operation (see Chapter XXVII).

Acute heart failure after operation is extremely rare and appears to react best to nikethamide in large doses given intramuscularly or in emergency by the intravenous route. This drug is also of great value if too much bromethol has inadvertently been administered.

Post-operative soreness and stiffness of the neck muscles can be greatly relieved by sipping some such mixture as :

> Aspirin, gr. 10.
> Phenacetin, gr. 5.
> Spir. Chlorof., m. 5.
> Mucil. Trag. Co., q.s.
> Aq., ad ℥ss.[12]

Most cases of auricular fibrillation revert spontaneously to their normal rhythm after operation. If this does not occur within a month, the change can usually be effected by means of quinidine sulphate.[13]

The gradual perfecting of the anæsthetic technique has contributed to the gratifying reduction in operative mortality from thyroidectomy during the past thirty years. Prior to 1918, the risk was so great that the operation was rarely performed for toxic goitre. Between the two wars, a series of 2,000 cases operated upon at St. Bartholomew's Hospital had a total mortality rate of just under 1 per cent.[14] Since 1939, 1,000 cases of thyroidectomy given the paraldehyde—nitrous oxide, oxygen—adrenaline—saline technique have been done with a mortality of two (0·2 per cent.). It is worth noting that the patients who gave rise to the most anxiety in the last series had been given thiouracil before the dangers of this drug had been fully realized.[15]

Obstructive Goitres present an entirely different problem, and the main concern of the anæsthetist is to provide an efficient airway throughout the operation. The commonest situations for tracheal obstruction are lateral compression in the neck from the two lobes of the thyroid gland and antero-posterior constriction in the thorax between the convexity of the spine behind and the tumour pushed back by the sternum in front. In addition, the whole trachea and larynx may be displaced sideways by a unilateral goitre. The inspection of a skiagram may help the anæsthetist in locating the site and nature of the obstruction. It should always be remembered that, although a large cervical swelling may be present, the difficulty in respiration may be due to an invisible retro-sternal prolongation of the tumour. Some of the malignant goitres belong to this group.

The actual anæsthetic technique is discussed in Chapter XXII.

Total Thyroidectomy for Congestive Heart Failure

This operation differs in several respects from that for toxic goitre. The patient is always an extremely bad risk and is usually brought to the theatre sitting up, cyanosed and dyspnœic. At first these cases were operated upon under local analgesia only, but this method is unsatisfactory in that it is generally impossible for the patient to lie down or to extend the head. The "follow-up service" of a well-known clinic has shown that this class of case does better with general than with local anæsthesia.[16] Cyclopropane-oxygen is the anæsthetic *par excellence* for this type of work.[17] It is quite dramatic to observe the improvement in the patient's condition when anæsthesia has been established. The colour changes to bright red, respiration becomes tranquil, the pulse improves and in a short time the normal thyroid position can be adopted. Since the gland is not enlarged, the slight increased vascularity from the cyclopropane is of no account. As a rule these patients should spend the immediate post-operative period in an oxygen tent.

Estimation of Basal Metabolic Rate

As already mentioned, a knowledge of the B.M.R. may be useful in assessing the operative risk and in estimating the dose of bromethol in patients suffering from toxic goitre.

The relationship of the B.M.R. to age has been discussed in Chapter II. Besides thyroid activity, other factors such as fear and fever affect the B.M.R. For example, it has been estimated that there is an increase of about 7·5 per cent. for every degree of temperature rise above normal.[18]

In order to ascertain the B.M.R., four methods have been employed. They depend upon measuring

(1) the heat output ;
(2) the oxygen consumption ;
(3) the carbon dioxide output ;
(4) both the oxygen consumption and the the CO_2 output.

Two techniques are now in general use. (*a*) The open-circuit technique. Some type of apparatus such as the Douglas bag is used. The patient wears a face appliance with appropriate valves, allowing him to breathe outdoor air, while all his expired air over a certain period is collected, measured and analysed.

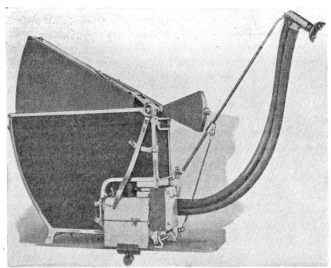

FIG. 125. Closed-circuit apparatus for estimating B.M.R. (McKesson).

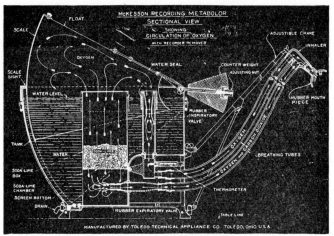

FIG. 126. Longitudinal section of apparatus in previous figure to show the mechanism.

(*b*) The closed-circuit technique. The patient inhales pure oxygen from the machine and exhales oxygen and carbon dioxide through a return pipe. The latter gas is absorbed in a soda-lime chamber, and it is evident that the total volume of oxygen will diminish as it is used up by the patient. The rate of absorption is accurately measured, and from this the B.M.R. can be calculated. The two methods agree closely in their results.[19]

The relatively difficult technique of direct estimation is a drawback, and many attempts have been made to calculate the B.M.R. indirectly from the blood pressure and pulse rate.

Read's formula is perhaps the best known,[20] B.M.R. $= 0\cdot683$ (P.R. $+ 0\cdot9$ P.P.)$-71\cdot5$, where P.R. represents the pulse rate and P.P. the pulse pressure.

Gale's formula is a modification of the above, viz. B.M.R. $=$ P.R. $+$ P.P. $-$ 111.[21] No calculations on these lines are, however, of sufficient accuracy to replace direct estimations.[22]

Thymectomy

The operation of thymectomy for the cure of myasthenia gravis has now been placed on a sound basis and the current theory is that removal of the thymus gland stops the secretion of some curare-like substance.[23] The surgical approach is usually by splitting the sternum, and although one or both pleuræ may be punctured, there is little technical difficulty as regards anæsthesia. A pre-operative enema is unnecessary and should be avoided as it can cause serious collapse in a patient suffering from severe myasthenia. An intravenous drip should, as a rule, *not* be set up as it increases bronchial secretions.[24] Premedication usually consists of neostigmine and atropine. Induction with intravenous thiopentone followed by cyclopropane given by the closed-circuit method with a face-piece is quite satisfactory. In the opinion of the writer and others,[25] the use of ether and the passage of an endotracheal tube are both contra-indicated as post-operative tracheitis may prove disastrous. No relaxant drug is necessary but it is worth remembering that these patients are abnormally sensitive to curare (and gallamine) and abnormally resistant to decamethonium (see Chapter XI). A fairly high mortality rate follows the operation owing to the prevalence of pulmonary collapse. This is due both to the fact that the thoracic cage is no longer intact and to the impaired power of coughing from muscular weakness. Intermittent inhalations of a CO_2-air mixture and large doses of neostigmine may tide over the crisis. Post-operative oxygen therapy is usually indicated and a pneumothorax should not be allowed to persist. If, on pre-operative examination, there are any signs at all of a respiratory infection or if there is a recent history of such, the anæsthetist would be well advised to suggest that thymectomy should be postponed.

References.

1. JOLL, C. A. " Diseases of the Thyroid Gland," 1932.
2. { HEWER, C. L. *Brit. Jour. Anœsth.*, 1931, April, p. 82.
   { KEYNES, G. *Brit. Med. Jour.*, 1934, May 12, p. 844.
3. CARLTON, H. *Pro. Roy. Soc., Med.* (An. Sec.), 1929, Nov. 1.
4. MEYER and ATANASOFF. *Med. Klin.*, 1931, No. 29.
5. HEWER, C. L. *Brit. Med. Jour.*, 1942, Aug. 29, p. 258.
6. HEWER, C. L., and KEYNES, G. *Brit. Med. Jour.*, 1937, Oct. 9, p. 724.
7. KLETZ, N. *Lancet*, 1933, Nov. 4, p. 1025.
8. GREEN, F. W. *Brit. Med. Jour.*, 1935, Oct. 26, p. 781.
9. CLAUSEN, R. J. *Lancet*, 1929, May 18, p. 1035.
10. HEWER, C. L. *Brit. Med. Jour.*, 1942, Aug. 29, p. 258.
11. JOLL, C. A. *Brit. Med. Jour.*, 1935, May 18, p. 1050.
12. Formula of Sir Thomas Dunhill.
13. HEWER, C. L. Adapted from Lecture to Liverpool Soc. of Anæsthetists, 1935.
14. KEYNES, G. *Pro. Med. Soc. Lond.*, 1947, March 10.
15. HEWER, C. L. *Pro. Roy. Soc. Med.* (An. Sec.), 1948, Dec. 3.
16. SISE, L. F. *Dept. of Anæsth. Lahey Clinic*, 1937, April.
17. HEWER, C. L. *Pro. Roy. Soc. Med.* (An. Sec.), 1935, Dec. 6.
18. HAUGEN, F. P. *Milit. Surg.*, 1941, July, p. 72.
19. ROBERTSON, J. D. *Lancet*, 1937, Oct. 2, p. 815.
20. READ, J. M. *Jour. Amer. Med. Ass.*, 1922, **78**, 24, p. 1887.
21. GALE and GALE. *Lancet*, 1931, *i*, p. 1287.
22. NEUMANN, H. *Klin. Woch.*, 1933, Sept. 16, p. 1444.
23. KEYNES, G. *Pro. Roy. Soc. Med.* (Neur. Sec.), 1942, Nov.
24. KEYNES, G. *Brit. Med. Jour.*, 1949, Sept. 17, p. 611.
25. KEYNES, G. *Brit. Jour. Surg.*, 1946, Jan., p. 201.

CHAPTER XXII

ANÆSTHESIA AND ANALGESIA FOR THORACIC SURGERY

Few branches of therapeutics have advanced further during the last twenty-five years than has thoracic surgery, the two World wars being largely responsible for this result. Previous to 1914 an intrathoracic operation was regarded as distinctly risky, whereas at the present time an exploratory thoracotomy can be performed with almost the same ease and safety as an exploratory laparotomy. This diminution in risk has been brought about, in part at least, by improved anæsthetic technique.[1]

With regard to *preliminary preparation* of the patient, drastic purgation is not only unnecessary but actually harmful. The patient should be directed to drink as much as he conveniently can for three days before operation, and most adults should be given a mild preliminary hypnotic such as pethidine and scopolamine. Induction, which is usually effected by means of intravenous thiopentone,[2] should not be started until the surgeon is actually ready to begin operating. It is quite possible for ten to fifteen minutes to be wasted at this stage.

Problems Involved. Thoracic operations present a variety of anæsthetic problems. In the first place, it is essential for the anæsthetist to realize the respiratory changes which occur when a pleural cavity is widely opened. These are mainly :

(1) Paradoxical Respiration. The normal negative intrapleural pressure is converted into atmospheric pressure on the affected side and the exposed lung tends to collapse. Furthermore the mediastinum moves over towards the opposite side thus tending to compress the other lung. On inspiration the lung on the sound side will fill with air drawn partially from the trachea and partially from the collapsed lung on the opposite side. The affected lung will thus become smaller on inspiration. When expiration occurs, the lung on the sound side sends its air partly up the trachea and partly into the opposite lung which consequently becomes bigger. This reversal of normal lung movements is known as paradoxical respiration and is a serious event since even the lung on the sound side is not working efficiently because of the vitiated air which it contains.[3] If the lung on the affected side is partly fixed by

336

adhesions to the chest wall paradoxical movements may be minimized.

(2) **Mediastinal Flap.** A further handicap to efficient pulmonary ventilation is the swing of the mediastinum towards the sound side during inspiration and this may be exaggerated by the hyperpnœa which follows on the inevitable retention of carbon dioxide. In long-standing disease the mediastinum may become relatively fixed in which case mediastinal flap will not be so pronounced.

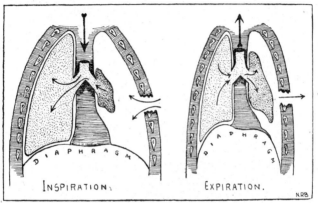

Fig. 127. Paradoxical respiratory movements resulting from an open pneumothorax (after M. D. Nosworthy).

It is not always appreciated that even if the pleura is intact interference with the thoracic cage as in sternum splitting for thymectomy (q.v.) or extensive rib resection as in thoracoplasty can result in paradoxical respiration and/or mediastinal flap.

The remaining major problem for the anæsthetist in thoracic surgery is the management of secretions. This is dealt with later.

Control of Open Pneumothorax

Various techniques have been tried to avoid the hazards of paradoxical respiration and mediastinal flap when the chest is open or when the integrity of the chest wall is impaired.

(1) **Continuous positive-pressure** anæsthesia was first used and as long ago as 1906 it was recognized that 6 mm. Hg was sufficient to maintain distension of the lungs in the presence of a pneumothorax.[4] In practice 8 mm. Hg should not, as a rule, be exceeded unless a bronchial fistula is present which acts as a safety-valve (Magill). A spontaneous pneumothorax has followed the employment of a pressure of 12 mm. Hg. At the close of a thoracotomy,

as the surgeon is on the point of closing the pleura, he may request the anæsthetist to apply positive pressure to expel air from the pleural cavity and reinflate collapsed lung. It should be realized that this method raises the intrabronchial pressure during both inspiration and expiration and this is accomplished by manual or other pressure on the rebreathing bag if a closed-circuit type of anæsthesia is being used. The Coxeter-Mushin absorber can be modified to suit this technique by hanging a 3 lb. weight from its projecting handle.[5] Continuous positive pressure allows spontaneous respiration to continue so that it does not entirely abolish paradoxical movements. Furthermore owing to the fact that the lungs never empty completely a CO_2 build-up may occur. Many anæsthetists consider that owing to its various dangers it should seldom or never be used.[6]

(2) **Assisted Respiration** in which the anæsthetist supplements the patient's breathing by applying positive pressure during inspiration only. This abolishes paradoxical movements and mediastinal flap and is thought by many to be the best technique for most major thoracic operations.

(3) **Controlled Respiration** which has already been described in Chapter I. Natural respiration is usually abolished by a combination of narcotic drugs depressing the respiratory centre, a relaxant paralysing the respiratory muscles and hyperventilation reducing the respiratory stimulus.[7] Passive ventilation can then be theoretically maintained by one of the followed methods.

(a) *Intermittent negative pressure* to the outside of the chest and abdomen as in the Drinker and Both respirators.

(b) *Intermittent positive pressure to the outside of the chest* and abdomen as in the Paul Bragg bag which is really an inflatable waistcoat. These two methods are obviously impracticable in thoracic surgery.

(c) *Intermittent positive pressure to the respired gases*, expiration taking place from the elastic recoil of the thoracic cage. This is done most simply by squeezing the rebreathing bag by hand. The manual method adds no complication and affords valuable information to the experienced anæsthetist who can judge the degree of relaxation of the respiratory muscles by the " feel " of the bag.

Various mechanical respirators have been invented to give automatic intermittent positive pressure the first practical one being the " spiro-pulsator " evolved by the Swedish surgeon Frenckner. The maximum and minimum pressures were usually set at 10 mm. Hg and nil respectively, but if the lung had to be kept distended throughout the cycle, pressures of 14 and 4 mm. were used.[8] A British machine, the " Blease pulmoflator " is now available.[9]

(d) *Intermittent positive and negative pressures applied to the respired gases* as in Moerch's and Pinson's apparatus.[10] It is said that the negative pressure whereby the gases are sucked out during expiration assists the venous return to the heart.[11] The range of safe pressures is said to be from +14 to —9 mm. Hg giving a total change of 23 mm. Hg. It is, however, by no means certain that alternative positive and negative pressures are in fact the best technique.

These mechanical respirators are necessarily complicated and expensive and must be combined with or used in conjunction with a closed-circuit gas-oxygen apparatus. It should be noted that in none do natural respiratory conditions obtain and it would appear that the risk of alkalosis from hyperventilation is greater than if simple manual control is used. On the other hand if the anæsthetist is working alone they do leave him freer to concentrate on other tasks.

Choice of Drugs and Methods

It is unfortunate that most thoracic surgeons make use of the diathermy inside the chest almost as a routine. This practice has ruled out the employment of cyclopropane which is otherwise an almost ideal anæsthetic, providing quiet shallow respiration with a high oxygen concentration and no irritation of the air passages. It is never justifiable to " take a chance " if an ignition risk is present as fatal explosions have demonstrated all too clearly.[12]

Induction of anæsthesia prior to a major thoracotomy is commonly effected by intravenous thiopentone and a small dose of a relaxant drug such as tubocurarine. The glottis and, if possible, the trachea, are well cocainized and a cuffed tracheal tube is passed through the mouth by direct laryngoscopy. The largest sized tube which will pass the glottis comfortably is used and this is generally a No. 10 Magill's tube. No attempt at blind nasal intubation should be made as such a tube may cause damage to the inside of the nose.[13] Unconsciousness is maintained by nitrous oxide with about 30 per cent. oxygen given in a closed circuit. As mentioned before, it is now felt by many anæsthetists that assisted respiration is usually preferable to completely controlled breathing. From time to time additional drugs will have to be given intravenously (preferably into the tubing of a saline or blood drip). If the pressure on the bag increases, a further dose of relaxant is probably necessary, while slight movements indicate the desirability of additional narcotics, usually thiopentone or pethidine. Considerable experience is required before an anæsthetist can maintain an even plane of relaxation and narcosis.

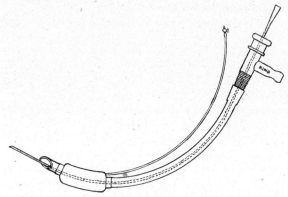

Fig. 128.   Rubber tracheal tube fitted with inflatable cuff and metal T-piece for passage of suction catheter through its lumen (Magill).

Respiratory Obstruction

Certain diseases for which thoracotomy is necessary may give rise to severe respiratory obstruction, of which the commonest is intrathoracic goitre. In certain large tumours the embarrassment may be such that respiration is only possible with the head held forward, any attempt at extension of the neck pulling up the tumour, which then compresses the trachea between the sternum in front and the vertebral column behind. In these cases, the maintenance of an efficient airway outweighs every other consideration and the following technique may be adopted. The pharynx and glottis are cocainized and anæsthesia induced by means of cyclopropane. If obtainable, helium should be added in the approximate proportions of cyclopropane 20 per cent., oxygen 30 per cent. and helium 50 per cent[31] (see Chapter IV). A fairly rigid tube must then be passed down the trachea beyond the site of obstruction. An ideal tube is one made of latex reinforced with a spiral wire embedded in its wall. This is virtually unkinkable and is inserted with a stylet inside it. Such a tube is often impossible to pass by blind nasal intubation and even direct-vision laryngoscopy may be extremely difficult. This manœuvre may have to be performed rapidly if there is no airway with the head extended until the tube is in position. On several occasions the author has overcome the difficulty by using a stiff blunt-ended catheter bent to a " coudé " curve. This may be manipulated through the glottis even though no part of it can be exposed by a laryngoscope. If, in an exceptional case, it proves impossible to insert a tracheal tube, anæsthesia will have to be maintained with the patient's head held in the position in which the least respiratory obstruction occurs until the sternum is split or the pressure relieved in some other way during the course of the operation.

When the patient is to be returned to bed, the tracheal tube should be removed cautiously, for if the trachea has been softened, it may be necessary to re-intubate. Tracheal collapse has caused fatalities after thyroidectomy.[24]

An occasional cause of respiratory obstruction during a thoracic operation is the presence of an unsuspected cyst of the lung. These cysts may have valvular openings, and if controlled breathing is practised, air may be forced into them at each bag pressure which cannot escape. The cyst may then attain a large size in a very short time with possibly disastrous results.

Control of Secretions

It may as well be admitted at the outset that the problem of controlling excessive secretions in " wet-lung " cases has not been

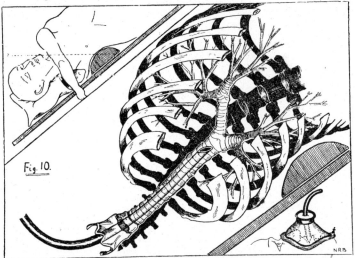

Fig. 10.

FIG. 129. Degree of Trendelenburg necessary to prevent secretion from left lung running into right bronchial tree. When the endotracheal tube is not fitted with a balloon, sputum will not be dammed back near the carina (after Nosworthy).

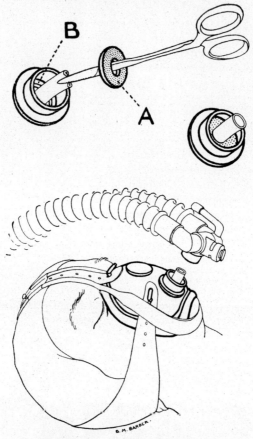

F I G. 130.   Morton's modification of McKesson face-
piece for " wet-lung " cases.   An orotracheal
tube is shown projecting from the outlet.
With aid of artery forceps, a sorbo rubber
washer A is threaded over the end of the tube
and pushed down until it rests on the flange B.
The closed-circuit adapter is then plugged in
and the rubber harness adjusted (*Brit. Med.
Jour.*).

entirely solved.   In every major thoracotomy provision should be
made for tracheal suction by passing a catheter through the tracheal
tube as shown in Fig. 128.   If a Teeman's catheter is used it is
often possible to suck out both bronchi by rotation of the solid end.

The various devices used to avoid flooding the tracheo-bronchial tree with fluid must now be considered.

(1) Posture. Most thoracic surgeons prefer to operate with the patient in the lateral position. For a left-sided operation it will then be necessary to tilt the operating table to at least 35° to the

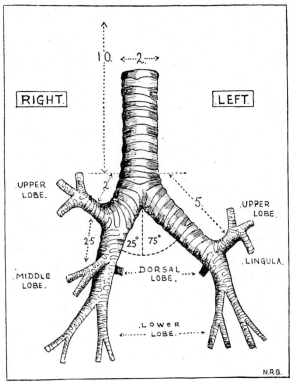

Fɪɢ. 131. Anatomy of normal adult tracheo-bronchial tree. Distances are in centimetres (modified from Nosworthy).

horizontal to prevent secretions spilling over to the right side. If the operation is on the right side a tilt of no less than 55° will be necessary (see Fig. 129). If this technique is adopted, a plain Magill's endotracheal tube should be used, the proximal end of which passes through a diaphragm on the face-piece. A London Hospital type prop can be threaded over the tube to prevent kinking by the teeth.[14] Reference to the caption of Fig. 130 will indicate how this manœuvre is accomplished. Intermittent tracheal suction should be used[15] at regular intervals as by the time that moist sounds can be heard in the trachea, the damage may have been done.[16]

If the surgeon can be persuaded to use the prone position advocated by Overholt[17] and Parry Brown,[18] the head-down tilt need not be nearly so steep (about 10°).

(2) Bronchial Blocking for Lobectomy. Before embarking on the introduction of blockers to the affected bronchi, the anæsthetist

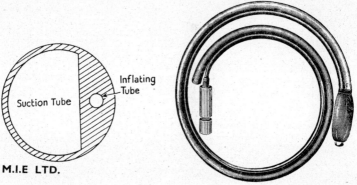

Suction Tube

Inflating Tube

M.I.E LTD.

Fig. 132.   Section through Magill's bronchial blocker.

Fig. 133.   Thompson's bronchial blocker.

must be familiar with the anatomy of the normal tracheo-bronchial tree and the probable abnormality resulting from the disease of any particular patient often made evident by a bronchogram.

There are two types of bronchial blockers or, more correctly, balloon suction catheters, in use at the present time. Both are fitted with inflatable cuffs and provision is made for aspirating secretions distal to them. Thompson's blocker has a cuff covered with a nylon net and was originally meant for inflation by water. Most anæsthetists, however, consider it safer to use air from a syringe. This blocker can only be used with the balloon placed in the main bronchus or distal to the upper-lobe bronchus and must be passed (with an inserted metal stylet) through an 11 mm. broncho-scope. For lower lobectomies, however, the cuff is usually held in position firmly. In right lower lobectomy the cuff should be pushed past the opening of middle lobe bronchus in which case the dorsal lobe bronchus will also be free. It should be realized that the Thompson blocker has to pass outside the cuff on the tracheal tube and this may cause some leakage. Magill's blocker is smaller and the cuff has no net. It is consequently easier to put into position and can sometimes be inserted into an upper lobe bronchus. It is possible to insert Magill's blocker through the lumen of the tracheal tube but this is a feat calling for considerable dexterity.

Tamponage of the involved secondary bronchus can also be performed and anæsthesia maintained by the endotracheal technique.

(3) One Lung Anæsthesia for Pneumonectomy. Blocking of the main bronchus of the affected side by means of tamponage[19] or one of the ballooned suction-catheters already described can be combined with an endotracheal tube to produce one-lung anæsthesia.

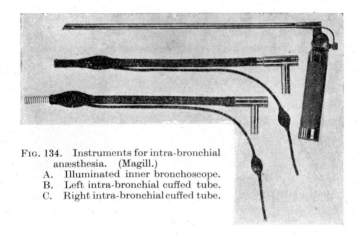

Fig. 134. Instruments for intra-bronchial
anæsthesia. (Magill.)
A. Illuminated inner bronchoscope.
B. Left intra-bronchial cuffed tube.
C. Right intra-bronchial cuffed tube.

Alternatively the sound bronchus can be intubated with a cuffed tube and one-lung anæsthesia maintained through it. This method was introduced by Waters,[20] and should be confined to pneumonectomy, as in lobectomy the portion of lung remaining may become infected. Owing to the difference in the angles of deviation of the two bronchi, " blind " bronchial intubation usually results in the tube passing down the right side, but the method is too uncertain for practical use. Magill's technique is to use a stiff inner cannula (A, Fig. 134) illuminated at its distal end by a battery in its handle. Outside this cannula is a cuffed and armoured intrabronchial tube. In accordance with anatomical differences between the two sides of the tracheobronchial tree (Fig. 131), a left intrabronchial anæsthesia is comparatively easy since the balloon can be accommodated in 5 cm. of the left main bronchus. On the right side, however, the main bronchus is much shorter and the orifice of the left main bronchus may be occluded by the balloon. Air will thus be trapped in the diseased lung so that collapse will not take place and unoxygenated blood will continue to circulate in it. Furthermore, it is very easy to push a right bronchial tube too far and block the right upper lobe bronchus. This will result in the patient breathing with two lobes only, with consequent dyspnœa and cyanosis. In order to overcome this difficulty, the right bronchial tube has an open wire spiral extending for an inch below the cuff (Fig. 134 C). This enables the tube to be pushed well home without obstructing the upper lobe bronchus. In addition to the normal asymmetry of the tracheo-bronchial tree areas of atelectasis from disease may give rise to various distortions.[3]

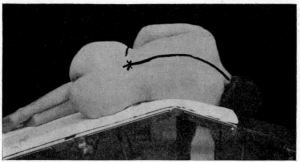

FIG. 135.   Patient in position for unilateral high spinal block for left thoracotomy. The line of the spinous processes and the site of the lumbar puncture are marked. Photo by C. Langton Hewer.

(4) Retention of Consciousness. If a purely local analgesia is used, the patient has some control over his coughing but paradoxical movements cannot be prevented. A simple block of the thoracic wall is insufficient for a thoracotomy and a *high spinal analgesia* is the only practicable method. High bilateral blocks have been attempted with light nupercaine by Etherington-Wilson's technique[21] (q.v.) or otherwise,[20] but the margin of safety is so small that this method must be considered dangerous and fatalities have resulted.[22] Unilateral blocks were first tried in America with hyperbaric procaine. This, however, necessitated turning the patient over and gave an inadequate duration of analgesia.[23] The writer has used unilateral spinal block with light nupercaine for thoracotomies about thirty times without mishap. The patient lies on his sound side with his back flexed laterally so that the highest point is the level of T. 5 (see Fig. 135). He also lies slightly over towards his face. The lumbar puncture is performed in the usual position and about 10 c.cm. of 1 in 1,500 nupercaine solution are injected. A motor and sensory block more or less confined to the affected side of the chest should result. The method has several advantages : the patient need not be moved for the operation, the fall in blood pressure is usually not marked owing to the few anterior roots paralysed, and the respiratory muscles affected will be confined to the inter-costals and some of the abdominal muscles on the affected side only. This results in much more effective coughing than is obtain-able with bilateral high blocks. Furthermore, the analgesia lasts from two and a half to three hours, which should be sufficient for the longest thoracotomy. It must be remembered that with all high blocks there is not much safety margin and the patient's position must be correct.

It is possible that *extra-dural spinal block* may prove to be a safer technique for this type of case.[25]

Thoracoplasty under local analgesia is an ordeal for most patients who prefer to be made unconscious.[26] In the writer's experience of about 500 such operations, the general upset, as judged by the post-operative pulse and respiration rates, is, on the average, greater after local than general anæsthesia but each case must be judged on its merits.

If it is decided that local (as opposed to spinal) *analgesia* should be used, fairly heavy premedication is desirable. The writer uses a solution of 1 in 2,000 amethocaine and 0·25 per cent. procaine with 1 in 500,000 adrenaline. The mixture is constituted as follows :

Sodium chloride 4·45 g. ⎫
Procaine   1·25 g. ⎬ in 500 c.cm. double distilled water.
Amethocaine   0·25 g. ⎭

This is sterilized and 1 c.cm. of 1 in 1,000 adrenaline solution is added from an ampoule. Analgesia develops rapidly and lasts for at least two hours.

The line of incision is infiltrated widely and deeply with this solution, care being taken to inject some well under the posterior border of the scapula. A unilateral paravertebral block correspond-ing with the ribs to be removed can also be carried out, but an intercostal block can be performed with greater precision by the surgeon under vision during the course of the operation. This procedure may be followed by some after-pain.[27] For first stage (upper) thoracoplasties a supra-clavicular brachial plexus block (q.v.) is also advisable. Lastly, subcuticular wheals, usually five, should be raised for the reception of the towel clips.

It must be remembered that thoracoplasty results in a mobile thoracic wall (like a " stove-in chest ") and consequently para-doxical respiration (q.v.) to a greater or lesser extent will follow operation according to the number and extent of ribs removed. It is thus most important that the affected side should be supported and immobilized with strapping after operation.

Minor Thoracic Operations

Such minor procedures as **thoracoscopy, phrenic crush** and the **induction of artificial pneumothorax** can be conveniently performed under local infiltration analgesia with 0·5 per cent. procaine and 1 in 250,000 adrenaline. The same remarks apply to the **drainage of acute empyema** in adults and to the **drainage of lung abscess.** The danger of general anæsthesia in such cases is the possibility of the pus rupturing through into the bronchial tree.

The usual technique is as follows : four intradermal wheals are raised, A, B, C and D, two in the intercostal space above and two in the space below the selected rib (Fig. 136). An infiltration of the subcutaneous tissues and muscles joining the wheals is then made. Finally, from the lower posterior wheal B, a deep injection is made

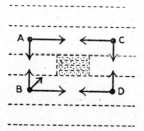

Fig. 136.   Local analgesia
for small rib resection.

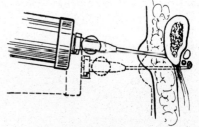

Fig. 137.   Diagram showing initial and
final position of needle in intercostal block (from *Anesthesiology*
after T. H. Sheldon).

under the lower border of the selected rib in order to block the intercostal nerve in its groove. The needle must not be advanced deeper than 0·5 cm. from the posterior surface of the rib, and the aspiration test must be negative before 2 c.cm. of analgesic solution are injected. When the rib is exposed, a subperiosteal injection minimizes the pain of stripping the periosteum. The patient should always be warned when the pleura is about to be opened or the sudden sucking noise may cause great alarm.

If it is proposed to use a sulphonamide as an antibiotic either locally or systemically, nupercaine should be substituted for procaine (see Chapter XIII).

Children are, as a rule, unsuitable for local analgesia and empyemata in them can be drained under cyclopropane.

Cardiac Investigations in Children

Cardiac catheterization has recently been introduced for obtaining samples of blood from the heart in order to investigate the nature of congenital cardiac lesions by the evidence supplied by gas analysis. For this procedure a cardiac catheter is passed via an antecubital vein into the right heart and pulmonary artery under X-ray control. At intervals the blood pressure is taken and samples of blood are withdrawn for gas analysis. Cardiac catheterization is unfortunately not so innocuous as was at first supposed and multifocal ventricular tachycardia and ventricular fibrillation with fatal results have occurred, presumably caused by initiation of impulses from the tip of the catheter. Young children should always be made unconscious for this investigation and basal narcosis with bromethol has been used successfully with infiltration of the site of introduction of the catheter with procaine.[28] The inhalation of oxygen has everything to recommend it from the physiological point of view as these children are usually anoxic in any event but some surgeons object on the grounds that false readings are given by the gas analysis of the blood. It has, however, been pointed out that for most investigations, it is the relative readings, with the tip of the catheter in different positions, which are much more important than the absolute ones.[29] If arrhythmia persists after the investigation, intravenous procaine or pronestyl (q.v.) is probably the most effective treatment.[30]

Angiocardiography may be combined with cardiac catheterization and is accomplished by withdrawing the catheter until only an inch or so remains in the vein. A rapid injection of a contrast medium (e.g. diodrast) is made and a series of skiagrams of the heart and great vessels are taken either in the antero-posterior or oblique positions. Unless the patient is deeply narcotized, vomiting, coughing, bronchospasm and collapse may occur and, in the writer's opinion, endotracheal nitrous oxide-oxygen and trichlorethylene is a satisfactory technique. If the explosion hazard of the X-ray apparatus could be ignored (as is said to be the case with modern plants) endotracheal ether-oxygen or cyclopropane-oxygen would be a preferable method. Difficulty is sometimes experienced in making an almost instantaneous injection of the diodrast. A preliminary injection of procaine often obviates the trouble.

Cardiac Surgery

The scope of cardiac surgery has increased greatly in the past few years and the following operations are becoming relatively common :

Cardiolysis or pericardiectomy for constrictive pericarditis (Pick's disease).

Closure of patent ductus arteriosus with a consequent immediate rise in diastolic pressure. Uninfected cases do better than those with bacterial endocarditis even with intensive treatment by antibiotics.[32]

Blalock's operation for anastamosing the pulmonary artery to the aorta or one of its main branches for such congenital cardiac diseases as pulmonary stenosis accompanied by an interventricular leak causing Fallot's tetralogy.

Crafoord's operation for coarctation of the aorta. In this condition there is a constriction at the level of the ligamentum arteriosum with the result that the upper half of the body has a higher blood pressure than the lower half. The operation consists in clamping the aorta above and below the stenosis, excising this and resuturing the two ends.

Valvulotomy for mitral stenosis.

Suture of cardiac wounds and the removal of foreign bodies embedded in the musculature or lying in one of the cardiac cavities are not common in civilian practice.

Anæsthesia for the performance of these operations can be carried out on the lines mentioned for an ordinary thoracotomy but several special factors may require consideration.

Cardiac Arrhythmias. Irregularity of the heart's action is frequently caused by surgical manipulation especially if the whole organ has to be twisted. If untreated, the arrhythmia may progress to ventricular fibrillation or actual standstill. The usual prophylactic measures employed are to give quinidine before and after operation and to use procaine during the surgical interference. Both these drugs reduce myocardial irritability and prolong the refractory period of the auricle, so diminishing the risk of premature contractions and fibrillations.[28] As a rule a 0·6 per cent. procaine drip is arranged to deliver about 1,000 mg. per hour in an adult. Some surgeons also inject 2 to 4 c.cm. 2 per cent. procaine into the pericardial cavity about five minutes before the pericardium is opened (e.g. during a valvulotomy) and then to apply swabs soaked in the same solution to the base of the auricular appendage.[33] This concentration should not be exceeded, as the writer has knowledge of a patient whose heart stopped instantaneously after an intra-pericardial injection of 4 per cent. procaine. Some observers have great faith in the ability of procaine to avert arrhythmias[34] but the writer has not been greatly impressed by it. In children the concentration of the procaine drip is reduced to 0·2 per cent. Recent work suggests that procaine amide (pronestyl) given in considerably larger doses may prove superior to procaine.

Anoxia. It is imperative to avoid anoxia, even for a brief period, in cardiac surgery, and for this reason it seems best to use either cyclopropane or ether and oxygen by a simple endotracheal method. In adults a cuffed tube can be passed but in young children this is replaced by a plain tube with a pharyngeal pack.[35] Sufficient relaxant to permit of controlled respiration is given. When administered in this way a low concentration of cyclopropane in oxygen can be used and with the procaine drip the gas rarely produces serious arrhythmias. Some anæsthetists, however, prefer to rely on ether and oxygen, a technique which has the advantage of relaxing the whole bronchial tree. Most surgeons are willing to forego the use of the diathermy in cardiac surgery in order to enable the above-mentioned inflammable drugs to be used. In the writer's opinion, this is distinctly preferable to the substitution of non-volatile drugs such as thiopentone and pethidine.

Fluid Loss. An intravenous drip should always be set up (often a double-drip with procaine as mentioned above) in case of sudden and severe hæmorrhage. Great care must be taken, however, not to overload the heart and cause pulmonary œdema so that the drip rate should be slow. Many patients with congenital cardiac lesions show compensatory polycythæmia and in these, blood should not as a rule be given but saline, plasma or a plasma substitute (q.v.).

After-treatment. Unless the patient is gravely shocked, it is usually advisable to carry out suction-bronchoscopy on completion of the operation. During transit from theatre to bed oxygen should be given usually by a B.L.B. mask and efficient oxygen therapy continued thereafter for as long as is necessary.

Sterilization of Anæsthetic Apparatus

The **sterilization of face-pieces** and breathing tubes after thoracic operations is most important to avoid cross-infection, particularly if sputum is present. Bacteriological examination of face-pieces removed from patients suffering from active phthisis showed contamination with the tubercle bacillus in 33 per cent. After simple rinsing in water 15 per cent. of the face-pieces were still infected, but after washing and immersion in a formaldehyde-alcohol solution all were sterile.[36] The recommended formula is :

Formaldehyde (38%)	..	..	210 c.cm.
Water	..	..	606 c.cm.
Alcohol (95%) ad	..	..	4,000 c.cm.

It is fortunate that the soda-lime canister acts as a most efficient bacterial filter so protecting the inspiratory side of a " circle " apparatus.

References

1. CHARNIER, A., and LOUBAT, E. " Traitement Chirurgical de la Tuberculose Pulmonaire," 1932, pp. 274 and 279.
2. HALTON, J. *Brit. Med. Jour.*, 1935, July 27, p. 159.
3. NOSWORTHY, M. D. { *Pro. Roy. Soc. Med.* (An. Sec.), 1940, Dec. 4. / *Pro. Roy. Soc. Med.* (An. Sec.), 1941, April 4. / *Anæsthesia*, 1951, Oct., p. 211.
4. TUFFIER, T. *Presse Medicale*, 1906, xiv, p. 57.
5. WYNNE, R. L. *Anæsthesia*, 1952, Jan., p. 46.
6. EATHER, K. F., *et al.* *Anesthesiology*, 1949, Mar., p. 125.
7. NOSWORTHY, M. D. *Anæsthesia*, 1948, July, p. 36.
8. ANDERSON, E., *et al.* *Acta Oto-Laryngol.*, 1939, 28.
9. MUSGROVE, A. H. *Anæsthesia*, 1952, April.
10. { PINSON, K. B., and BRYCE, A. C. *Brit. Jour. Anæsth.*, 1944, Jan., p. 2. / PINSON, K. B. *Anæsthesia*, 1949, April, p. 79.
11. MOERCH, E. T. *Anæsthesia*, 1948, Jan., p. 4.
12. *Brit. Med. Jour.*, 1949, Jan. 15, p. 117.
13. MAGILL, I. W. *Lancet*, 1943, Jan. 23, p. 125.
14. MORTON, H. J. V. *Brit. Med. Jour.*, 1945, Jan. 6, p. 16.
15. BEECHER, H. K. *Jour. Thorac. Surg.*, 1940, Dec., p. 202.
16. MAGILL, I. W. *Pro. Roy. Soc. Med.* (An. Sec.), 1941, April 4 (discussion).
17. ORTON, R. H. *Med. Jour. Australia*, 1949, Feb. 12, p. 189.
18. BROWN, A. I. P. *Thorax*, 1948, Sept., p. 161.
19. CRAFOORD, C. { *Acta. Chir. Scand.*, 1938, Suppl. 54. / " On the Technique of Pneumonectomy in Man," 1938.
20. WATERS, R. M., and GALE, J. W. { *Jour. Thorac. Surg.*, 1932, April, p. 432. / *Anesth. & Anal.*, 1932, Nov. -Dec., p. 283.
21. GURD, F. B., *et al.* *Jour. Thorac. Surg.*, 1938, June, p. 506.
22. GURD, F. B. *Ann. Surg.*, 1939, Nov., p. 872.
23. SHIELDS, H. J. *Anesth. & Anal.*, 1935, Sept.-Oct., p. 193.
24. PETERSON, M. C., and ROVENSTEINE, E. A. *Anesth. & Anal.*, 1936, Nov.-Dec., p. 300.
25. DURRANS, S. F. *Anæsthesia*, 1947, July, p. 106.
26. YOUNG, F. H. *Brit. Med. Jour.*, 1936, Apr. 4, p. 683.

27. HEWER, C. L.   *Post. grad. Med. Jour.*, 1935, Jan., p. 11.
28. MILLAR, E. J.   *Pro. Roy. Soc. Med.* (An. Sec.), 1951, Nov. 2.
29. ANSTRUTHER-SMITH, J.   *Brit. Med. Jour.*, 1950, Mar. 25, p. 705.
30. MICHEL, J., *et al.*   *Circulation*, 1950, **2**, p. 245.
31. SISE, L. F.   *Jour. Indiana State Med. Ass.*, 1937, Apr., p. 180.
32. GILLIES, J.   *Pro. Roy. Soc. Med.* (An. Sec.), 1945, May 4.
33. { BAKER, C., *et al.*   *Brit. Med. Jour.*, 1950, June 3, p. 1283.
{ SELLORS, T. H., and BELCHER, J. R.   *Lancet*, 1950, Dec. 30, p. 887.
34. BURSTEIN, C.   *Anesthesiology*, 1946, March, p. 113.
35. RINK, E. H., *et al.*   *Guy's Hosp. Rep.*, **97**, Nos. 1 and 2.
36. LIVINGSTONE, H., *et al.*   *Surgery*, 1941, March, p. 433.

CHAPTER XXIII

ANÆSTHESIA AND ANALGESIA FOR ABDOMINAL SURGERY

Upper and Lower Abdominal Operations—Gynæcological Surgery—Intestinal Obstruction—Acute Abdominal Conditions in Children—Toxæmia—Jaundice

THERE is considerable divergence of opinion as to the best anæsthetic technique for major abdominal surgery. It is universally admitted, however, that the nearer the incision is to the diaphragm the greater are the difficulties encountered.

In **upper abdominal operations** the wound is made in the area in which respiratory movement is at its maximum, so that it is desirable that the anæsthetic should produce as little additional excursion as possible. Secondly, in order to obtain the best exposure, the recti and other abdominal muscles should be completely relaxed. This desirable result may be difficult to obtain owing to the fact that severe traction on the peritoneum and diaphragmatic attachments may result in reflex laryngeal spasm. Furthermore, operative trauma in the upper abdomen gives rise to more shock than is the case in the lower abdomen and pelvis. Lastly, prolonged operations upon upper abdominal viscera tend to be followed by more pulmonary complications than do those on other parts of the body (see Chapter XXV).

It will be seen, therefore, that the ideal anæsthetic for upper abdominal surgery should afford : (i) minimal respiratory movements ; (ii) absolute muscular relaxation ; (iii) protection from operative shock ; and (iv) absence of post-operative pulmonary complications.[1]

Until the introduction of the muscle relaxants the methods which fulfilled these conditions most closely were :

(i) Endotracheal nitrous oxide-oxygen-ether with subsequent hyperventilation with carbon dioxide-air.[1, 2, 3] For many years the writer used a modified insufflation technique for this work. A fairly large blunt-ended catheter was employed and the expiratory valve closed. A certain amount of rebreathing took place and the excess gases escaped around the catheter. Extremely quiet respiration was possible with this technique. Alternatively, an ordinary rubber tracheal tube can be passed and a semi-open circuit used with a T-piece and a short length of open-ended wide-bore tubing. In this case also, respiration should be quiet and shallow. For bad-risk patients, the writer has found endo-tracheal cyclopropane preferable. The closed-circuit method minimizes heat-loss and the post-operative condition is most gratifying. Partial gastrectomy for carcinoma in the aged (75-85) has proved practicable upon several occasions with this technique.

In the last few years, however, the general opinion is that in fairly muscular subjects less damage is done by securing relaxation with blocks or specific relaxants than in " pushing " the narcotic used to produce unconsciousness to the plane necessary for muscular relaxation. The following three techniques have had some vogue.

(ii) Spinal block, preferably with nupercaine (see Chapter XV). This method probably conforms most closely to the " abdominal silence " and " negative intra-abdominal pressure " so beloved by surgeons. It also provides contracted intestines.

(iii) Field block of abdominal wall with splanchnic or mesenteric block or intraperitoneal procaine (see Chapter XIV).

(iv) Bilateral thoracic (6 to 12) and posterior splanchnic blocks[4] combined with infiltration of the line of incision. The thoracic nerves are blocked at a point four fingers' breadth from the mid-line. The needle is felt to impinge upon the selected rib and is made to slide beneath its lower border. It is then advanced not more than 1 cm. and 10 c.cm. of 1 in 1,000 amethocaine solution are injected, the needle being kept moving backwards and forwards.

The last three methods can be usefully combined with an intra-venous injection of a short-acting barbiturate given just before the local block or by a very light cyclopropane anæsthesia. The majority of patients object to being completely conscious during an abdominal operation. Intravenous morphine usually gives better sedation with less excitement than the barbiturates, but it should not be used in combination with high spinal block or serious respiratory depression may occur. Continuous oxygen inhalation may be indicated during long abdominal operations performed under local analgesia. For further details of technique the reader is recommended to peruse the excellent monograph by N. R. James entitled " Regional Analgesia for Intra-abdominal Surgery " (1943).

(v) The introduction of the muscle relaxants has changed the whole position regarding anæsthesia for upper abdominal surgery. The intravenous injection of one of these drugs gives perfect muscular relaxation within a very short time, and the general narcosis is used for little more than keeping the patient unconscious. Various methods can be used and from experience of over 500 partial and total gastrectomies, the writer can recommend the following technique. After light premedication a Ryles' tube is passed through the nose in the ward and this is kept *in situ* during and after operation, suction being applied as required. Induction of anæsthesia is by intravenous thiopentone, maintenance being effected either by nitrous oxide-oxygen and minimal trilene or ether or by cyclopropane. A preliminary dose of 5 mg. tubocurarine is given intravenously and intubation is carried out, preferably with a

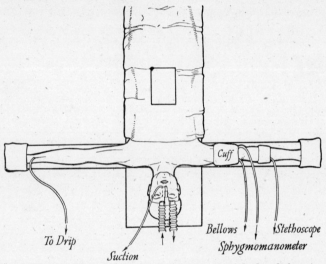

FIG. 138.   General set-up for gastric operation in right-handed patient.

cuffed tube. The patient is then placed on the operating table with his arms bandaged to a double splint which passes behind the sorbo rubber mattress. This position gives unhampered respiration and ready accessibility to each arm.[5] It is important to see that the parts of the splint projecting from the table are well padded and that the centre part is unpadded so that the arms are not forced backwards. Furthermore the hands should be allowed to assume their natural position as forced supination and external rotation undoubtedly predisposes to brachial plexus palsy.[6] Arm splints should not be used if a Trendelenburg tilt sufficiently steep to necessitate shoulder rests is required.

For right-handed patients an intravenous drip is set up in the left forearm and the blood-pressure apparatus fixed on the right arm (Fig. 138). By this time the surgeon will have reached the peritoneum and unless relaxation is adequate (which is unlikely) a further dose of 10 mg. of " tubarine " is given into the intravenous drip. Within two minutes the full effect should be apparent and the respiratory exchange should be carefully watched. Breathing may have to be " aided " by pressure on the rebreathing bag during inspiration or fully " controlled " if diaphragmatic paresis is marked. In no case must any anoxia be permitted. It cannot be too strongly stressed that it is quite unjustifiable to use a muscle relaxant unless the anæsthetist has the means and skill to control pulmonary ventilation. If the operation is prolonged, further doses of curare may be required, but inadequate relaxation towards the end is better treated by a small intravenous dose of pethidine. When the parietal peritoneum is being closed a momentary tightening of the abdominal musculature is dealt with by a very small dose of thiopentone, the effects of which will have worn off before the skin is sutured. If, by some mischance, such as the discovery of an inoperable growth, the patient is still curarized at the conclusion of the operation, prostigmine and atropine should be given. Before the tracheal tube is removed, the trachea and bronchi should be sucked out by means of a Teeman's catheter.

It might be mentioned that a recent series of 200 consecutive partial gastrectomies for ulcer has been recorded[7] with one death (mortality 0·5 per cent.). Most of these operations were performed with the anæsthetic technique just described.

Some anæsthetists prefer to keep curarized patients only just unconscious with nitrous oxide-oxygen and occasional small doses of thiopentone but, in the writer's opinion, hiccup is much more likely to develop if the surgeons exercise traction on the œsophagus. This complication is a distressing one as it may hamper the surgeon greatly. All kinds of remedies have been tried, two of the most successful being a small intravenous dose of methedrine, or the introduction of amyl nitrite vapour into the anæsthetic circuit.[27] If patients are kept at a reasonably deep plane of narcosis and relaxants are used sparingly, hiccup is rarely seen and the blood pressure and pulse rate readings are much more constant.

If an open inhalation technique must be used, a preliminary cocainization of the glottis tends to obviate reflex laryngeal spasm. Caution should be exercised if a preliminary basal narcotic is employed, as there is no doubt that respiratory depressants given in large doses before long abdominal operations do tend to increase pulmonary complications.[8]

It has been shown that the rigid dorsal decubitus tends to make the abdominal muscles tense as the weight of the legs rotates the pelvis downwards. If, however, a hard cushion (as illustrated) is used to raise the knees 6 to 8 inches off the table, abdominal relaxation is greatly facilitated.[9] In the writer's opinion, this advantage

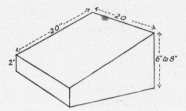

Fig. 139.   Knee-cushion for abdominal surgery (Fitzwilliam's).

is more than counterbalanced by the increased risk of venous stasis and pulmonary embolism. He prefers to have the patient's legs flat with their weight supported by an oblong sorbo pad placed underneath the tendo Achillis. There is then no compression of the veins of the calf.

If severe shock has occurred or is anticipated during a prolonged upper abdominal operation, a pint of gum-saline at 105° F. can be introduced into the peritoneal cavity just prior to its complete closure. The writer has been most favourably impressed with this procedure. The absorption of fluid appears to be more prolonged than is the case with pure saline, and the absence of thirst after operation is most marked. This latter feature is of particular benefit after gastric operations, where little or no fluid can be given by mouth for some time.

Comparatively **minor procedures in the upper abdomen,** such as gastrostomy, can generally be performed under local infiltration analgesia only.

Operations involving the opening of the thoracic cavity such as transthoracic gastrectomy and the repair of diaphragmatic hernia have been considered in Chapter XXII.

Lower abdominal operations do not demand such complete muscular relaxation and can usually be performed efficiently under nitrous oxide-oxygen with either minimal ether or a medium acting relaxant such as gallamine, or with an abdominal wall field block and light cyclopropane. Long operations, which may be followed by severe shock, such as abdomino-perineal resection of the rectum,[10] are frequently done with spinal block. The same technique is often used for prostatectomy,[11] but many surgeons dislike it on account of the tendency towards reactionary hæmorrhage when the blood pressure subsequently rises. The writer has found that equally good results are obtained with light general anæsthesia with tubocurarine and that this causes less anxiety both during operation and afterwards. In the synchronous-combined type of rectal excision, great blood-loss may occur from the two wounds during the first half-hour of operation. The rate of drip of the transfusion can be speeded up to a continuous stream during this period.

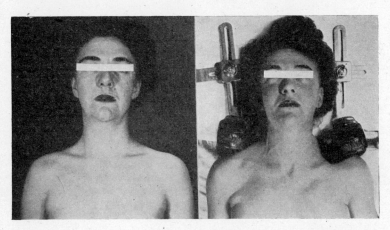

FIG. 140. Patient lying horizontal on operating table. (*Photos by Photographic Dept. of St. Bartholomew's Hospital.*)

FIG. 141. Same patient after one minute in 45° Trendelenburg slope. Note œdema of face, chemosis and congestion of cervical veins.

Gynæcological operations usually present no difficulty as regards relaxation, but the steep Trendelenburg position so often adopted may lead to complications. An immediate rise in blood pressure occurs and the head and neck frequently become congested and œdematous, especially if the shoulder rests are incorrectly adjusted. (The writer is aware of a case of retinal detachment which immediately followed a gynæcological operation performed with a steep head-down slope.[12]) Furthermore respiration is embarrassed and calls for more exertion than usual on account of the difficulties under which the diaphragm must function. Not only must this muscle perform its normal work of producing negative pressure in the thorax, but it must also push up the abdominal viscera which are now resting against it both by the force of gravity and also by abdominal packs often reinforced by retractors or by an assistant's hand. It has been found that a tilt of 30° causes a reduction in

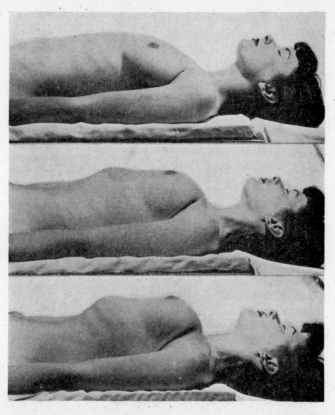

FIG. 142.   Patient lying (1) horizontal, (2) in 20° head-down tilt, (3) in 45° head-down tilt.   Note alteration in contour of thorax and abdomen associated with the rise in diaphragm and compression of lungs.   (*Photos by Photographic Dept. of St. Bartholomew's Hospital.*)

vital capacity of about 15 per cent. and this is due mainly to the compression of the lungs from the high diaphragm.

The technical difficulties in maintaining a steep tilt in a fat patient are considerable.   Shoulder rests occasionally cause postoperative brachial plexus palsy and the incidence is increased if one or both arms are abducted and if the patient is curarized.[6]   Pelvic rests are a good alternative if the operating table is fitted to take them. If not, some of the patients' weight can be taken by her legs if the knees are bent, but as mentioned before this increases the risk of stasis in the veins of the calf. A considerable amount of friction can be brought into play between the skin of the patient's back and the rubber mattress which should be securely strapped to the table. If the surface of the mattress is corrugated, friction alone will hold a patient in a moderate tilt. The writer has been well pleased with experiments carried out with this method, the only difficulty encountered being the reduction in friction if the corrugations become wet from perspiration or other cause. For this reason shoulder rests should always be employed as an additional precaution against the patient slipping. The anæsthetist should see that the head-down slope is not adopted before it is necessary, is as slight as is compatible with the surgeon's work, and is not maintained after the peritoneal closure. When placing the patient flat once more, the slope should be altered in stages or a severe fall in blood pressure may occur. During the period of tilting, it is probable that saliva and mucus may have collected in the naso-pharynx and any secretions should be removed by a nasal suction catheter before the horizontal position is resumed.[28]

Operations for acute intestinal obstruction are always an anxiety to the anæsthetist. Spinal block is thought by some to be the best method[13] (see Chapter XV), but in the opinion of the author and others[14] the endotracheal technique with a gauze pack or inflated cuff is safer, as no further lowering of blood pressure occurs and the inspiration of septic material is avoided. If possible a Ryle's tube should be passed through the nose before operation and suction applied before the induction of anæsthesia. The tube can be kept in position throughout and after operation, suction being used intermittently as required. Even if no suction pump is available, an aural or bladder syringe or even a 20 c.cm. " Record " syringe can be pressed into service. If, for any reason, preoperative gastric siphonage is impossible, or if there is a possibility that the stomach contains semi-solid material, a full-size stomach tube should be passed before the induction of anæsthesia is begun. If the patient will not co-operate, it is better to start with an inhalation method as vomiting is less likely to be followed by dire results before intubation has been accomplished, than if intravenous thiopentone were used. At the end of the operation, a full tracheo-bronchial toilet should be carefully performed to make sure that, in spite of all precautions, no stomach contents have entered the respiratory passages. An excellent article on this subject can be perused by the reference.[15]

If the intestinal obstruction is known to be due to a strangulated inguinal hernia, the operation can frequently be performed successfully under local analgesia. After infiltration of the skin and subcutaneous tissues, an attempt should be made to deposit solution in the area surrounding the internal ring by means of a needle introduced at the top of the scrotum and passed along the spermatic cord.[16]

High intestinal obstruction produces alkalosis and a reduction of the chlorides in the blood. Consequently, in such cases, a preoperative intravenous infusion of sodium chloride should be given, preferably by the drip method.[17]

Observation on anæsthesia for **acute abdominal conditions in young children** is not conclusive as to the desirability of any particular technique. Some observers consider that general anæsthesia gives better results than local or spinal analgesia[18] while at a large children's hospital the results of Rammstedt's operation under general and local methods over a period of many years were indistinguishable.[19] However this may be, the three essential factors to ensure a low mortality in such cases are : (a) speed in operating ; (b) conservation of body heat ; (c) administration of adequate fluids. These points are dealt with under " shock ".

If general narcosis is to be used, an open endotracheal technique is probably the best, e.g. ether and oxygen using Ayre's T-piece.

In local analgesia[20] it is usual to " crucify " the baby previously by binding its limbs to a padded wooden cross splint. A nurse can give the infant a comforter to suck dipped in equal parts of port and glycerine. The infiltration of the abdominal wall should be undertaken with not more than 15 c.cm. of 0·33 per cent. procaine with 1 in 600,000 adrenaline solution. This contains 50 mg. procaine which should be regarded as the maximum dose for a baby weighing 7 lb. It is extremely easy to give an overdose to infants, e.g. a fatality has occurred with 20 c.cm. of 1 per cent. procaine.[21] The chief difficulty with simple infiltration is the closure of the peritoneum in a fairly lusty infant who is crying. Pushing out of the viscera may result in considerable shock.

In cases of **grave toxæmia,** e.g. old perforations or appendicitis with general peritonitis, the use of toxic drugs such as chloroform or ether should be eschewed or at any rate reduced to a minimum. At the same time there is no doubt that many of the patients whose deaths have, in the past, been attributed to the toxic effects of anæsthetic drugs have really died of septicæmia. It has been found that on making a blood examination a pure culture of *Streptococcus faecalis* can frequently be obtained.[22] Spinal analgesia has been advocated for this type of operation,[23] but the writer has been disappointed in the results obtained, and considers that cyclopropane or nitrous oxide-oxygen with minimal ether or infiltration is preferable.

It has been demonstrated that the absorption of toxic matter from the peritoneum takes place chiefly through the diaphragmatic lymphatics and the venules of the omentum. The rate of absorption by the former route varies with the respiratory activity. Consequently, any method of anæsthesia which causes deep breathing should be avoided in cases of peritonitis.[24]

Jaundiced patients should always be given calcium in the pre-operative period. This not only shortens the clotting time of the blood but also protects the tissues from the toxic effects of bilirubin and abnormal liver products, such as methyl guanidine.[25] Calcium can be given in various forms but di-calcium phosphate with viosterol and calcium gluconate are favourite preparations.[26]

Vitamin K is also given as a rule for several days before operation in subcutaneous doses of about 10 mg. (e.g. as " Synkavit " Roche, 10 mg. per c.cm.). The reason for this procedure is that as vitamin K is fat-soluble, it is not absorbed from the bowel if bile is absent. Consequently the formation of prothrombin in the liver will be impeded so that increased bleeding can be expected during operations for the relief of obstructive jaundice. Vitamin K analogues such as menaphthone and acetomenaphthone can be employed.

In the writer's experience transfusion with *fresh* blood during operation definitely diminishes capillary oozing in jaundiced patients but stored blood appears to have no effect.

References

1. HEWER, C. L. *Brit. Med. Jour.*, 1926, Aug. 14.
2. TANNER, W. E. *Post-Grad. Med. Jour.*, 1932, Jan., p. 25.
3. GRIFFITH, H. R. *Anesth. & Anal.*, 1932, Sept.-Oct., p. 207.
4. JAMES, N. R., and BURGE, H. W. *Brit. Med. Jour.*, 1941, Dec. 21, p. 906.
5. WILSON, W. E. *Pro. Roy. Soc. Med.* (An. Sec.), 1944, Nov. 3.
6. EWING, M. R.
   KILON, L. G. *Lancet*, 1950, Jan. 21.
   Annotation.
7. HOSFORD, J. *Brit. Med. Jour.*, 1949, May 28, p. 929.
8. HEWER, C. L. *Brit. Med. Jour.*, 1930, Nov. 29.
9. FITZWILLIAMS, D. C. L. *Lancet*, 1934, Nov. 24, p. 1161.
10. CATTELL, R. B. *Jour. Amer. Med. Ass.*, 1936, Dec. 19, p. 2011.
11. THOMSON-WALKER, J. *Brit. Med. Jour.*, 1923, *i*, p. 137.

12. DALY, A. S.   1944.   Personal Communication.
13. McGAVIN, L. H.   *Brit. Med. Jour.*, 1911, *ii*, p. 1638.
14. HOWARD JONES, W.   *Brit. Med. Jour.*, 1933, Jan. 21, p. 119.
15. MORTON, H. J. V., and WYLIE, W. D.   *Anæsthesia*, 1951, Oct., p. 190.
16. POWER, R. W.   *Brit. Med. Jour.*, 1934, May 3, p. 787.
17. THALHIMER, W.   *Anesth. & Anal.*, 1928, Jan.-Feb.
18. SINGTON, H.   *Brit. Med. Jour.*, 1923, Nov. 3, p. 787.
19. COPE, R. W.   *Pro. Roy. Soc. Med.* (An. Sec.), 1948, Feb. 6.
20. { LEVI, D.   *Post-Grad. Med. Jour.*, 1936, Oct., p. 417.
     { BROWNE, D.   *Pro. Roy. Soc. Med.* (Sec. Paed.), 1951, Apr. 27.
21. McQUAID, J. N. W., and PORRITT, B. E.   *Lancet*, 1950, Feb. 4, p. 201.
22. BROWN, H.   *Pro. Roy. Soc. Med.* (Med. and Surg. Sec.), 1932, Nov. 2.
23. RAYNER, H. H.   *Pro. Roy. Soc. Med.* (Med. and Surg. Sec.), 1932, Nov. 2.
24. MENGLE, H. A.   *Arch. of Surg.*, 1937, May, p. 839.
25. MINOT, A. S., and CUTLER, J. T.   *Jour. Clin. Invest.*, 1928, **6**, p. 369.
26. BLISS, R. A., and MORRISON, R. W.   *Jour. Amer. Pharm. Ass.*, 1935, **24,**
     p. 280.
27. { FAJARDO, J.   *Lancet*, 1952, Feb. 2.
     { LEE, J. A.   *Lancet*, 1952. Feb. 16.   } Correspondence.
     { HENDRIE, J., and KAUFMAN, L.   *Lancet*, 1952, Mar. 1.
28. HEWER, C. L.   *Lancet*, 1952, Oct. 25, p. 826.   (Correspondence).

CHAPTER XXIV

ANÆSTHESIA AND ANALGESIA IN OBSTETRICS— RESUSCITATION OF THE NEW-BORN

" Natural " Childbirth

BEFORE discussing the various methods of relieving the pain of childbirth, it is only fair to say that one school of thought maintains that normal labour (vertex presentation with anterior occiput and no mechanical obstruction) can be virtually painless even among civilized races.[1] The obvious fact that it usually is not is explained by supposing that fear causes a sympatheticotonia which makes the circular fibres of the cervical sphincter contract. In turn the longitudinal fibres of the upper uterine segment increase their tension to overcome the obstacle and thus the threshold of pain is crossed. " A tense woman means a tense cervix and a long and painful labour." This is probably an over-simplification of a complicated problem, but there is no doubt that antenatal teaching and emphasis on " relaxation " at crucial times of the labour can work wonders with a co-operative patient. Unfortunately this technique makes very heavy demands on the doctor's time and patience, and in these days it often cannot be practised.

Methods of Pain Relief

It is probable that every known type of anæsthetic, analgesic and amnesic has been used to mitigate or eliminate the pain of natural and operative childbirth.

For those who wish to see how the various drugs can be administered for this type of work, the following alphabetical list of references is given, with no expression of opinion on their merits and demerits :

Acetylene.[2]
Adaline.[3]
Bromethol.[4]
Chloral hydrate.[3]
Chloroform.[4]
Cyclopropane.[5]
Dial-urethane.[6]

Di-ethyl ether by inhalation[7] and rectal instillation.[8]
Di-vinyl ether.[9]
Ethyl alcohol.[10]
Ethyl chloride.[2]
Ethylene.[11]
Heroin.[12]
Hexobarbitone.[13]
Hypnosis and suggestion.[2]
Intravenous procaine.[14]
Isopropyl chloride.[15]
Morphine and scopolamine.[18]
Nembutal.[16]
Nitrous oxide and air[17] or oxygen.[3]
Paracervical field block.[19]
Paraldehyde and benzyl alcohol.[20]
Pernocton.[21]
Pethidine.[22]
Physeptone.[23]
Rectidon.[24]
Sacral and caudal blocks.[25]
Sodium amytal.[26]
Sodium soneryl.[27]
Spinal block.[23]
Synergistic techniques.[29]
Thiopentone.[30]
Trichlorethylene.[31]
" Voluntary " relaxation.[1]

The advantages of relief of pain in labour are obvious in the case of the mother, but recent work tends to show that the child also benefits. The precise time that the fœtus begins to feel pain is not known, but it has been established that immediately after birth the baby normally suffers from mild shock from the trauma of delivery. If the mother is anæsthetized, the shock to the infant is diminished, and it has been shown that the loss of weight sustained in the first few days after birth is also lessened.[32]

Criteria for Choice of Method

It is now generally considered desirable to provide almost instantaneous analgesia for the duration of the pains leaving the patient conscious but placid between them. Prolonged periods of semi-narcosis have been shown to be undesirable for both mother and child. Actual anæsthesia is preferable when delivery is taking place and until the expulsion of the placenta. Finally, the drugs employed must not reduce the force of the uterine contractions nor have any toxic effects on mother or child.

Chloroform Analgesia

It will readily be seen that the popular practice of giving **chloroform** " à la reine "* does not conform to the requirements given above, although it seems probable that the normal risk of primary cardiac failure in light chloroform anæsthesia is diminished in labour.[33] The condition does occur, however, while cases of delayed chloroform poisoning have, also, been described after delivery.[34] These are most likely to occur if labour is prolonged or if the patient is dehydrated from vomiting or is suffering from toxæmia. If the condition is established the only treatment likely to be of any use is intravenous glucose with insulin. There is no evidence to show that methionine is of any value.[35]

Chloroform is still employed largely by general practitioners, who usually fit up some type of Junker's apparatus and mask, so that the patient, by pumping herself, can get some slight analgesia. If this method must be used, the modified bottle of Dr. Mennell (illustrated) is probably the safest pattern. The tubes cannot be connected wrongly, the bottle cannot be upset and is difficult to overfill. The strength of vapour is insufficient to produce full surgical anæsthesia.[36]

Chloroform capsules have been suggested for the use of midwives working without a doctor. These capsules each contain 20 minims of chloroform, and are designed to be crushed and placed under a mask in order to produce analgesia.[37] In the opinion of the writer and others, encouragement should not be given to this enterprise. Apart from the impossibility of a single midwife

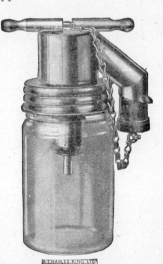

Fig. 143. Mennell's modified Junker bottle for obstetrical analgesia.

* So called in 1853, when Queen Victoria gave birth to her seventh child Prince Leopold, under chloroform analgesia administered by John Snow.

remaining sterile while administering chloroform, it is, indeed, para-doxical for a drug to be abandoned by expert anæsthetists owing to its toxicity, but to be encouraged for use by unqualified persons.[38] The conclusion formulated by a report of the British (now Royal) College of Obstetricians and Gynæcologists is that " chloroform by any method should not be used by midwives acting alone."[39]

It is now established that the replacement of chloroform by **trichlorethylene** (see later) results in a better analgesia with less toxicity.

Nitrous oxide-oxygen analgesia and anæsthesia

It is impossible in the scope of this book to consider all the various methods individually, but it is probable in spite of many new drugs and methods that the desiderata enumerated above are fulfilled most closely by **nitrous oxide-oxygen analgesia and anæsthesia**,[3, 40, 41] and a short description of this technique will now be given.

An intermittent-flow apparatus is the most suitable, the small obstetric model McKesson being a compact type. As soon as the pains become severe the mixture control is set at 25 per cent. oxygen, 75 per cent. nitrous oxide, the face-piece is placed in position and the patient directed to take three deep breaths, holding the third one at the end of inspiration and at the same time " bearing down ". It will be found that relief from pain is nearly always complete : if it is not, four breaths should be substituted for three at the next application. After being shown the method, the average intelligent woman will grasp the idea and can use the machine herself. There is no waste of gas as the flow is automatically cut off as the face-piece is removed. When the head is beginning to pass over the perineum, the anæsthetist takes charge and keeps the patient fully under nitrous oxide-oxygen until the placenta is expelled and any necessary suturing is finished. When continuous anæsthesia is substituted for intermittent analgesia, the oxygen percentage can be increased considerably. Some gynæcologists are of opinion that it is psychologically better for the patient to be conscious during delivery, and if she definitely expresses a wish to this effect it should be respected if possible.

Although nitrous oxide and oxygen cannot be administered in Great Britain by an unsupervised midwife, a simple automatic apparatus has been devised which delivers a constant mixture (usually 75 per cent. N_2O and 25 per cent. O_2). This is very suitable for institutions and incorporates a safety device so that if the oxygen supply runs out or fails, the nitrous oxide is automatically cut off.[42]

It has been shown that prolonged inhalation of mixtures containing less than 15 per cent. oxygen may lead to inadequate oxygenation of the fœtal blood.[43]   On the other hand, it has been shown

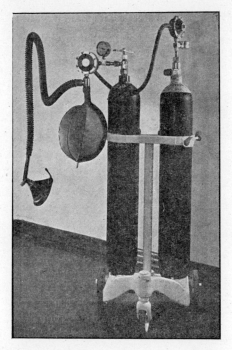

FIG. 144. " Calmator " automatic nitrous oxide-oxygen apparatus showing chamber above reservoir bag. (Seward, *Pro. Roy. Soc. Med.*)

that at the moment of delivery the blood in the umbilical cord has a higher oxygen content than the mother's venous blood, and it is possible for the mother to be cyanosed without any appreciable fœtal anoxia.[44]   So long as the placenta is normal, a reservoir of oxygen in combination with hæmoglobin estimated at about 40 c.cm. is present.   This safety-factor enables the fœtus to survive short periods of severe maternal anoxia.

It has been shown by internal hysterograms that while chloroform, ether and other anæsthetics have an inhibiting effect on

uterine contractions,[45] nitrous oxide-oxygen either has no effect
or tends to increase them.[46] These findings have been confirmed
by external hysterography,[47] and are borne out in actual practice,
as labours conducted under N_2O—O_2 are generally slightly shorter
than normal.[8]

The method described above gives, in the author's opinion, the
best all-round results in obstetrics, its main advantages being :

(i) There is no toxic effect on mother or child unless gross anoxia
is permitted. As a matter of fact, " gas " babies almost always
cry lustily the moment they are delivered. The absence of toxicity
is of special value in cases of pregnancy toxæmia. In this connection it is interesting to note that continuous nitrous oxide-oxygen
anæsthesia has been used successfully for the treatment of eclamptic
fits.[48]

(ii) Labour is not prolonged and is often shortened.

(iii) Relief from pain in the early stages of labour is almost
instantaneous without the production of unconsciousness, so that
the patient's full co-operation is secured.

(iv) The incidence of subinvolution, hæmorrhage and inertia is
not increased (Rucker).

(v) With proper technique the method is completely successful
in 100 per cent. of cases.

The only disadvantage that can fairly be alleged against nitrous
oxide-oxygen for labour is the necessity for an anæsthetist of
sufficient experience to use it. The increased expense of materials
is negligible, the cost per case in hospital of gases used being
estimated at two shillings.[49] From the patient's point of view the
method is ideal, and it is found in practice that once a woman has
experienced its advantages she will almost always insist upon it for
subsequent deliveries.

It sometimes happens that the patient complains of severe
backache between the pains, in which event *continuous* gas analgesia
with a closed-circuit apparatus is invaluable.

Analgesia with hydrocarbon Gases and Oxygen

Ethylene-oxygen and **cyclopropane-oxygen** have also been used
for intermittent analgesia in labour and have the advantage of a
higher oxygen percentage.[50] In the case of the latter combination,
fœtal movements *in utero* are not diminished and may be actually
increased during inhalation.[51]

Nitrous oxide-air Analgesia

If an anæsthetist is not available, the next best technique for normal labour is possibly **nitrous oxide-air analgesia.** This method was first tried out in Liverpool in October, 1933, by Minnitt, who adapted a McKesson oxygen-therapy apparatus for the purpose.[52] The standard apparatus designed by Minnitt is extremely portable and weighs 15 lb. without gas, while the " Minnitt Minor " light-weight type scales only $12\frac{1}{2}$ lb. with one 50-gallon nitrous oxide cylinder. The machine consists of a reducing valve and an inter-mittent-flow device delivering about 45 per cent. N_2O in air through a flexible tube to a face-piece. The latter is fitted with an air-hole which the patient normally closes but which allows pure air to be inspired should the finger pressure relax.[53] It is important that the mask should be applied to the face at the very first indication of a pain and should remain in position until the pain is quite over. At the time of actual delivery, the patient should be inhaling gas and air continuously and should be instructed *not* to bear down.[54] A trace of trichlorethylene vapour added to the gas-air mixture renders the analgesia much more certain. A (Rowbotham's) bottle can be plugged into the circuit to effect this.[31]

This technique is naturally inferior to gas and oxygen in that full anæsthesia is unobtainable for the actual delivery or for perineal suture. On the other hand, the apparatus is practically foolproof, and has already been used extensively by midwives in hospital. It is hoped in the future to extend its application more widely to domiciliary practice. A resolution passed by the Central Midwives Board for England and Wales permits gas-air analgesia to be administered by midwives, trained in its use subject to certain conditions. Since July, 1946, it has been obligatory for all pupil midwives to take a course of instruction and to be found proficient before being enrolled as certified midwives. The portable model of the Minnitt apparatus costs about 12 guineas and 50-gallon cylinders can be supplied delivered and collected at a flat rate charge of 3*s*. 6*d*. In a series of 1,065 cases it has been estimated that the actual cost of gas used per case was 2*s*. 6*d*.[55] As regards efficiency, it is stated that in 250 labours conducted under gas-air analgesia without premedication, 44 per cent. of patients had no pain what-ever, 53 per cent. experienced great relief, and 3 per cent. some relief.[56] No anæsthetic mortality has been recorded in over 3,000 administrations.[57]

Delay in obtaining analgesia is sometimes due to the fact that when the face-piece is laid aside after a pain, air dilutes the mixture in the breathing tube. This can be avoided by introducing a non-return valve near the face-piece[58] (see Fig. 145).

Moir considers that a quicker onset of analgesia ensues by using a limited quantity of **pure nitrous oxide** for each pain, and has designed an apparatus so that two consecutive breaths only are available. This is provided by a bag of $\frac{5}{8}$-gallon capacity, which automatically shuts off the gas supply when full. A carburettor jet is interposed between the reducing valve of the cylinder and the

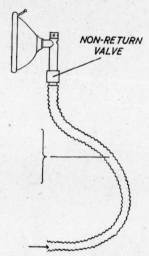

NON-RETURN VALVE

Fig. 145. Site of non-return valve in breathing tube. (A. H. Galloy, *Lancet*, 1950.)

bag, which so limits the gas flow that the bag takes one minute to refill.[59] On further investigation, however, it has been shown that many labour pains exceed 100 seconds' duration and that this technique may not give a sufficiently long analgesia.[60] In order to overcome this difficulty, Elam has designed an ingenious apparatus which on the first few inspirations delivers pure gas but which follows this with a gas-air mixture.[61] The same effect is obtained by a simple attachment fitted to Minnitt's machine (see Fig. 146). It must be clearly understood that this modification does not conform to the requirements of the C.M.B. and the apparatus so modified must only be used under medical supervision.

For further information on this subject, the reader is referred to

" Gas and Air Analgesia " by R. J. Minnitt (1949, Baillière, Tindall & Cox) and " Relief of Pain in Childbirth " by W. C. W. Nixon and S. G. Ransom (1951, Cassell).

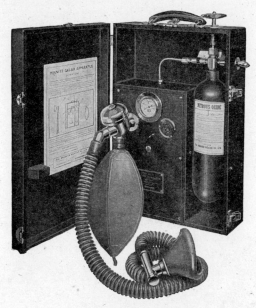

Fig. 146. Latest type portable model of Minnitt's apparatus with attachment so that a gas, gas-air sequence is delivered.

Whatever type of gas inhalation is adopted, it is most important that the stomach should be kept empty. Neglect of this obvious precaution has been the cause of many deaths from asphyxia and from aspiration pneumonia particularly when actual narcosis has been established.[62]

Analgesia with Trichlorethylene and Air

Trichlorethylene and air can be used to produce analgesia in a similar way to nitrous oxide and air with the advantages of lighter apparatus and no gas cylinders. Marrett's inhaler (see Fig. 42) is very efficient for this purpose[63] and complete narcosis can be produced if an anæsthetist is present. An Oxford ether vaporizer can be used in the same way[64] (75 per cent. on the ether calibration being equivalent to approximately 1·5 per cent. trichlorethylene).

Recently, smaller and simpler machines have been devised, such as Freedman's and the " cyprane ". The patient uses the inhaler

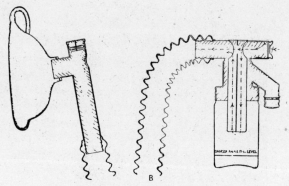

Fig. 147. Inhaler for trichlorethylene analgesia in midwifery (Freedman).

herself and under no circumstances can any liquid enter the face-piece. The inhaled mixture is about 0·65 per cent. trichlorethylene

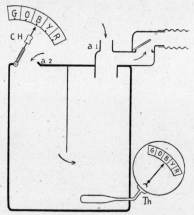

Fig. 148. Diagram showing principle of " Emotril " inhaler. (Epstein and Macintosh, *Brit. Med. Jour.*)

in air (by weight). This will cause analgesia only, but, as an added precaution, the patient must cover an air-hole with her finger as in Minnitt's apparatus. If unconsciousness should occur, the finger

would slip off and pure air would be inhaled.[65] Complete amnesia
has been noted after 20 per cent. of administrations.[66] A Committee of the Royal College of Obstetricians and Gynæcologists has

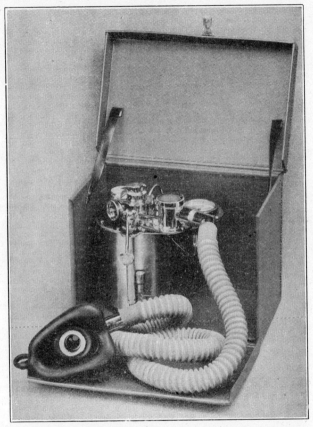

Fig. 149. " Emotril " analgesia inhaler for trichlorethylene
with hand-operated temperature compensator. (Epstein
and Macintosh, *Brit. Med. Jour.*)

made an exhaustive study of 2,354 patients given trichlorethylene
with Freedman's inhaler in sixteen hospitals.[67] The method was
found to be most effective, only 7 per cent. of mothers being
dissatisfied with the relief obtained, and there was no evidence of
increased risk to mother or child. Two observers thought that

there might be a possibility that unsupervized midwives might use the drug for a longer period than was customary in this series, and two thought that the fœtal heart rate was occasionally affected. In view of the generally favourable findings, it is disappointing that the Council of the College did not recommend the technique for use except under the supervision of a doctor.

To maintain a really constant vapour concentration with draw-over inhalers, account must be taken of the atmospheric temperature. In the Oxford vaporizer, this is done by means of a chemical thermostat (see Chapter VI). Another method of securing constant vapour concentration is to vary the size of the air inlet with the temperature. This can be done automatically by means of a thermostat as in the " Airlene " inhaler or by hand control as in the " Emotril " apparatus. The variable air inlet a2 is controlled by the lever CH which travels round a dial marked off into five segments of different colours. The thermometer Th has a similarly coloured dial and it only remains to set the control lever to the same colour as that on which the thermometer needle rests. The air inhaled by the patient through the fixed inlet a1 and the variable orifice a2 will now contain 0·5 per cent. trichlorethylene vapour over a wide range of temperature provided that some of the liquid drug remains in the container.[68] A " weak " mixture of 0·35 per cent. trichlorethylene can also be obtained. (Fig. 148.)

Non-volatile Analgesics

If no apparatus of any kind is available, it may be necessary to have recourse to narcotic and analgesic drugs, but it must be remembered that these do not fulfil all the requirements of an ideal obstetrical anæsthesia as set out above. The **nembutal-chloral** combination has had some vogue recently.[69] The initial dose of nembutal, gr. 3, followed in ten minutes by chloral hydrate, gr. 30, is given to primiparæ when the os is 2/5 to 3/5 dilated with regular pains, and to multiparæ when the os is 1/5 to 2/5 dilated. These doses are repeated after two hours, and, if necessary, small subsequent doses may have to be given, but 7½ gr. of nembutal and 120 gr. of chloral should not be exceeded in twelve hours. Some inhalation anæsthesia may be necessary when the head passes over the perineum. In sixty consecutive labours with this technique 62 per cent. were painless with perfect amnesia, and in no case were any ill-effects noted in mothers or babies. On the other hand, restlessness occurred in 20 per cent., while the first stage was prolonged in 40 per cent. and the second stage in 50 per cent. A somewhat similar technique, using **oral nembutal combined** with **hypodermic scopolamine,** has also been fairly successful,[70] as has **oral nembutal combined with rectal paraldehyde.**[71]

A serviceable and simple method is that using **oral thiopentone.** Four gr. are given by mouth as soon as the pains are definitely established. A further 3 gr. are given after half an hour and the dose is repeated after another hour. If the effects of the drug wear off, 2 to 3 gr. are repeated at hourly intervals, the *total* quantity varying from 10 to 20 gr. A small dose of scopolamine given simultaneously with the first dose of pentothal sodium will enhance the amnesia.[72] **Thiopentone** (acid) by mouth in rather higher dosage has also proved effective.[73]

Pethidine (demerol, dolantal, dolantin, isonipecaine, meperidine)

$$C_6H_5-C-COOC_2H_5$$

$$H_2C \diagup\ \diagdown CH_2$$

$$H_2C \diagdown\ \diagup CH_2$$

$$N$$

$$CH_3$$

is the ethyl ester of 1-methyl-4-phenyl-piperidine-4-carboxylic acid and was synthesized in 1939 by Eisleb and Shaumann. The drug is related chemically to atropine and the hydrochloride is now being used extensively as an analgesic in the first stage of labour. An initial dose of 100 mg. is usually given intramuscularly and this can be repeated at two to three hourly intervals up to a maximum of 400 mg. Although the fœtal respiration is not depressed as much as with morphine, it is unwise to give a dose of pethidine within three hours of delivery. Analgesia is generally fairly good but occasionally vomiting is a troublesome complication.[73] In Great Britain since April 1st, 1950, unsupervised midwives can employ pethidine subject to various safeguards. Besides its use alone, pethidine has been combined with other methods, such as the inhalation of trilene or with an injection of scopolamine gr. 1/150 followed possibly by one other equal dose unless the os is more than three-quarters dilated. This latter technique usually affords some degree of amnesia as well as analgesia.[74]

Physeptone (amidone, dolophine, " Höchst 10820 ", methadon and **miadone)** is al 2-dimethylamino 4-4-diphenyl-heptan-5-1-hydrochloride with the structural formula :

$$
\begin{array}{c}
\text{(C}_6\text{H}_5)_2 \\
|\\
\text{C}\\
\text{CH}_2\qquad \text{C}=\text{O}\\
\text{CH.CH}_3\quad \text{CH}_2\\
\text{N}\qquad\quad \text{CH}_3\\
(\text{CH}_3)_2
\end{array}
$$

Its analgesic potency is said to be approximately equal to that of morphine and about ten times that of pethidine.[75] The side-effects such as giddiness and blurred vision are less than with pethidine, while nausea and vomiting occurred less frequently than with morphine.[76] The drug appeared most promising as an obstetrical analgesic, but unfortunately it has a pronounced depressing action on the infant's respiration so that great caution is necessary.[77]

" **Twilight sleep** ", first employed by von Steinbüchel and Gauss in 1902, has **morphine and scopolamine** as active agents. Its original popularity has largely disappeared, owing to frequent failure of analgesia, prolonged· labours, occasional violent excitement and narcotized babies.[8] The effect of morphine on infants has been examined in Canada, and in 320 deliveries after the drug had been given to the mothers, 120 infants showed some signs of narcosis, 25 showed deep narcosis, and 6 were completely apnœic for over twenty minutes.[78] The result of another investigation carried out at the Boston Lying-in-Hospital was even more striking, the opinion being expressed that " we do not believe that morphine or any of its derivatives should be used during labour, as they have a marked effect in delaying the initial respirations of the infant ".[34] **Scopolamine** alone has its advocates, one series of 2,000 administrations showing good results.[78] In this technique, however, amnesia is all that can be expected.[80] The pure lævo-rotatory alkaloid should be used (see Chapter II). An initial light chloroform anæsthesia, followed by repeated scopolamine injections, has also been tried.[81]

If it is desired to use **bromethol,** the drug is given rectally at the termination of a pain, in the case of primiparæ when the os is fully dilated, and in multiparæ at three-quarters' dilatation. The dosage is 0·075 gm. per kilogramme body weight (see Chapter II). The rectum must first be emptied by an enema, and if a pain occurs during the injection, the catheter is withdrawn and the anus closed by pressure on the buttocks to prevent return. Labour may be prolonged, owing to the diminution in strength and frequency of the uterine contractions,[82] while depressed respiration in the child frequently persists for some time after birth.[83]

Local Analgesia

Local analgesia has the advantage that it avoids the " transplacental narcosis " of the infant.

If nerve-blocking is to be used, it must reach as high as the segmental level of T.11 to abolish all pain but not higher or the imperfectly understood motor innervation of the uterus may be adversely affected. Bilateral **paravertebral block** is possible but not generally practicable. **Fractional caudal block** is the method now usually employed.[84] This technique unfortunately had a sensational " boosting " in the American lay press which had the temporary effect of discrediting it. Nevertheless in spite of some difficulties and dangers,[85] there seems a definite place for fractional caudal analgesia in labour.[86] The alternative methods for carrying out this procedure are discussed in Chapter XIV together with the possible complications of the method *per se*. The main objection is that it alters the whole course of labour.[87] The patient has no urge to bear down or to use her abdominal muscles in the second stage so that this is prolonged and interference with the normal flexion of the head and rotation of the occiput result in an unusual number of persistent occipito-posterior presentations (e.g. 12 per cent. against 4 per cent. controls in 1,200 cases).[88] The incidence of forceps deliveries is also greatly increased (70 per cent. against 12 per cent.).[89] Several fœtal deaths have apparently been due to the injection of the drug.[90] On the whole, however, it is probable that if the technique is carefully carried out by a skilled team in the obstetric unit of a modern hospital, infant mortality and morbidity will be reduced in comparison with other methods of analgesia.[91] It is also of value in the control and treatment of eclampsia.

In an emergency some relief can be obtained by **infiltration** with nupercaine on each side of the mid-line half-way between the anus and the anterior edge of the perineum.[92]

Spinal analgesia has not proved very satisfactory in labour.   The reason appears to be that the action of the longitudinal muscle fibres of the uterus is inhibited, while that of the circular fibres is increased.   This leads to a violently contracting uterus with poor expulsive power.[75]   The method is also not without danger.[93]   The difficulty of procuring sufficiently long analgesia can be overcome by fractional spinal block (q.v.) but this method greatly increases the incidence of operative deliveries.[94]   Spinal analgesia in relation to Cæsarian section is discussed below.   Spinal block can be useful in the treatment of post-partum hæmorrhage due to uterine atony.[95] Presumably the spasmodic contraction of the circular muscle fibres mentioned above, arrests the bleeding.

Anæsthesia for Cæsarian Section

A great deal has been written on the most desirable method of anæsthesia for Cæsarian section[96] but in the writer's experience perfectly simple methods are quite satisfactory.   The problem is the removal of a large abdominal tumour with the undesirability of obtaining an anoxic or narcotized baby.   A satisfactory technique is—premedication with atropine, gr. 1/75 hypodermically, induction with intravenous thiopentone to the point of unconsciousness only, and maintenance with cyclopropane-oxygen.   If this gas is not available, nitrous oxide with not less than 25 per cent. oxygen and minimal trichlorethylene or ether can be substituted.[97]   A small amount of a supplementary anæsthetic is certainly better for the baby than the anoxia inevitable without it.   It is now established that curare passes very slowly, if at all, from mother to fœtus, so there seems no reason for withholding its use.[98]   This, however, is probably *not* the case with decamethonium.[99]   Although some gynæcologists object to a thiopentone induction, the writer has never seen ill-effects from it when used in the way described.   Directly the baby is delivered, omnopon gr. $\frac{1}{6}$ and scopolamine gr. 1/150 can usefully be given hypodermically to the mother.   This not only gives a calmer post-operative recovery but usually leads to a most desirable retrograde amnesia.

The above technique must only be taken as a suggested one for the average case with a mother in good condition and the fœtus not distressed.   If these conditions are not present, each case must be taken individually, together with the type of operation proposed. For example, the lower segment Cæsarian section takes much longer and requires greater relaxation than the classical upper segment operation.

Some patients definitely express a wish to be conscious during the operation and if they are neither anæmic nor shocked, a spinal block can be considered. The method has rather unjustly acquired an evil reputation due to various errors in technique.[100] Maternal mortality has usually been due to respiratory embarrassment from splinting of the diaphragm by the tumour mass. The antidote to this is early and continuous inhalation of oxygen. Foetal deaths appear to be due to excessive uterine contraction before delivery[101] and the intrathecal injection should not be made until the last possible moment. In a fairly recent series of cases the very high maternal mortality of 3·3 per cent. and fœtal mortality of 4·7 per cent. were recorded, although it is only fair to say that the figures of other workers were considerably less. Gynæcologists are themselves divided upon the desirability of spinal block for Cæsarian section but are usually strongly biased in one direction or the other. Two eminent teachers have stated their views in these trenchant words : " There is, we fear, in this country, a considerable number of young, healthy, pregnant women who stand condemned to death by spinal analgesia for Cæsarian section." In the writer's opinion this is as unwarranted as saying that spinal block should always be used.

Alternative methods of local analgesia are lumbar or caudal peridural block (q.v.).

Resuscitation of the New-born

It sometimes falls to the lot of the anæsthetist to attempt the revival of an apparently dead baby. It is customary to distinguish between blue and white asphyxia, but there is no rigid line of demarcation between the two types. In blue asphyxia, respiration is usually ineffective, either from fluids in the air passages or from a drugged or damaged respiratory centre. In white asphyxia the chief characteristics are shock and cardiac failure. It is really a more severe form of the blue variety.

It is probable that the three fundamental causes of neonatal asphyxia are intrauterine trauma, fœtal anoxia and maternal narcosis.[102] The initial gasp after birth opens up the bronchial tree and some of the alveoli, but the cause of this gasp is still wrapped in mystery. One of the less unlikely theories is that immediately after delivery the placental circulation is impaired by the contracting uterus. This results in a diminution of the oxygen and an increase in the carbon dioxide tension in the baby's blood, the latter factor stimulating the respiratory centre to action.[103] The former (anoxic) factor probably plays no part in the initiation of breathing as babies born in blue asphyxia do not readily breathe.[102] Sensory stimuli from the skin may also play their part. It is known that some respiratory movements occur *in utero* (Snyder and Rosenfeld) and some physiologists regard the chief change at birth as simply the replacement of the liquor amnii by air in the respiratory passages. However this may be, it is essential to discover if the child has or has not made attempts to breathe after delivery. In the latter case, it is not only futile but dangerous to make any attempt at artificial respiration, since no air will enter the solid fœtal lung either by the elastic recoil of the chest or by safe pressures applied in the trachea. On the other hand, if a small, soft rubber tube is passed into the trachea and oxygen insufflated through it *at a very low pressure* the baby's colour usually improves and breathing may start. These effects are probably due to oxygen diffusing through the mucous membrane of the trachea and bronchi and a reflex stimulation being produced.[104]

The question of giving **respiratory stimulants** to a baby suffering from neonatal asphyxia is an unsettled one. It used to be customary to inject lobeline gr. 1/20 or nikethamide 0·5 c.cm. into the umbilical vein and to " milk " it towards the umbilicus. If given at all these drugs must be well diluted as serious effects such as sciatic paralysis have followed undiluted injections.[105] Some pharmacologists deprecate the use of analeptics altogether on the ground that unless they achieve spontaneous respiration immediately they will increase anoxia by raising the metabolic rate.

Electrical stimulation of the phrenic nerve can prove successful in starting an infant's respiration but is still in the experimental stage[106] although it was used in animals as long ago as 1783.[107] The active electrode is a silver plated probe covered in lint soaked in a saturated solution of sodium chloride. This is placed on the motor point of the phrenic nerve which, with the head turned towards the opposite side, is just behind the junction of the middle and lower thirds of the sterno-mastoid muscle. The baby lies on the large indifferent electrode.[108] A somewhat complicated apparatus supplies the electric current intermittently. Both lungs are aërated, that on the unstimulated side being ventilated by movements of the mediastinum.[109] In adults, spontaneous respiration stops when electrical stimulation begins but this is not the case in infants.

Other routine general measures in the treatment of asphyxia neonatorum are the removal of liquor, mucus and other fluids from the respiratory passages by gentle suction, keeping the infant warm and laying it in a head-down slope of about 45°. The more vigorous procedures sometimes adopted such as swinging the baby by its feet, slapping its back and dashing cold water over it are more likely to do harm than good.

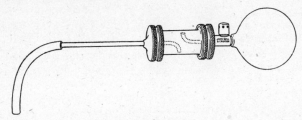

FIG. 150. Hand-operated mucus extractor for infants. (Barns, *Brit. Med. Jour.*)

If a baby is not breathing, it goes against an anæsthetist's instincts and training to do nothing after the simple measures already mentioned. It is well to reflect in such circumstances that in 1870 Paul Bert demonstrated that the new-born have the power of anaerobic metabolism[115] and this has recently been confirmed.[116]

When respiration has begun, oxygen can be added to the inspired air by a nasal catheter. The addition of about 5 per cent. carbon doxide usually increases the respiratory exchange but some workers deprecate this on the grounds that there is already an increased CO_2 tension in the blood.[110] Small and feeble babies frequently derive great benefit from prolonged inhalation of 50 per cent. oxygen. This can be conveniently carried out by modifying a standard " Hess " incubator[111] or by using a simple " perspex " hood. The required percentage of oxygen can be maintained by a flow of about 1 litre per minute. Carbon dioxide is absorbed by soda-lime contained in a wire-mesh holder.[112] Some obstetricians consider that " rocking " is of benefit in establishing regular and effective respiration. It is not always appreciated that while periodic breathing is often associated with anoxia in the adult this is not the case in infants and is quite common.[117]

If a baby is apparently still-born it is worth trying an intracardiac injection of 10 minims of 1 in 1,000 adrenaline solution. Several cases of resuscitation have been recorded although no cardiac activity whatever could be detected at birth.[113] In the writer's opinion the rapid injection of 3 c.cm. sterile normal saline into the left ventricle would be a more rational procedure (see Chap. XVII).

It is also worth noting that intra-uterine asphyxia can be success-fully treated temporarily by means of leptazol injections into the mother's vein.   The fœtal pulse rate usually rises within twenty-five seconds and the improvement lasts about five minutes.[114]

References.

1. Technique of READ, C. D.   See *Brit. Med. Jour.*, 1949, Apr. 16, pp. 651 and 669.
2. { KROGER and DELEE.   *Amer. Jour. Obst. & Gyn.*, 1943, **46**, p. 655.
   { GAUSS, C. J.   *Brit. Jour. Anæsth.*, 1929, p. 142.
3. MCILROY, A. L.   *Brit. Med. Jour.*, 1930, Oct. 4, p. 550.
4. SPENCER, H. R.   *Pro. Roy. Soc. Med.* (An. Sec.), 1922, Nov. 3.
5. BOURNE, W.   *Lancet*, 1934, July 7, p. 20.
6. RUND, E. H.   *Amer. Jour. Surg.*, 1934, p. 288.
7. FEATHERSTONE, H. W.   *Pro. Roy. Soc. Med.* (An. Sec.), 1922, Nov. 3.
8. BURROWS, J. R.   *Anesth. & Anal.*, 1933, July-Aug., p. 149.
9. BOURNE, W.   *Lancet*, 1934, March 17, p. 566.
10. COOKE, S.   *Lancet*, 1944, Sept. 23, p. 423.
11. DAVIS, C. H.   *Pro. Assoc. Anæsth. U.S. & Canad.*, 1927, May.
12. ROSS, J.   *Brit. Med. Jour.*, 1944, Jan. 8, p. 59.
13. SAMUEL, M.   *Deut. med. Woch.*, 1933, **8**, p. 286.
14. ALLEN, F. M.   *Amer. Jour. Surg.*, Dec., p. 283.
15. MACDONALD, T. J. C.   *Brit. Jour. Anæsth.*, 1950, April, p. 92.
16. TAIT, F. S.   *Pro. Roy. Soc. Med.* (An. Sec.), 1931, March 7.
17. MINNITT, R. J.   " Gas and Analgesia," 1949, 4th edit.
18. Introduced by KRONIG and GAUSS in 1907.
19. PRIBRAM, E.   *Klin. Woch. Berlin*, 1927, July 2.
20. KANE, H. F., and ROTH, C. B.   *Anesth. & Anal.*, 1937, May-June, p. 121.
21. SHEPHERD, H. L.   *Pro. Roy. Soc. Med.* (An. Sec.), 1931, March 7,
22. SPITZER, W.   *Brit. Med. Jour.*, 1944, Feb. 5, p. 179.
23. THORP, R. H.   *Nature*, 1947, **159**, p. 679.
24. BRAMMER, H.   *Schmerz-Narkose-Anæsth.*, 1935, June, p. 45.
25. OLDHAM, S. P.   *Brit. Jour. Anæsth.*, 1927, p. 35.
26. FEATHERSTONE, H. W.   *Pro. Roy. Soc. Med.* (An. Sec.), 1931, March 7.
27. *Rep. Med. Res. Counc.*, 1934-35.
28. ASTLEY, G. N.   *Brit. Jour. Anæsth.*, 1927, p. 35.
29. GWATHMEY, J. T., *et al.*   *Brit. Jour. Anæsth.*, 1921, p. 62.
30. HORSLEY, S.   *Lancet*, 1936, March 21, p. 690.
31. MINNITT, R. J.   *Practitioner*, 1942, Oct., p. 244.
32. COLE, W. C. C.   *Surg. Gyn. & Obst.*, 1939, Feb., p. 179.
33. LEVY, G.   *Pro. Roy. Soc. Med.* (An. Sec.), 1922, Feb. 3.
34. AVERETT, L.   *Amer. Jour. Obst. & Gyn.*, 1934, Jan., p. 109.
35. SHEEHAN, H. C.   *Brit. Jour. Anæsth.*, 1950, Oct., p. 204.
36. MENNELL, Z.   *Practitioner*, 1933, April.
37. RIVETT, L. C.   *Brit. Med. Jour.*, 1933, Oct. 28, p. 778.
38. BEATTIE, L.   *Lancet*, 1933, July 1, p. 36.
39. *Brit. Med. Jour.*, 1936, Feb. 8, p. 273.
40. BOYLE, H. E. G., and HEWER, C. L.   *Jour. Obst. & Gyn.*, 1924, **31**, No. 2, p. 264.
41. WILLIAMS, L.   *Lancet*, 1932, Oct. 8, p. 804.
42. SEWARD, E. H.   *Pro. Roy. Soc. Med.* (Sec. Obst. and Gyn.), 1949, March 18.
43. EASTMAN, N. J.   *Amer. Jour. Obst. & Gyn.*, 1936, April, p. 563.
44. MINNITT, R. J.   *Pro. Roy. Soc. Med.* (An. Sec.), 1934, May 4.
45. BOURNE, A. W., and BURN, J. H.   *Brit. Med. Jour.*, 1930, *ii*, p. 87.

46. McMechan, F. H. *Brit. Med. Jour.*, 1926, Dec. 11, p. 1111.
47. Dodek, S. M. *Surg. Gyn. & Obst.*, 1932, July, p. 45.
48. Allen, T. W. *Lancet*, 1936, July 25, p. 189.
49. King, J., and Morgan, J. *Lancet*, 1931, Aug. 15, p. 346.
50. Caine, A. M. *Amer. Jour. Surg.*, 1936, Dec., p. 463.
51. Smith. *Surg. Gyn. & Obst.*, 1939, **69,** p. 584.
52. Minnitt, R. J. *Lancet*, 1934, June 16, p. 1278.
53. Minnitt, R. J. Paper read at Liverpool Medical Institution, 1934, Feb. 22.
54. Minnitt, R. J. *Brit. Med. Jour.*, 1937, Sept. 11, p. 538.
55. *Brit. Med. Jour.*, 1936, Oct. 31, p. 887.
56. Elam, J. *Brit. Med. Jour.*, 1934, Dec. 29, p. 1196.
57. *Brit. Med. Jour.*, 1936, Feb. 8, p. 273.
58. Galley, A. H. *Lancet*, 1950, Aug. 12, p. 256.
59. Moir, C. *Lancet*, 1937, March 13, p. 615.
60. Barry, H. *Brit. Jour. Anœsth.*, 1937, April, p. 132.
61. Elam, J. *Jour. Obst. & Gyn. Brit. Emp.*, **46,** No. 1, p. 61.
62. { Hall, G. C. *Jour. Amer. Med. Ass.*, 1940, March 2, p. 728.
    { Morton, H. J. V., and Wylie, W. D. *Anœsthesia*, 1951, Oct., p. 190.
63. Edwards, W. *Brit. Med. Jour.*, 1943, Dec. 18, p. 795.
64. Heyworth, P. S. A. *Brit. Med. Jour.*, 1949, Mar. 12, p. 442.
65. Freedman, A. *Lancet*, 1943, Dec. 4, p. 696.
66. Barrat, A., and Platts, S. H. B. *Brit. Med. Jour.*, 1946, July 6, p. 10.
67. { Reynolds, F. N. *Brit. Med. Jour.*, 1949, Mar. 26, p. 537.
    { *Lancet*, 1949, Feb. 19, p. 312.
68. Epstein, H. G., and Macintosh, R. R. *Brit. Med. Jour.*, 1949, Nov. 12, p. 1092.
69. O'Sullivan, J. X., and Craner, W. W. *Lancet*, 1932, Jan. 16, p. 119.
70. Irving, F., *et al. Surg. Gyn. & Obst.*, 1934, Jan., p. 1.
71. Rosenfield, H., and Davidoff, R. *Surg. Gyn. & Obst.*, 1935, Feb., p. 235.
72. MacPhail, *et al. Canad. Med. Ass. Jour.*, 1937, Nov., p. 471.
73. { Gallen, B., and Prescott, F. *Brit. Med. Jour.*, 1944, Feb. 5, p. 176.
    { Spitzer, W. *Brit. Med. Jour.*, 1944, Feb. 5, p. 179.
74. Roberts, H. *Brit. Med. Jour.*, 1948.
75. Hewer, A. J. H., and Keele, C. A. *Lancet*, 1947, Aug. 23, p. 281.
76. Thorp, R. H. *Nature*, **159,** p. 679.
77. Prescott, F., and Ransom, S. C. *Lancet*, 1947, Oct. 4, p. 501.
78. Shute, E., and Davis, M. E. *Canad. Med. Ass. Jour.*, 1933, Sept., p. 252.
79. Van Hoosen, B. *Anesth. & Anal.*, 1928, May-June.
80. Barnett, T. *Brit. Med. Jour.*, 1934, May 26, p. 940.
81. Clark, J. *Brit. Med. Jour.*, 1934, Sept. 8, p. 468.
82. Morgan, G. N. B. *Brit. Med. Jour.*, 1932, July 2, p. 10.
83. Wahl, F. A. *Arch. für Gynäk.*, 1934, May 23.
84. Hingson, R. A., and Edwards, W. B. *Anesth. & Anal.*, 1942, Nov.-Dec., p. 501.
85. Gluck and Rochberg. *Amer. Jour. Obst. & Gyn.*, 1943, **45,** p. 645.
86. Adams, C., *et al. Jour. Amer. Med. Ass.*, 1943, May 15, p. 152.
87. Browne, F. J. *Brit. Med. Jour.*, 1945, May 26, p. 746.
88. Siever. *Jour. Amer. Med. Ass.*, 1944, **125,** p. 327.
89. Fitzgerald, *et al. Amer. Jour. Obst. & Gyn.*, 1944, **48,** p. 94.
90. Minnitt, R. S. *Pro. Roy. Soc. Med.* (An. Sec.), 1943, Oct. 1.
91. { Hingson, R. A. *Brit. Med. Jour.*, 1949, Oct. 8, p. 777.
    { Galley, A. H. *Anœsthesia*, 1949, Oct., p. 154.
92. Moss, E. P. *Brit. Med. Jour.*, 1934, Feb. 3, p. 215.
93. Laffont and Fulconis. *Bull. Soc. d'Obstét. et de Gyn. de Paris*, 1932, Oct., p. 548.

94.   HINEBAUGH, M. C., and LANG, W. R.   *Ann. Surg.*, 1944, Aug., p. 143.
95.   HANSEN, J. L.   *Acta. Obstet. et Gyn.*, 1943, vol. xxii, Fasc. 4, p. 305.
96.   Discussion.   *Pro. Roy. Soc. Med.* (Sec. Obst. and Gyn.), 1947, March 21.
97.   HEARD, K. M.   *Surg. Gyn. & Obst.*, 1940, **70,** p. 657.
98.   YOUNG, M.   *Lancet*, 1949, June 18, p. 1052.
99.   ELLERKER, A. R.   *Brit. Med. Jour.*, 1950, Aug. 12, p. 398.
100. { FAIRFIELD, L.   *Pro. Roy. Soc. Med.*, (Sec. Obst. and Gyn.), 1937, Nov. 19.
      MONTGOMERY, T. L.   *Jour. Amer. Med. Ass.*, 1937, May 15, p. 1619.
      WALKER, A. H. C., and MATTHEWS, S.   *Brit. Med. Jour.*, 1950, April 22, p. 938.
101. MACINTOSH, R. R.   *Brit. Med. Jour.*, 1949, March 5, p. 409.
102. LUCAS, H. B.   *Pro. Roy. Soc. Med.* (Sec. Obst. and Gyn.), 1950, Feb. 17.
103. WILSON, R. A.   *Pro. Roy. Soc. Med.* (Sec. Obst. and Gyn.), 1937, Apr. 16.
104. BLAIKLEY, J. B.   *Pro. Roy. Soc. Med.* (Sec. Obst. and Gyn.), 1950, Feb. 17.
105. HUDSON, F. P., *et al.*   *Brit. Med. Jour.*, 1950, Jan. 28, pp. 223 and 237.
106. CROSS, K. W.   *Pro. Roy. Soc. Med.* (Sec. Obst. and Gyn.), 1950, Feb. 17.
107. By C. W. HUFELAND of Göttingen.
108. CROSS, K. W., and ROBERTS, P. W.   *Brit. Med. Jour.*, 1951, May 12, p. 1043.
109. SARNOFF, S. J., *et al.*   *Jour. Thorac. Surg.*, 1950, **19,** p. 929.
110. EASTMAN, H. J.   *Bull. Johns Hopkins Hosp.*, 1932, Jan., p. 39.
111. BOOTHBY, W. H.   *Pro. Staff Mtgs. Mayo Clinic*, 1934, Feb. 28, p. 129.
112. MACCLANCY, P. C. D.   *Brit. Med. Jour.*, 1947, Dec. 13, p. 970.
113. EMANUEL.   *Lancet*, 1933, July 1.
114. DORR, H.   *Inschr. Geburtsh. Gynäk.*, 1938, Feb., p. 129.
115. BERT, P.   " Leçons sur la Physiologie comparée de la Respiration," 1870.   Baillière, Paris.
116. WILSON, *et al.*   *Paediatrics*, 1948, **1,** p. 581.
117. GRAHAM, B. D., *et al.*   *Paediatrics*, 1950, **6,** p. 55.

CHAPTER XXV

ANÆSTHETIC SEQUELÆ

Nausea—Vomiting—Headache—Parotitis—Ophthalmic Complications—
Cerebral Complications—Nerve Palsies—Pulmonary Complications—
Recovery Rooms.

A CONSIDERABLE number of undesirable symptoms may follow
the administration of general and local anæsthetics. Some of these
are preventable, such as conjunctivitis, pharyngitis and laryngitis,
whilst others, if not inevitable, are more difficult to avoid.

Nausea and Vomiting

Vomiting is rare after nitrous oxide, intravenous anæsthesia
and a pure local analgesia, but is unfortunately common after an
anæsthesia incorporating any of the more toxic volatile drugs
such as ether. The accompanying nausea is often more unpleasant
than the act of vomiting. Patients vary greatly in their liability
to these disturbances. One person may be a notoriously bad sailor
and will vomit repeatedly at the slightest provocation. Another
may undergo a two hours' operation under open ether anæsthesia
without even feeling sick. Females vomit more often than males
after operation.[1] Certain **prophylactic measures** definitely reduce
the incidence of nausea and vomiting. These are :

(i) Suitable preparation so that the patient arrives in the
anæsthetic room with no solid contents in the stomach.

(ii) The administration of glucose for twenty-four hours before
operation, and of glucose in an enema after operation. (But see
Chapter I for dangers of oral glucose.)

(iii) The post-operative administration of insulin (usually 10
units) in addition to the glucose if a considerable amount of ether
has been used.[2]

(iv) The administration of a basal narcotic[3] (with the possible
exception of bromethol) or the induction of anæsthesia with an
intravenous barbiturate. Enquiry should be made as to previous
experiences with morphine and its derivatives before incorporating
them into the premedication as these drugs are very prone to
cause vomiting in susceptible patients. The substitution of
pethidine eliminates this cause.

(v) The use of minimal quantities only of toxic drugs such as chloroform and ether.

(vi) Hyperventilation for a *short* time with CO_2 after the completion of long operations which have necessitated the use of much ether.[2]

(vii) The elimination to a large extent of the psychic factor by suitable suggestion made during the induction of anæsthesia.[4]

(viii) Recent work has suggested that much earlier post-operative feeding than usual results in less vomiting, distension and " gas pains ". The food should *not* contain milk, orange juice or fats.

Kemp considers that **vomiting after ether anæsthesia** can be greatly diminished by

(*a*) A meat-free diet for a week before operation supplemented by additional carbohydrates, vitamins, calcium and $1\frac{1}{2}$ oz. of lactose daily.

(*b*) 10 minims of Lugol's solution daily for five days before operation.

(*c*) Hospitalization for three days to attain " physical and environmental equilibrium ".[5]

A great variety of drugs have an effect on minimizing the vomiting of pregnancy[6] and of radiation sickness[7] and trials have been made of them with disappointing results.[8] Pyridoxine was said to be an exception[9] but further work failed to confirm any significant results.[10]

The **treatment** of vomiting which is actually occurring is largely empirical. The patient may be turned over on to his right side (to aid the flow of gastric contents into the duodenum) and a variety of remedies may be administered by mouth, such as iced soda water, strong black coffee, chloretone, etc. Gastric lavage with warm sodium bicarbonate solution was suggested as long ago as 1892 and may be most effective.[10] Nicotinic acid has been found to relieve vomiting due to sulphonamides, radiation therapy and pellagra but unfortunately appears to have little effect on post-operative sickness.[11] The oral administration of from 5 to 20 minims of 1 in 1,000 adrenaline to 1 ounce of water is, however, said to have a beneficial effect. It can safely be repeated in an adult.[12] Counter-irritation, such as a mustard leaf on the epigastrium, may effect a cure. It must not be forgotten that the vomiting may be due to causes other than the anæsthetic, e.g. to the manipulation of abdominal viscera, to dilatation of the cervix,[1] to swallowed blood after nose and throat operations, or to the effects of radium needles. Cases of acute intestinal obstruction have been missed because the vomiting was attributed to a previous anæsthetic. The " pernicious " type of vomiting characteristic of delayed chloroform poisoning is of grave omen, but recoveries have been reported by the prompt exhibition of glucose and insulin.

Headache

Headache is occasionally an annoying sequel to general anæsthesia. The usual remedies are indicated, whilst in addition it is said that activated vegetable charcoal, e.g. " carboserin ", given by mouth has a rapid effect. Headache following spinal analgesia is discussed in Chapter XV.

Parotitis

Parotitis occasionally follows operation, and it is thought by some that the inhibition of secretion by atropine may be a causative factor.[3]

Ophthalmic Complications

Conjunctivitis and **corneal abrasions** may follow unskilled anæsthesia usually of the open mask type. The former is often due to insufficient lubrication during deep narcosis in which the lachrymal secretion is diminished. The latter may follow frequent trials of the corneal reflex. Both conditions are much more likely to occur if the patient has exophthalmos (see Chapter XXI).

Diminished intra-ocular tension may follow the prolonged application of an ill fitting face-piece pressing on the globes.[13] This may be aggravated by excessive pressure, e.g. by using a rubber face-piece retainer which is interleaved with canvas. The diminished tension is followed by a reactionary rise and this may be the cause of the occasional attacks of **acute glaucoma** seen after operation. These were formerly ascribed to atropine used for premedication.[3]

Cerebral Complications

Cerebral changes due to anoxia have already been noted (see Chapter III). Recently, a new type of encephalopathy which may follow any type of general anæsthesia has been reported. It is characterized by the onset of light coma without localizing signs in the nervous system some hours after apparent recovery. The usual necropsy findings are cerebral congestion, some areas of softening and multiple subarachnoid hæmorrhages. The cause is obscure but the condition differs significantly from ordinary cerebral thrombosis.[14]

Nerve Palsies

Apart from various palsies following spinal block (q.v.) and trichlorethylene with faulty soda-lime (q.v.) brachial plexus palsy is not very uncommon after operation. This is usually due to pressure from shoulder rests in obese, curarized patients placed for some time in a high Trendelenburg position or from improper splinting of an abducted arm in breast operations or for transfusion.[16] The precautions necessary to guard against this complication have already been discussed. In a five-year review of 30,000 operations, there were 31 cases of nerve palsies, 11 of which affected the brachial plexus.[17]

Pulmonary Complications

The onset of pulmonary complications after operation has been the subject of observation and research for many years, the Society of Anæsthetists having had a discussion upon it in 1900. It is unfortunate that after so much progress in the arts of surgery and anæsthesia, the occurrence of these complications still remains relatively frequent.

The usual **types** of lung trouble after operations are small areas of atelectasis, massive collapse, bronchitis, broncho-pneumonia and pulmonary embolism.

The **operations** following which pulmonary complications are commonest are long abdominal procedures, particularly those in the upper abdomen,[18] such as gastrectomy and cholecystectomy.[19] Operations for the cure of hernia are also notorious for being followed by coughs. The infrequency of complications after orthopædic operations is evidenced by a series of 11,200 cases with one pneumonia.[20] The author has been greatly struck by the rarity of chest complications following nose and throat operations performed under endotracheal anæsthesia, and also following partial thyroidectomy.

The **frequency** of these complications is difficult to determine, but it is probable that, if really accurate records are kept, the incidence is considerably higher than was formerly supposed. For example, the following figures were accepted as typical some years ago : 0·42 per cent. in 2,400 cases (Corner and Crouch)[21] ; 1·1 per cent. in 441 cases (Smith)[22]; 1·51 per cent. in 7,900 cases (Alma Vedin)[23] ; 2·6 per cent. in 3,729 cases (Whipple).[24] Two more recent analyses utilizing the most modern record systems and including even mild " coughs " show the much higher figures of 6 per cent. in 7,874 cases[25] and 8·9 per cent. in 7,065 cases.[26]

The influence of sex, age, habits and season is marked, as all observers are agreed that post-operative pulmonary complications are much more frequent in men than in women.[27] One authority, indeed, maintains that they are twice as common in the male sex.[19]

During the late war, several observers have recorded the curious fact that Service patients are more liable than civilians.[28] This may be partly due to heavy smoking which is all too common in the Services leading to habitual chronic laryngitis and tracheitis. In one investigation into 1,257 abdominal operations under nitrous oxide-oxygen-ether anæsthesia, in adults, it was found that in " heavy " smokers (more than ten cigarettes or $\frac{1}{2}$ oz. tobacco per day) the total morbidity rate was about six times as high as that for non-smokers. Even temporary abstentions from smoking before operation appears to have some beneficial effect.[29] Older patients are, on the average, more susceptible than younger,[30] as is the case in respiratory diseases generally. In this country the incidence is much higher in the winter months, as would be expected.

The **types of anæsthesia** which are most frequently followed by pulmonary disease are not so easy to state except that as a general rule the deeper the plane of narcosis, the greater the incidence. At first sight it might be thought that ether was the main culprit and that the substitution of chloroform, or, better still, local analgesia, would reduce the incidence to vanishing point. Unfortunately this is not the case, as was pointed out by Mikulicz in 1898[31] and confirmed by all recorders since.[3, 19] It is true that ether is an irritant of the respiratory passages, and, if given by a poor technique in unsuitable cases, may initiate or aggravate respiratory diseases, but on the whole it seems doubtful whether there is any appreciable difference in this respect between any of the modern methods of anæsthesia or analgesia if they are properly administered and chosen to suit the individual case.[30, 32] For instance, endotracheal techniques were at one time suspected of an increased incidence of sequelæ, but subsequent careful investigation shows this view to be false[18] except after such operations as thyroidectomy and thymectomy (q.v.).

The main **causes** of post-operative lung complications seem to be :

(*a*) Impaired respiratory movements after operation. This is very obvious if a partly curarized patient is sent back to bed. It has been shown that the vital capacity one day after a laparotomy may be only 50 per cent. of the pre-operative capacity.[33] This is accompanied by sluggish venous drainage and resulting anoxia.[34] It is clear that diminished movement of the diaphragm by itself does not lead to lung trouble, as no untoward events follow deliberate paralysis of half this muscle from avulsion of the phrenic nerve nor from the induction of artificial pneumothorax.[35] The super-added factors appear to be (i) the lowering of the patient's resistance to infection. Recent work on animals has shown that during the period of narcosis with ether and with bromethol, resistance to pneumococcal infections is negligible even in animals rendered highly immune by the intravenous injection of anti-pneumococcal serum. Local phagocytosis at the site of infection is greatly reduced.[36]   (ii) The presence of pathogenic organisms in the lungs either before operation or aspirated during operation (see (b)), or conveyed by the diaphragmatic lymphatics. It is also probable that the shallow respiration, coupled with the patient's reluctance to cough, causes some of the bronchioles to be blocked with exudate or œdema, with the result that " apneumatosis " occurs.[37]   The rate at which various gases are absorbed by the alveoli beyond the block also has a bearing on local pulmonary collapse and is discussed under cyclopropane anæsthesia.

The administration of certain drugs after operation also diminishes respiratory movements. There is no doubt that the *indiscriminate* use of basal narcotics or large doses of morphine increases the incidence of pulmonary complications,[3, 38] and it is possible that the substitution of post-operative intravenous procaine may diminish them (see Chapter X).

Certain postures which may be necessary during operation impede respiration. Examples are the " bridged " gall-bladder position and a steep Trendelenburg tilt, with the stomach and intestines packed tightly against the diaphragm. The vital capacities in different postures have been estimated as in the subjoined table, 100 per cent. being the highest reading obtained in the sitting position.[39]

> Reverse Trendelenburg, 91 per cent.
> Dorsal, Prone and Left Lateral, 90 per cent.
> Right Lateral, 88 per cent.
> Gall bladder bridge (Lilienthal), 87 per cent.
> Trendelenburg, 85 per cent.
> Lithotomy, 82 per cent.

the use of widely extended mechanical retractors for some time in the upper abdomen does not conduce to free respiration during and after operation.

(b) The inspiration of infected material which may originate in the teeth, tonsils, nasal sinuses, stomach, or even in the small intestine in cases of obstruction. This cause of pulmonary complications is largely preventable and is due to poor technique.

(c) The irritating effects of certain anæsthetic vapours (chiefly di-ethyl ether) on the respiratory passages, especially in the presence of an existing infection. This irritation produces excessive secretion in the pharyngeal and bronchial mucosa which can be demonstrated by laryngoscopy[40] and bronchoscopy[36] respectively. (Curiously enough it would seem that the tracheal mucosa is not irritated to the same degree and does not produce excessive mucus.[40]) If the bronchial secretion becomes viscid, some of the bronchioles may become blocked[41] as already noted under heading (*a*). The excretion of irritant drugs through the lungs as well as their inhalation can give rise to morbidity. For example, fatal pulmonary complications have followed both the rectal and the intravenous administration of ether.[42] The chilling effect of a long open ether anæsthesia may have a deleterious action (see Chapter VI). Ether vapour should always be well diluted, as it has been shown in animals that concentrated doses may produce petechial hæmorrhages and pulmonary œdema (Poppert). In lesser concentrations volatile narcotic drugs paralyse the vaso-motor control of the blood vessels of the lungs.[43] Impurities in ether can also play a part in the production of pulmonary complications. It has been shown that pure ether in the usual anæsthetic concentration has little effect on ciliary action, but the addition of minute quantities of aldehydes and peroxides causes paralysis.[44]

(*d*) Patients who are allowed to remain in a profound degree of shock for a considerable time frequently develop pulmonary complications,[45] so that the causes of operative shock (see Chapter XVII) must be included. Considerable research had been carried out lately both in animals and in man upon pulmonary complications following severe aseptic operations performed under pure local analgesia. Post-mortem examination revealed lesions which macroscopically resembled infarcts and microscopically showed (i) atelectasis with dilated vessels, and (ii) alveoli distended with blood. There is some evidence to show that these lesions are caused by autogenous polypeptides produced by the operative trauma and disseminated by the blood stream.[46]

(*e*) A certain proportion of lung infection has been shown to be embolic in nature. Pulmonary embolism is considered later in this chapter.

(*f*) Acute pulmonary œdema very occasionally follows a simple administration of nitrous oxide in elderly and debilitated patients.

(*g*) Direct trauma from misplaced needles during paravertebral and brachial plexus blocks not infrequently gives rise to pneumothorax.

The **prophylactic measures** available against lung complications can be summarized as follows :

(*a*) Preliminary attention to the mouth to clear up any existing dental or tonsillar sepsis[47] and the adoption of an anæsthetic technique which precludes any possibility of the inhalation of septic material. If there are any moist sounds in the air-passages at the end of operation, aspiration of the tracheo-bronchial tree by a suction catheter is usually indicated.

(*b*) The postponement of non-urgent operations upon patients known to be suffering from colds, or who have recently recovered from any respiratory infection, however slight. This precaution is especially needed during the winter months.[48] If the patient can be seen a day or so before operation, excessive smoking should be stopped (see above) and the institution of breathing exercises, with the stress on expiration, should be undertaken if there is reason to fear lung complications. These exercises should be resumed as soon as possible after operation and the patient should be encouraged to cough. A trained physiotherapist can be invaluable for this work as it has been shown that ordinary " breathing exercises " are valueless.[79]

(*c*) Caution in the administration of powerful narcotics before and immediately after operations, particularly those involving the upper abdomen.

(*d*) The employment of a minimal amount of ether, particularly for patients liable to respiratory diseases. In such cases the required relaxation should be obtained by other inhalation agents such as cyclopropane or by an intravenous relaxant, or by suitable nerve- or field-blocking. If an appreciable amount of ether has to be used, the inhaled vapour should be approximately at body temperature, premedication should include an adequate dose of atropine or scopolamine,[49] and " de-etherization " with carbon dioxide should be practised at the conclusion of the anæsthesia. This last procedure should be carried out in a steep Trendelenburg position if there appears to be mucus present in the bronchial tree.[3] It has also been suggested that feeble patients in a semi-conscious condition could be placed in a Drinker's respirator so that pulmonary ventilation could be improved for some time after operation.[50] There is some statistical evidence to show that chemotherapy with the sulpha drugs has some prophylactic effect,[51] but this was not the case with procaine penicillin.[79]

(*e*) The anti-shock measures described in Chapter XVII. Rapidity and gentleness in the surgical technique are particularly important when dealing with viscera immediately below the diaphragm. There is no doubt that mechanical retractors, particularly those of the frame type, cause bruising of the tissues and tend towards diminished respiratory movements after operation. The maintenance of body temperature during and after operation should not be neglected.[49] Exposed viscera should be protected by hot packs and all instruments should be warmed. In smaller hospitals the transit of the patient from theatre to bed often leaves much to be desired. The use of air-conditioned recovery rooms is of great value in the prevention of pulmonary complications (see later).

(*f*) The use of binders and bandages, which do not impede the respiratory movements of the bases of the lungs,[49] but which give sufficient support to the abdominal wall to enable the patient to cough. Tight many-tailed bandages which tend to " ride up " on the chest, should be suspect if the respiratory rate is rising after operation.[52]

The repeated injection of small doses of atropine *after* operation is a practice which has practically died out. Mucus inhibits bacterial growth and is favourable to efficient ciliary action.[38] Atropine not only inhibits the secretion of mucus, but renders it more viscid and more difficult to cough up.[53] The drug is thus extremely useful before operation, but should not, as a rule, be employed afterwards. It is said that " autohæmo injection " is a useful prophylactic against pulmonary complications. Immediately after operation 20 c.cm. of blood are taken from a vein and reinjected intramuscularly.[54]

The **treatment** of post-operative pulmonary complications when established is most important. The commonest initial lesion is an area of atelectasis caused by a plugged bronchus or bronchiole and every effort should be made to dislodge the mechanical plug. If the patient is co-operative, he should be turned on to his sound side, the approximate position of the mucus plug is then firmly pressed and he is told to cough. This simple procedure is often successful. Semi-conscious or unco-operative patients can usually be made to cough by the following device. Intravenous thiopentone is given until the patient is drowsy. The syringe is then detached from the needle and 5 c.cm. of nikethamide solution is injected as quickly as possible from a fresh syringe. Occasionally the spasms of coughing which follow this technique are undesirably violent and in at least one instance have caused a hernia. A better method (in the author's opinion) is to give nitrous oxide and oxygen until the patient is drowsy and then to turn on ether vapour at maximum concentration for one inspiration. Voluntary coughing under the analgesic effect of intravenous procaine has also been used successfully. If these attempts have not availed to dislodge the obstruction and produce aeration of the lung, suction bronchoscopy[38] carried out under local analgesia (see Chapter XX) will probably be advisable. Deep breathing can be ensured by five-minute inhalations of CO_2-air at four-hourly intervals.[55] Oxygen should not be used instead of air as it is more absorbable. Carbon dioxide in solution becomes carbonic acid, and this is thought to exert a bactericidal action on the pneumococcus.[56] On the other hand, the acid mucus will paralyse ciliary action temporarily, so that prolonged administration should be avoided.[38]

If the pulmonary lesion has advanced to the stage of infection, the exhibition of adequate doses of the sulphonamides or penicillin should be started without delay. The somewhat anomalous treatment by intramuscular injections of ether originally introduced by Bier is said to be effective in certain cases.[57]

The effects of general anæsthesia on **allergic** patients has been studied recently, and it has been shown that with a proper technique no added risk is incurred.[58] It is a remarkable fact that **asthmatics** nearly always take general anæsthetics well, and the attacks are usually less severe for a considerable time after operation. This observation has been turned to practical account, and severe and intractable cases of asthma have been treated by general anæsthesia with beneficial results.[59]

Pulmonary Embolism

Pulmonary embolism is still responsible for most of the unexpected tragedies following apparently successful operations. It usually occurs in patients over thirty from two to fourteen days after an abdominal section. There is no evidence to show that there is any seasonal or epidemic incidence[69] or that the type of anæsthesia or analgesia has any effect. Slow surgery, however, is certainly a factor. In a large general hospital there have been twenty-two fatal cases of pulmonary embolism in a series of 29,000 consecutive operations of all kinds, giving a mortality of 0·07 per cent.[61]

It has now been established that the common sites for the formation of an embolus are the deep veins of the calf and foot[62] (98 per cent. according to Bauer). It was formerly thought that the internal iliac vein was the commonest situation owing to stagnation of its contents caused by the crossing of the internal iliac artery, but more careful work has shown this to be unlikely. It also appears that a fibrinolysin always present in the plasma can be activated —possibly by trauma—and certainly by an anxiety state, an interesting example of the effect of the mind on the body.[62]

Prophylactic treatment should include the placing of a sorbo rubber bar under the tendo Achillis on the operating table if the patient is lying in the supine position and early and frequent movements of the leg muscles to empty the deep veins of the calf and foot after operation. Blocking of the foot of the bed diminishes venous congestion of the leg. The use of a knee-pillow to maintain the Fowler's position is to be avoided.[63] Breathing exercises under the supervision of a physiotherapist are useful and the patient should be got up reasonably soon after operation, but too much of a fetish has been made of this. If a patient cannot be sat up he should be turned at intervals into the right and left lateral positions[64] and not left to lie immobile in a soft comfortable bed.[65] Anti-coagulant treatment has been tried with thyroid extract,[54, 66, 67] atropine with ephetonin[68, 69] and calcium chloride[70] but none of these measures are effective. Dicoumarin, however, when taken by mouth definitely diminishes the production of prothrombin by the liver within 24 to 48 hours. One technique is to give a single oral dose of 300 mg. on the first day after operation, 200 mg. on the second day and 100 mg. on each successive day until the prothrombin time exceeds 27 seconds. Subsequent doses are given to maintain this level[71] but it must be remembered that dicoumarin is a cumulative drug.

When pulmonary embolism is about to occur, there may be premonitory symptoms, such as irregular temperature. From a statistical study of 1,665 cases of post-operative thrombosis and pulmonary embolism, it has been shown that two or more distinct episodes may occur separated by an interval of from four to ten days. It seems reasonable to infer that heparinization of all patients who manifest symptoms of an initial non-fatal embolism would reduce the mortality rate.[72] It is said that 300 mg. of heparin in 1,000 c.cm. normal saline given by an intravenous drip over twelve hours are sufficient to prevent fresh clotting without affecting clots already formed. The clotting time should be estimated and the heparin continued until the dicoumarin, which should have been given when heparin was started, takes effect.[73] The cause of death is probably not wholly mechanical but is in part due to the intense stimulation of abnormal reflexes in the autonomic nervous system.[74] This probably explains the fact that relief of pain and diminution of cyanosis have followed stellate ganglion block. This procedure would seem to be worth doing in severe cases of embolism which are not immediately fatal.[75] As a last resort Trendelenburg's operation for embolectomy may be attempted.

Post-operative Recovery Rooms

There is no doubt that a high proportion of deaths occurring in the immediate post-operative period are due to inefficient handling of patients by porters, orderlies and nurses so that conditions such as respiratory obstruction and circulatory depression are allowed to occur. Of 307 post-operative deaths investigated in America, it was estimated that about half were due to these causes.[76] In many new hospitals, recovery rooms have been installed under the charge of their Department of Anæsthesia, and this type of fatality has virtually disappeared in consequence.[77] It is indisputable that such rooms are most valuable. They should be installed in close proximity to the operating theatres and must be properly heated and provided with the apparatus necessary for oxygen therapy, suction, intravenous fluids and other resuscitative measures.[78]

References

1. DAVIES, R. M. *Brit. Med. Jour.*, 1941, Oct. 25, p. 578.
2. { MINNITT, R. J. *Pro. Roy. Soc. Med.* (An. Sec.), 1932, Dec. 2.
    { SMITH, G. F. R. *Brit. Jour. Anæsth.*, 1934, July, p. 138.
3. DAWKINS, C. J. M. " Incidence of Anæsthetic Complications and their Relation to Basal Narcosis." Murray, London.
4. { WILSON, S. R. *Pro. Roy. Soc. Med.* (An. Sec.), 1927, Feb. 4.
    { HOLLANDER, B. *Pro. Roy. Soc. Med.* (An. Sec.), 1932, Feb. 5.
5. KEMP, W. H. *Anesth. & Anal.*, 1936, Nov.-Dec., p. 285.
6. HESSELTINE, H. C. *Amer. Jour. Obst. & Gyn.*, 1946, **51,** p. 82.
7. VAN HELTERN, H. L. *Radiology*, 1946, **47,** p. 377.
8. BERGMANN, W. *Canad. Med. Ass. Jour.*, 1947, **56,** p. 554.
9. { VERNIER, L., and STODSKY, B. *Anesthesiology*, 1950, **11,** p. 212.
    { HILL, F. W. *Anæsthesia*, 1951, Jan., p. 52.
10. LENEVITCH. *Ann. Univ. Med. Sci.*, 1892, **3,** Sec. P, p. 13.
11. MUSHIN, W. W., and WOOD, H. M. *Brit. Med. Jour.*, 1944, May 27, p. 719.
12. CRAWFORD, B. G. R. *Brit. Med. Jour.*, 1944, June 17, p. 826.
13. BRITTAIN, I., and G. J. C. *Brit. Med. Jour.*, 1945, March 31, p. 442.
14. HUNTER, A. R. *Lancet*, 1949, June 18, p. 1045.
15. SINCLAIR, R. N. *Glasgow Med. Jour.*, 1948, Nov., p. 378.
16. { EWING, M. R. *Lancet*, 1950, Jan. 21, p. 99.
    { KILOH, L. C. *Ibid.*, p. 103.
    { RAFFAN, A. W. *Brit. Med. Jour.*, 1950, July 15, p. 149.
17. DHUNER, K. G. *Anesthesiology*, 1950, May, p. 289.
18. CAMPBELL, S. M., and GORDON, R. A. *Canad. Med. Ass. Jour.*, 1942, April, p. 347.
19. KING, D. S. *Surg. Gyn. & Obst.*, 1933, Jan., p. 43, *et seq.*
20. JORDAN, W. R. *Pro. Roy. Soc. Med.* (An. Sec.), 1923, Dec. 8.
21. *Trans. Soc. of Anæsth.,* 5.
22. *Brit. Med. Jour.,* 1922, April 1.

23. Paper read at Women's Med. Soc. of New York City, 1921, April 20.
24. *Surg. Gyn. & Obst.*, 1918, Jan.
25. ROVENSTINE, E. A., and TAYLORD, I. B. *Amer. Jour. Med. Sci.*, 1936, **191**, p. 807.
26. KING, D. S. Massachusetts General Hospital.
27. FULLER, C. J. *Lancet*, 1930, Jan. 18, p. 117.
28. BIRD, H. M., *et al. Brit. Med. Jour.*, 1943, June 19, p. 754.
29. MORTON, H. J. V. *Lancet*, 1944, March 18, p. 368.
30. GRIFFITHS, H. F. *Brit. Jour. Anœsth.*, 1934, April, p. 107.
31. Quoted by ROVSING. "Abdominal Surgery," 1914, p. 85.
32. { CORYLLOS, P. N. *Jour. Amer. Med. Ass.*, 1929, July 13, p. 98.
      SAUNDERS, E. W. *Ann. of Surg.*, 1931, Nov., p. 931.
      KING, D. S. *Surg. Gyn. & Obst.*, 1933, Jan., p. 43.
33. CHURCHILL, E. D., and McNEIL, D. *Surg. Gyn. & Obstet.*, 1927, **44**, p. 483.
34. CHASE, H. C. *Int. Abst. Surg.*, 1941, **73**, p. 106.
35. CHURCHILL, E. *Arch. of Surg.*, 1925, **2**, p. 489.
36. PICKRELL, K. L. *Anesth. & Anal.*, 1940, Sept.-Oct., p. 272.
37. DARLING, H. C. R. *Med. Jour. Australia*, 1932, July 23, p. 104.
38. NEGUS, V. E. *Pro. Roy. Soc. Med.* (An. Sec.), 1933, May 5.
39. CASE, E. H., and STILES, J. A. *Anesthesiology*, 1946, Jan., p. 30.
40. ARKELS, C. S. *Afr. Med. Jour.*, 1945, **19**, p. 223.
41. BAND, D., and HALL, D. S. *Brit. Jour. Surg.*, 1932, **19**, p. 387.
42. *Trans. Soc. of Anœsth.*, 2.
43. FEATHERSTONE, H. W. *Brit. Med. Jour.*, 1932, Oct. 1, p. 628.
44. MENDENHALL, W. *Anesth. & Anal.*, 1933, Nov.-Dec., p. 264.
45. GREEN, H. N. *Pro. Roy. Soc. Med.* (An. Sec.), 1946, Dec. 6.
46. DUVAL, P., and BINET, L. *Presse méd.*, 1936, **92**, p. 1800.
47. BROCK, R. C. *Guy's Hosp. Rep.*, 1936, p. 191.
48. FEATHERSTONE, H. W. *Pro. Roy. Soc. Med.* (Combined Meeting), 1925, Feb. 4.
49. LAMB, D. *Brit. Med. Jour.*, 1922, Nov. 11, p. 916.
50. MACINTOSH, R. R. *Lancet*, 1940, Dec. 14, p. 745.
51. COLSTON, J. A. C., and SATTERTHWAITE, R. W. *Southern Med. Jour.*, 1942, Nov., p. 1006.
52. BOWEN, W. H. *Brit. Med. Jour.*, 1944, Oct. 23, p. 573.
53. RINK, E. H. *Pro. Roy. Soc. Med.* (Joint Mtg.), 1938, March 2.
54. HANNAN, J. H. *Brit. Med. Jour.*, 1932, May 21, p. 959.
55. MACKENZIE, J. R. *Brit. Med. Jour.*, 1932, March 26, p. 561.
56. HENDERSON, Y. *New England Jour. of Med.*, 1932, Jan. 28.
57. { BIER. *Münch med. Woch.*, 1925, May 19.
      HAYWARD, E. *Zentralb. f. Chir.*, 1928, Oct. 16, p. 2501.
58. ANDRE, R. H. *Anesth. & Anal.*, 1937, March-April, p. 65.
59. TROSIER, J., *et al. Bull. et Mem. de la Soc. med. des Hôpitaux de Paris*, 1931, March 2.
60. PILCHER, R. *Anesth. & Anal.*, 1938, Sept.-Oct., p. 104.
61. WATSON, C. G. *Pro. Roy. Soc. Med.* (Combined Meeting), 1925, Feb. 4.
62. MACFARLANE, R. G. *Lancet*, 1937, *i*, p. 10 and 1946, *ii*, p. 862.
63. BEARD, J. *Anœsthesia*, 1947, Jan., p. 28.
64. MOYNIHAN, Lord. "Abdominal Operations," 4th edition, **1**, p. 54.
65. PLLWES, B. *Canad. Med. Ass. Jour.*, 1939, Sept., p. 271.
66. By WALTERS of the Mayo Clinic.
67. { FRASER, I. *Brit. Med. Jour.*, 1932, April 9, p. 569.
      BRAITHWAITE, L. R. *Brit. Jour. Surg.*, **19**, p. 337.
68. BANKOFF, G. *Brit. Med. Jour.*, 1934, Feb. 3, p. 189.
69. PILCHER, R. *Lancet*, 1939, April 1, p. 752.
70. MUFF, E. *Schweiz. med. Woch.*, 1937, July 10, p. 643.
71. HERMANN, L. G. *Surg. Clin. N. Amer.*, 1945, **28**, p. 1167.
72. *Pro. Mayo Clinic*, 1940 and 1941.

73. BEARD, J. *Anæsthesia*, 1947, Jan., p. 28.
74. DE TAKATS, C. *Bull. New York Acad. Med.*, 1944, **20,** p. 623.
75. BAGEANT and RAPPEE. *Anesthesiology*, 1947, **8,** p. 500.
76. Philadelphia Anesthesia Study Commission, 1947.
77. { LOWENTHAL, P., and RUSSELL, A. S. *Anesthesiology*, 1951, **12,** p. 470.
    { *Pro. Mayo Clinic*, 1951, **26,** p. 290.
78. ANDERSON, C. D. *Anesthesiology*, 1951, **12,** p. 604.
79. PALMER, K. N. V., and SELLICK, B. A. *Lancet*, 1952, Feb. 16, p. 345.

CHAPTER XXVI

PSYCHOLOGICAL ASPECTS OF ANÆSTHESIA AND ANALGESIA

Suggestion—Hypnosis—Personal Factor

THE psychological aspects of anæsthesia have not received much attention in the past, but in the last few years have come greatly to the fore. The patient rightly regards a serious operation as one of the most important events in his life, and not only appreciates real kindness and sympathy from his anæsthetist, but is also in a state which readily responds to **suggestion**. It has been observed for many years that suggestion can profoundly modify the induction of anæsthesia, and, indeed, suitable subjects can be rendered anæsthetic by **hypnosis** alone. Operations were, in fact, beginning to be performed in large numbers under hypnotic anæsthesia when the properties of the more reliable anæsthetics, chloroform and ether, were discovered, and these tended to absorb the whole attention of the surgeons then practising.[1] It is worth noting that during the Japanese occupation of Singapore at the beginning of 1945 the stocks of anæsthetic drugs became extremely low and attempts were made to use hypnotism. Some success was achieved in minor operations.[1]

The late S. R. Wilson did a great deal to demonstrate the physiological basis on which these phenomena rest.[2] It has been shown[3] that there is localization in depth as well as on the surface of the cortical grey matter, the three cell layers being (a) the supragranular or " intelligence " layer, constituting the conscious brain and governed by the laws of reason, argument, etc. ; (b) the granular or " artistic " layer, concerned with subconscious memory, music, etc. ; (c) the infragranular or " instinctive " layer. The two lower layers together constitute the subconscious brain and obey the laws of reflex action which have been fully investigated by such workers as Sherrington and Pawlow. It follows then that if interference from the supragranular layer can be inhibited we are left with a subconscious brain which will blindly accept any suggestion made to it. The various means at our disposal for inhibiting the conscious brain are :

(i) Psychological methods, e.g. by temporary distraction.

(ii) Certain drugs, e.g. barbiturates.

(iii) Sub-anæsthetic concentrations of narcotic gases.

In recent years basal narcosis, or, at any rate, sedation, has been used almost universally before general anæsthesia for major surgery, and thus the psychic factor has been largely eliminated (see Premedication). Even if preliminary narcotics are not used the anæsthetist can still render the induction of anæsthesia pleasant by suggestion and can even modify after-effects. The psychical part of post-operative vomiting, for example, which is so marked in certain nervous and hysterical types of patients, can often be entirely eliminated by suitable suggestion made during the induction of anæsthesia with nitrous oxide and oxygen. It is even held by some authorities that a strong suggestion of muscular relaxation made during the induction period will minimize the dosage of anæsthetic subsequently necessary to obtain adequate relaxation.[4] It need hardly be said that for suggestion to be effective an absolutely quiet induction room is essential and no interference with the patient can be permitted by well-meaning nurses or others.[5] As a matter of fact, a good anæsthetist does actually employ suggestion, whether he consciously realizes it or not. It has been aptly remarked[6] that " personality (in the anæsthetist) is non-toxic, and does not throw any strain on the (patient's) heart, liver or kidney, nor does it depress respiration ". This is more than can be said of many types of premedication. Suggestion also plays a large part in operations performed under local analgesia only,[7] and in certain countries the " **psycho-anæsthetist** " is a regular institution. For example, Pitkin describes his " auburn-haired vamp who has the faculty of making a woman forget that she is in the operating room—and makes the men feel that the operation could go on for ever if she would only remain with them ! ".[8] If pure local analgesia is to be used, the whole operating team must co-operate wholeheartedly. Even now it is not very uncommon for the surgeon to make his incision at the same time asking in a loud voice, " Do you feel that ? " There is no doubt that local analgesia applied indiscriminately and with no attempt at suggestion does frequently result in psychic shock and actual insanity has occurred as a result. It is the duty of the psycho-anæsthetist to prevent " psychic trauma " by suggestion, by drugs, and, if necessary, by inhalation of nitrous oxide or cyclopropane. In America, earphones are often supplied to patients undergoing operations under local analgesia so that they can listen to recorded **music.**[9] Their tastes are ascertained beforehand and selections from " classical ", " semi-classical " and " popular " tunes can be supplied.[10] Apart from its psychological aspects, pre-anæsthetic fear has two physical consequences. Firstly, it increases the amount of adrenaline in the circulation and this is known to be a predisposing factor in the causation of ventricular fibrillation. Secondly, the metabolic rate is raised, which is the exact opposite to the ideal condition if a nitrous oxide-oxygen anæsthesia is to be superimposed.[11]

The Personal Factor

It is, perhaps, insufficiently appreciated how differently individuals react to identical stimuli, and, indeed, the same individual varies from time to time. For example, such factors as a delicate upbringing, culture, education, artistic temperament, fatigue and cold will produce surprising variations in the response to suggestion and the amount of anæsthetics required.[12]

Dawkins has estimated that the average length of time necessary to produce anæsthesia with nitrous oxide in fair-haired patients was fifty-two seconds, and in red-haired ones sixty-eight seconds.

Drug addiction affects the susceptibility of patients to anæsthetics. The difficulty in inducing anæsthesia in alcoholics is well known and this has been quantitatively estimated in mice.[13] Addiction to morphine and cocaine, however, *increases* the susceptibility of animals to ether anæsthesia.

It has been shown that while women are more likely to vomit after operation, men are much more prone to the severe forms of post-operative complications.[14]

Special care should be taken with children as a badly given anæsthetic may affect their mental outlook for a very considerable time. Adequate premedication is most important while deception and trickery of any kind should be eschewed.[15]

The weather also has a marked influence. For example, the lower the relative humidity, the shorter is the induction time. Again, as the barometric pressure falls, the induction time increases.[16]

The extreme variability of action of drugs such as the barbiturates on patients who appear very similar has already been noted. Considerations such as these show the futility of any fixed technique or dosage.

In busy hospital practice, the preliminary investigation of the patient from the anæsthetic aspect is often unsatisfactory and in Great Britain the **anæsthetic out-patient clinic** has been started by several institutions with great success.[17] Apart from a routine check-up, patients are encouraged to ask questions and have the whole pre-operative technique thoroughly explained to them. The personal factor can here be assessed by the anæsthetist and the most suitable methods of induction and maintenance of anæsthesia decided upon.[18]

Reference has already been made to **anæsthetic rooms.** Although most hospitals subscribe to these in theory, they leave much to be desired in practice. A good deal of thought has been devoted to their design, the London County Council having agreed that their minimum area should be 196 sq. ft. if serving one operating theatre only. Further points to be noted are that the exit from the theatre must not be through the anæsthetic room nor should the theatre ever be visible to a waiting patient. The corridor outside the anæsthetic room should be at least 7 ft. wide so that trolleys can be turned easily into the door.[19] The anæsthetic room must be used solely as such and not as a store room, passage or social club room for students and nurses. A useful arrangement is to divide the anæsthetic room into two compartments by a washable curtain. The part into which the conscious patient is wheeled should be homely and look exactly like an ordinary room including pictures, curtained windows and a vase of flowers. After the induction of anæsthesia by an intravenous barbiturate, the patient is wheeled into the other compartment of the anæsthetic room where the gas-oxygen machine and other apparatus is ready for action.[20]

References

1. { HOLLANDER, B. *Pro. Roy. Soc. Med.* (An. Sec.), 1932, Feb. 5.
   { SAMPIMON, R. L., and WOODRUFF, M. F. *Med. Jour. Austral.*, 1946, March 23, p. 393.
2. WILSON, S. R. *Pro. Roy. Soc. Med.* (An. Sec.), 1927, Feb. 4.
3. By CAMPBELL, BRODMANN, BOLTON and others.
4. HORNABROOK. *General Practice*, 1932, March 15, p. 365.
5. RAWLINGS, N. W. *Brit. Jour. Anæsth.*, **7**, p. 127.
6. CRAMPTON, H. P. *Pro. Roy. Soc. Med.* (An. Sec.), 1934, **28**, p. 94.
7. BUXTON, D. W. *Brit. Jour. Anæsth.*, **7**, p. 69.
8. PITKIN, C. P., quoted by MAXON, L. H. " Spinal Anæsthesia," 1938.
9. JARMAN, R. *Pro. Roy. Soc. Med.* (An. Sec.), 1948, Nov. 5.
10. *Lancet* (Annotation). 1950, June 24, p. 1162.
11. STEWART, J. D. *Brit. Jour. Anæsth.*, 1939, Jan., p. 41.
12. STACEY, J. E. *Brit. Med. Jour.*, 1935, p. 820.
13. ABREU, B. E., and EMERSON, G. A. *Anesth. & Anal.*, 1939, Sept.-Oct., p. 294.
14. GORDH, T. *Pro. Roy. Soc. Med.* (An. Sec.), 1949, Dec. 2.
15. *Brit. Med. Jour.* (Edit.), 1943, Dec. 25, p. 820.
16. DAWKINS, C. J. M. *Brit. Med. Jour.*, 1938, July 30, p. 244.
17. LEE, J. A. *Anæsthesia*, 1949, Oct., p. 169.
18. HOWAT, D. D. C., and GREEN, R. A. *Pro. Roy. Soc. Med.* (An. Sec.), 1951, May 4.
19. WARD. " The Design and Equipment of Hospitals." London, p. 213.
20. OSTLERE, C. *Anæsthesia*, 1950, April, p. 91.

CHAPTER XXVII

OXYGEN THERAPY

PRIESTLEY discovered oxygen in 1774 and soon afterwards
suggested that it might be "peculiarly salutary to the lungs in
certain morbid cases". Its inhalation for therapeutic purposes
was initiated by Thomas Beddoes, in 1799, who opened a "Pneumatic Institute" at Bristol with Sir Humphry Davy as director.
Effective oxygen therapy was largely popularized by Haldane, who
demonstrated its efficiency in pulmonary œdema from gassing
during the 1914-18 war.[1]

Physiological Principles

Man normally breathes air containing 20·96 per cent. oxygen,
and at sea level 95 per cent. of his arterial hæmoglobin exists as
oxyhæmoglobin, whilst the dissolved oxygen in the plasma amounts
to 0·24 per cent.

If a normal individual inhales pure oxygen, *all* the hæmoglobin
is present as oxyhæmoglobin and the plasma oxygen reaches
2·2 per cent. At rest the average adult requires about 300 c.cm.
of oxygen per minute but in strenuous exercise this can reach
3,000 c.cm. At sea-level this means that 90 litres of air must be
passed through the lungs in each minute and at the same time the
lungs must be perfused with 25 litres of blood or nearly 1 pint per
second.[47]

It has been shown by arterial puncture and blood analyses that
in a great variety of pathological conditions the oxygen saturation
of the blood is definitely diminished, and that, if this can be restored
to normal, great improvement in the patient's condition results.
This, then, is the object of oxygen therapy.

The next point to decide is whether the inhalation of high
percentages of oxygen itself results in any harm. Paul Bert in
1878[2] and Lorrain Smith in 1899[3] thought that the gas should
not be given in concentrations higher than 60 per cent. It was
stated that rabbits subjected to nearly pure oxygen inhalation for
some days eventually succumbed to pulmonary œdema. This
statement retarded the development of effective oxygen therapy,
but it is now recognized that it is fallacious to suppose that an

anoxic patient will react in the same way as a normal rabbit.[4] Furthermore, it now seems doubtful whether the original experiments were conclusive. In order to elucidate this point, rabbits, guinea-pigs and rats have been exposed to pure oxygen for sixteen hours per day. At the end of fifty consecutive days no ill-effects were observed. As regards the effect of the gas on healthy human beings, continuous inhalation of 100 per cent. under normal pressure for twenty-four hours (no mean feat !) sometimes produces temporary substernal distress but there is no significant change in pulse rate, blood pressure or blood counts.[5] It can, therefore, be assumed that injury to the lungs from oxygen inhalation at atmospheric pressure is highly improbable. At high pressures, however, the gas is not so innocuous. Paul Bert showed in 1878 that convulsions may occur when oxygen is breathed under high pressures. This subject is of importance in divers who can carry on much longer using oxygen rather than compressed air and no bubbles of nitrogen rise to the surface to betray their presence to possible enemy observers. It has been recognized in the Navy for some years that it is dangerous for divers to breathe pure oxygen at a pressure of three atmospheres,[6] although healthy men can submit to even this severe test for three hours without distressing symptoms. During the fourth hour, progressive contraction of the visual fields occurs.[7] As a result of repeated exposures to the pure gas under high pressure, certain divers eventually develop an idiosyncrasy.[8] The Admiralty Experimental Diving Unit carried out many experiments in 1942 to 1944 in preparation for attacks on enemy ships such as the *Tirpitz*. It was found that there was extreme variation in tolerance and a much lower tolerance under water than in compressed air. For example, convulsions have occurred at a depth of only 40 feet.[9] These untoward effects do not, however, concern us as regards oxygen therapy, but it has recently been observed that in certain stages of congestive cardiac failure due to chronic disease of the lungs (cor pulmonale) oxygen therapy can cause a sharp rise in cerebrospinal pressure, occasionally with disastrous results. The reason for this is obscure.

Indications

Anoxia due to any irremovable cause is the indication for the administration of oxygen.

The causes of anoxia can be classified as follows[10] :

(*a*) Obstructive. Mechanical respiratory obstruction may prevent an adequate amount of air from entering or leaving the lungs or may impede alveolar diffusion. This class will include such cases as obstructive goitre, glottic œdema and pneumonia.

(b) Non-obstructive.

  (i) Increased metabolic rate as in acute thyrotoxicosis.[11]

 (ii) Deficient circulation as in failing heart, shock, etc. (**Stagnant anoxia**).

(iii) Deficient amount of oxygen in the inspired air as at high altitudes. In aviation it has been found that added oxygen is beneficial even at such moderate heights as 10,000 feet[12] unless a pressurized cabin is used.

(iv) Decreased oxygen-carrying capacity of the blood as in anæmia and in sulphonamide and carbon monoxide poisoning (**Anæmic anoxia**).

 (v) Decreased capacity for using oxygen by the tissues as in extreme cachexia, cyanide poisoning, overdose of toxic anæsthetics and rheumatic myocarditis[13] (**Histotoxic anoxia**).

At this point it might be mentioned that " **Anoxic anoxia** " although often used, is a bad term and simply indicates that when the blood returns from the lungs inadequately oxygenated, it cannot meet the requirements of the tissue cells.

One of the less pleasing amenities promised during the next war is the employment of " nerve gases ". For security reasons, full details of these compounds cannot be given but it can be stated that at atmospheric pressure they are liquids with boiling points between 150° C. and 250° C. The vapours are colourless, odourless and practically indetectible. These poisons are absorbed readily by the inhalation of vapour or by contact of the liquid with skin or mucosa. They are intensely toxic, and act by the inhibition of cholinesterase with consequent accumulation of acetylcholine. Acute poisoning leads to asphyxia with death from anoxia. The treatment is (1) large doses of atropine intramuscularly (e.g. gr. 1/32) and (2) immediate and prolonged artificial respiration if the respiratory exchange is inefficient. The Ministry of Supply advocates a hand bellows for this purpose but intermittent oxygen inflation would be more efficient if the apparatus was available.[48]

Oxygen therapy has also been used successfully in the treatment of such conditions as surgical emphysema, air embolism and acute distension of the stomach and small intestine.[14] The *rationale* of this procedure is as follows : Collections of gas trapped in the body consist chiefly of nitrogen. If the patient breathes pure oxygen for some time, the partial pressure of nitrogen in the alveolar air will fall. The blood-nitrogen concentration will also fall so that this gas will pass from any trapped collections to the blood and will be removed by the lungs.

Methods

The various methods whereby oxygen can be effectively administered are of comparatively recent development, and it is still no uncommon sight to see a cyanosed patient gasping for breath

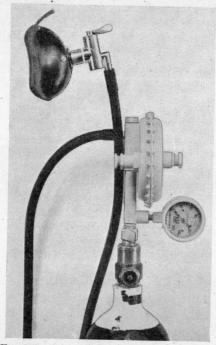

Fig. 151. Oxygen inflator (" The Oxford")
for patients who are not breathing.

a foot away from a glass funnel which discharges a feeble stream of oxygen (sometimes bubbling through brandy), the medical attendant being under the delusion that he is using oxygen therapy. It has been shown that no advantage whatever accrues from such a technique unless the gas flow is very high and the funnel is actually touching the patient's face.[15] The methods of proved efficiency will now be considered.

(a) **Face-piece.** If a patient has stopped breathing his chest must be rhythmically inflated by oxygen under pressure. The "emergency oxygen valves" on many types of anæsthetic apparatus are ideal for this purpose. Alternatively the special reducing valve shown can be attached to an oxygen cylinder. The screw at the side of the valve adjusts the pressure up to 45 mm. Hg. The face-piece is held firmly on the patient's face and the lever above it is turned to " ON ". When the chest is expanded it is turned back and the elastic recoil of the thorax causes deflation.[16] This sequence

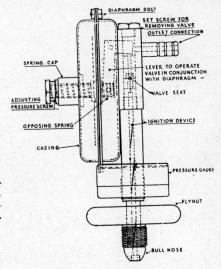

Fig. 152.   Oxygen   inflator ("The Oxford"). The dia-gram shows internal con-struction of reducing valve.

can be produced automatically by an apparatus such as the " pneumatic balance resuscitator " which in effect provides inter-mittent positive pressure.[17]

If the patient is unconscious but still breathing, pure oxygen can be supplied from any gas-oxygen apparatus or from a simple attachment to an oxygen cylinder as shown (Fig. 153).

In cases of emergency, an efficient oxygen inhaler can be made from a civilian or civilian duty respirator and an Association football bladder, size 4 or 5. A hole is cut in the latter opposite the inlet and is stretched so that the bladder overlaps the canister and is reinforced by a rubber band (Fig. 154). The oxygen flow is adjusted so that the bladder is about half full at the end of inspiration.[18]

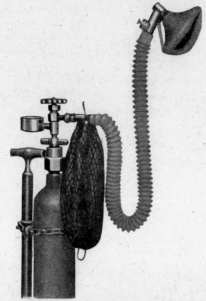

Fig. 153. Oxygen inhalation attachment
to cylinder (Magill's) for patients
who are breathing but unconscious.

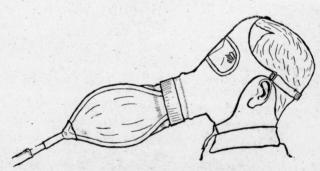

Fig. 154. Emergency oxygen inhaler made
from Government respirator and football bladder. (Marriott, *Brit. Med.
Jour.*)

The face-piece method is obviously unsuitable for prolonged administration and is not well tolerated by a conscious patient.

(*b*) **Nasal Inhaler.** A nasal inhaler, such as is used for dental anæsthesia (see Fig. 155), can be employed with an intermittent-flow apparatus. A mixture containing from 60 per cent. to 100 per cent. oxygen can be inhaled continuously provided that the patient keeps his mouth shut. The amount of rebreathing must be adjusted according to the percentage of CO_2 that is desirable. This type of

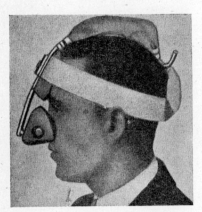

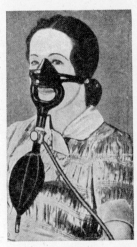

FIG. 155.   Nasal oxygen inhaler. (Christie, *Lancet*.)

FIG. 156.   B.L.B. oxygen inhaler (Oxygen Therapy Equipment Ltd.).

inhaler can be worn night and day without much discomfort, and even at high concentrations the oxygen consumption should not exceed 100 gallons per hour.

A specially modified nasal inhaler has been devised by R. Christie. The extremely thin-walled bag is made of goldbeater's skin. Even if no special effort is made to breathe through the nose, good results are claimed at a flow of 3 to 4 litres per minute.[19]

The " B.L.B." inhaler is of similar type and was widely used during the late war. Either a nasal or oronasal mask can be used and a variable proportion of air is admitted by rotating a sleeve which uncovers one, two or three holes. Partial rebreathing takes place into a small rubber bag. An oxygen flow of 3 litres per minute with two air-holes open should give an alveolar concentration of about 40 per cent., while it should be possible to step up the oxygen percentage to 90 with a flow of 6 to 8 litres per minute and all holes shut.[20]   Unfortunately this apparatus has several drawbacks.   At low oxygen flows the resistance to breathing is considerable and the CO_2 concentration may exceed 2 per cent.

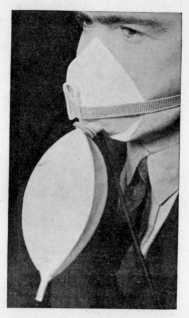

Fig. 157.   Polythene mask and
latex bag in position.   (Kent,
Lancet.)

Furthermore, the variation in oxygen concentration of the inspired air is as high as 18 per cent., fluctuating with the depth of respiration.[21]   Various modifications of the B.L.B. inhaler are in use[22] such as the very light plastic mask developed for high-altitude flying and made of polythene[23] (Alkathene, I.C.I.).   See Fig. 157.

In order to obviate the disadvantages of flow-meters, an injector has been devised to fit on to the oxygen cylinder so that the desired mixture with air is obtained at the source of supply.   No flow-meter is required and valves are provided so that no rebreathing occurs,

the bag simply acting as a reservoir.[24] It seems probable that some
such arrangement will soon become standard practice.

(c) **Nasal Catheter.** The *simplest* technique for effective oxygen
therapy is undoubtedly by means of nasal catheters.[25] Good results

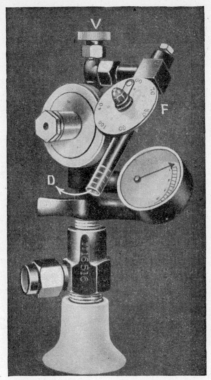

FIG. 158. Injector unit to supply adjust-
able mixtures of oxygen and air
(M.I.E. Co.).
V. Fine adjustment valve. F. Control
disc. D. To humidifier. (Cowan &
Mitchell, *Brit. Med. Jour.*)

are obtained by using two small lubricated rubber catheters A
(Fig. 159) passed about 3 inches inside the nose. These are connected to the catheter carrier B, fixed by a head band or a spectacle
frame (Fig. 160). Thick-walled pressure tubing C conveys the
oxygen from a reducing valve E via a combined flow-meter and

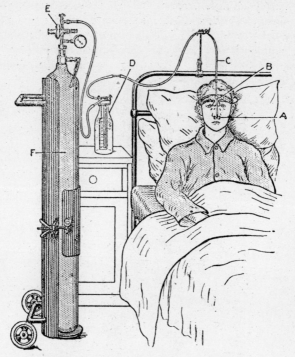

FIG. 159. Apparatus for the administration of oxygen by nasal
catheters. (Marriott and Robson, *Brit. Med. Jour.*)

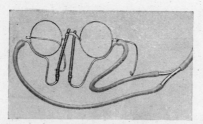

FIG. 160. Spectacle-type nasal catheter
carrier (Tudor-Edwards).

humidifier D. Gas-flows of 4 to 16 litres per minute are stated to
give oxygen percentages in the alveolar air of about 30 to 60
respectively, and little difference is noted whether the mouth is open
or shut.[26]

A more efficient technique is to use a single nasal catheter whose tip is in the oro-pharynx. The appropriate length of insertion is the distance between the nostril and the tragus of the ear. The catheter should be inserted while the oxygen is flowing to just beyond the estimated distance. It is then withdrawn until swallowing no longer occurs.[27] The rather large oxygen flow can be

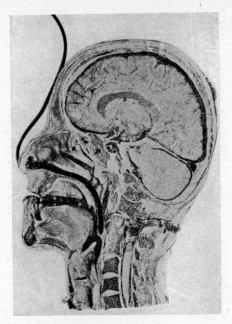

Fig. 161. Sagittal section showing correct position for naso-pharyngeal catheter (after Waters).

considerably reduced by combining a nasal catheter with a light aluminium box mask, as shown in Fig. 162.

A combined reducing and fine-adjustment valve R leads the oxygen through a bobbin-type flow-meter F and humidifier W to the catheter, which may be placed either 3 inches inside the nose or outside it and directed against the middle of the top of the mask. The opening for the nose and mouth is shown at C. The lower part of the mask is open. When the catheter is intranasal, the alveolar oxygen at 4, 5, 6 and 7 litres per minute is given at 40 per cent.,

50 per cent., 60 per cent., and 70 per cent. respectively. If the catheter is outside the nose, the system is not quite so efficient.[28] In an emergency a mask can be constructed quickly from light cardboard. The most recent type has the shoulders of the mask rounded off, thus improving vision and making the apparatus more comfortable to wear.[29]

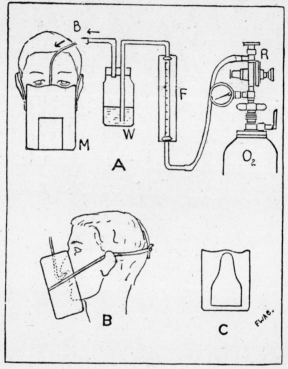

FIG. 162.   Nasal catheter combined with mask.   (Campbell, *Brit. Med. Jour.*)

It will have been noticed that most of the devices described require flow-meters and reducing valves. In cases of emergency it is possible to treat two patients with only one flow-meter and valve by using a special Y-tube, the upper arms of which contain resistances consisting of pinhole openings in brass discs. The lower limb of the Y is connected by pressure tubing to the cylinder reducing valve while the two upper limbs supply the selected apparatus to the patients. A single flow-meter is interposed in one circuit and each patient will receive practically the same volume of oxygen per minute. This idea might be of great use in Service or air-raid practice particularly if a large number of gassed patients had to be treated simultaneously with limited equipment.[30]

(*d*) **Oxygen Box.** An oxygen box is a simple and efficient device if no tent is obtainable. A box, measuring about 28 × 18 × 18

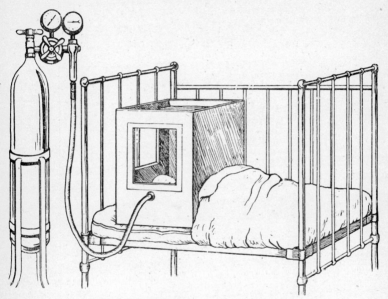

Fig. 163. Oxygen box (after Burgess).

inches, is used with either an open or closed top and with one side replaced by a curtain to fit around the patient's neck (Fig. 163). An oxygen inlet is arranged near the bottom and a flow of 4·5 to 5 litres per minute gives a continuous concentration of 40 per cent. to 60 per cent. at the level of the patient's nose, in spite of free upward diffusion with the top open. In the closed condition, a flow of only 1 litre per minute will provide a concentration of 70 per cent. oxygen after 3 hours. Adequate control of temperature can be obtained by the use of an ice container within the box.[31] The oxygen box is of great use for babies with asphyxia neonatorum and for premature infants[32] (see p. 383).

(*e*) **Oxygen Tents.** Oxygen tents are extremely useful for delirious patients and those who will not tolerate a nasal catheter or inhaler. Tents vary from simple mica hoods to those embodying extremely intricate mechanism. Fig. 164 shows the simplest possible type, in which the gas enters the top of the hood by a jet which causes a pleasant breeze to play upon the patient's face, increases the concentration near the nose, and helps to cool the internal atmosphere. If the flow-meter is set at 5 litres per minute an oxygen concentration of 60 per cent. to 70 per cent. is obtained. An electric fan playing on the outside of the hood also assists in cooling. Carbon dioxide escapes through the rubberized fabric,

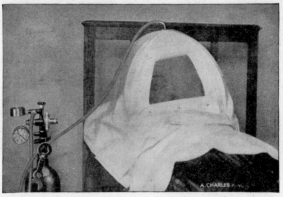

Fig. 164.   Simple type of oxygen tent for emergency use.

and should not exceed 1 per cent. even after prolonged use. It is found, however, that with this simple type of tent moisture tends to accumulate, and the patient, after a time, feels confined and oppressed. Two minutes' relief after every half hour is generally given and the inhalation also has to be interrupted when medicine and food are administered.

For these reasons the more elaborate types of tent have been designed. Although of many different patterns, these usually incorporate the following features :

(1) Positive ventilation is secured either by a pump driven by an electric motor, or preferably by an injector on the oxygen feed,[33] or by the up and down movements of a small gasometer worked by an oxygen motor.

(2) Definite regulation of the temperature and humidity of the internal atmosphere is obtained by an ice chamber and thermostat.

A hygrometer is usually incorporated, and the relative humidity should normally be kept below 50 per cent.

(3) Regulation of the CO_2 percentage is secured by a soda-lime chamber. If $O_2 + CO_2$ mixtures are desired, this filter is cut out and CO_2 added from a separate cylinder.

(4) Provision is made for securing samples of the internal atmosphere for gas analysis. It is essential that the oxygen concentration be estimated from time to time as leakage is frequently a cause of ineffective therapy.[32]

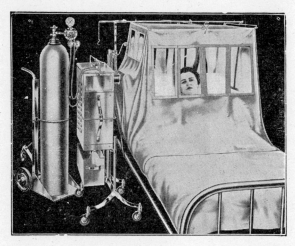

FIG. 165. Typical motorless oxygen tent (Heidbrink).

(5) The transparent windows must always be made of non-inflammable material, such as cellulose acetate. Neglect of this precaution (e.g. the use of cellulose nitrate or celluloid) has led to disasters.

(6) The interior of the tent must be sterilizable.

The chief disadvantages of oxygen tents are the high cost of maintenance, and the fact that some patients experience a type of claustrophobia when confined within them.[34] The cost of running tents can be considerably reduced by using commercial oxygen instead of the highly purified gas prepared for anæsthetic purposes. The only impurity in the former product is nitrogen, and since an atmosphere containing less than 70 per cent. oxygen is usually employed, this is of no importance. The cost can also be cut down by having hospital wards piped for oxygen with a control valve near each bed. This enables batteries of very large cylinders to be kept in a remote room and also eliminates the depression often experienced by patients when looking at oxygen cylinders. The Medical Block of St. Bartholomew's Hospital is piped in this way.

(*f*) **Oxygen Chambers.** Oxygen chambers are collapsible structures which will admit a bed, so that the patient does not feel so confined as he does in a tent.

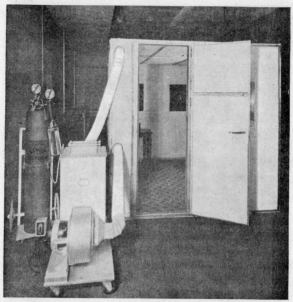

Fig. 166.   Transportable oxygen chamber (Barach).

The conditioning of the internal atmosphere is carried out on the same principles as oxygen tents. These chambers can be transported when packed, and have been in use in England since before the 1914-18 war.[35]

(*g*) **Oxygen Rooms.** Oxygen rooms are permanent structures which must be incorporated in hospitals or nursing homes. Patients can be nursed for indefinite periods without any interruption of the optimum oxygen concentration. In the room illustrated, thermal circulation is obtained by the brine coils on the left, which cool and dehumidify the atmosphere, and the heating radiator is on the right. Carbon dioxide is absorbed by the soda-lime trays seen just below the brine coils.

(*h*) **Oxygen Wards.** Certain large hospitals have found it economical to accommodate several patients at once in an oxygen therapy unit.[36] The obvious disadvantage of oxygen wards is the

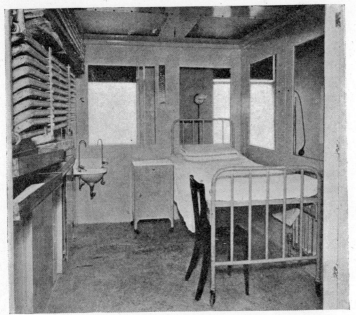

Fig. 167.   Oxygen room at Columbia Hospital, Milwaukee.

impossibility of regulating the conditions so that each patient has the optimum atmosphere.

Technique of Oxygen Inhalation

The patient's condition should first be noted with special reference to cyanosis, air hunger, pulse and respiration rates, blood pressure and mental state. It must, of course, be realized that cyanosis is not necessarily a sign of anoxia, the distinction being discussed in Chapter III. Pure oxygen should then be administered (in practice this will not exceed 98 per cent.) until maximum improvement has taken place. If none occurs within eight hours, the oxygen can be abandoned as useless. The oxygen percentage is then gradually reduced until the minimal amount is found which will maintain the patient's condition at the highest level. This concentration is continued until recovery from the disease permits a lower percentage to be employed. This process is continued until atmospheric air can be inhaled without deterioration in condition. This technique requires hourly charting of pulse, respiration and blood pressure for considerable periods, but the dramatic results obtained when the treatment is scientifically carried out more than justify the extra trouble entailed.[37]

Subcutaneous Administration of Oxygen. Oxygen has been administered subcutaneously for some years,[38] but recently doubts have been thrown upon its efficacy. It has been shown that the efficiency of the lungs in saturating the blood with oxygen is from fifteen to twenty times greater than that of the whole subcutaneous region of the body. At first sight, therefore, it seems problematical whether subcutaneous oxygen could have much value.[39] There is no doubt, however, that clinically considerable improvement in a patient's condition may ensue,[40] and in hæmoptysis[41] and acute asthma[42] this method is said to yield brilliant results. Subcutaneous oxygen is also of definite value in acute inflammatory conditions where it is possible to inject the gas into or over the affected part. For example, many cases of intractable sciatica and other forms of neuritis have been cured in this way.[43] Oxygen has also been used successfully in injecting infected joints in order to promote synovial secretion and to prevent adhesions,[44] while infiltration for gas gangrene has caused spectacular improvement.[45]

Technique. Some such apparatus as the " oxygenateur " of Dr. Bayeux, of Paris, is generally used, the average dose being 500 c.cm. If the patient's circulation is poor, it is advisable to distribute the gas by injecting 200 to 300 c.cm. in different areas. The dose should not be repeated until all the gas has been absorbed, as shown by the absence of crepitations.

Intravenous Administration of Oxygen. It is possible to inject intravenously about 10 c.cm. of commercial " medical " oxygen per minute or 20 c.cm. of the pure gas prepared by electrolysis of a 10 per cent. solution of sodium hydroxide. This is under 10 per cent. of the basal requirement and the flow cannot be increased without risk of gas embolism. Nevertheless, improvement has been recorded in cases of pneumonia.[46]

Surface Application of Oxygen. The exposure of certain surface lesions such as chronic ulcers of the leg to an atmosphere of oxygen is said to be very beneficial.[8]

References

1. HALDANE, J. S.   *Brit. Med. Jour.*, 1917, *i*, p. 181.
2. BERT, P.   " La Pression Barometrique," 1878, Paris, p. 764.
3. SMITH, L.   *Jour. Physiol.*, 1899, **24,** p. 19.
4. EVANS, J. H.   *Anesth. & Anal.*, 1927, **6,** p. 57.
5. COMRIE, J. H., *et al.   Jour. Amer. Med. Ass.*, 1945, **128,** p. 710.
6. DUDLEY, S. F.   *Pro. Roy. Soc. Med.* (United Serv. Sec.), 1935, April 8.
7. BEHNKE, A. R., *et al.   Amer. Jour. Physiol.*, 1936, Jan. 1, p. 436.
8. BEHNKE, A. R.   *Anesthesiology*, 1941, May, p. 245.
9. DONALD, K. W.   *Brit. Med. Jour.*, 1947, May 17 and 24.
10. Modified from " Index of Differential Diagnosis," by H. French, 1923, p. 156.
11. JOLL, C. A.   *Brit. Med. Jour.*, 1935, May 18, p. 1050.
12. BARACH, A. L.   *Jour. Amer. Med. Ass.*, 1937, May, p. 1868.
13. POULTON, E. P.   *Lancet*, 1939, Aug. 3, p. 305.
14. FINE, J., *et al.   Amer. Jour. Digestive Dis. & Nutrition*, 1935, Aug., p. 361.
15. HILTON, R.   *Brit. Med. Jour.*, 1928, *i*, p. 441.
16. MACINTOSH, R. R., and PRATT, C. L. C.   *Lancet*, 1939, Jan. 28, p. 206.
17. ADELMAN, M. H., *et al.   Anesthesiology*, 1949, Nov., p. 673.
18. MARRIOTT, H. L.   *Brit. Med. Jour.*, 1940, Oct. 19, p. 519.
19. CHRISTIE, R.   *Lancet*, 1938, Oct. 15, p. 880.
20. BOOTHBY, LOVELACE and BULBULIAN.   *Staffs Mtgs. Mayo Clinic*, 1938, Oct. 12.
21. BARACH, A. L., and ECKMAN, M.   *Anesthesiology*, 1941, **2**, p. 421.
22. CARD, W. I.   *Lancet*, 1944, Feb. 5, p. 177.
23. KENT, B. S.   *Lancet*, 1946, Sept. 14, p. 380.
24. COWAN, S. L., and MITCHELL, J. Y.   *Brit. Med. Jour.*, 1942, Jan. 24, p. 118.
25. BOURNE, G.   *Lancet*, 1922, *ii*, p. 23.
26. MARRIOTT, H. L., and ROBSON, K.   *Brit. Med. Jour.*, 1926, Jan. 25, p. 154.
27. WATERS, R. M., *et al.   Hospitals*, 1936, March.
28. CAMPBELL, J. A.   *Brit. Med. Jour.*, 1936, June 20, p. 1245.
29. CAMPBELL, J. A.   *Brit. Med. Jour.*, 1938, June 11, p. 1260.
30. WRIGHT, T. M., and CHRISTIE, R. V.   *Brit. Med. Jour.*, 1943, March 6, p. 287.
31. BURGESS, A.   *Anesth. & Anal.*, 1933, Sept.-Oct., p. 220.
32. { BARACH, A. L.   *Jour. Amer. Med. Ass.*, 1936, Feb. 29, p. 725.
     { JACKSON, C. R. S.   *Brit. Med. Jour.*, 1951, Nov. 10, p. 1129.
33. POULTON, E. P.   *Lancet*, 1933, Feb. 4, p. 246.
34. JOLL, C. A.   *Brit. Med. Jour.*, 1935, May 18, p. 1050.
35. HILL, L.   *Lancet*, 1933, Feb. 18, p. 384.
36. DAVIDSON, A. E.   *The Modern Hospital*, 1933, Feb.
37. EVE, F. C.   *Brit. Med. Jour.*, 1939, July 1, p. 20.
38. BURKARD, A. F.   *Med. World*, 1932, March.
39. SINGH, I.   *Quart. Jour. Exper. Physiol.*, 1932, **22**, p. 193.
40. SIMON, O. B.   *Anesth. & Anal.*, 1934, Nov.-Dec., p. 233.
41. LATINNE, A.   *Bruxelles-Médicale*, 1934, Dec., **23**, p. 219.
42. EVANS, J. H., and DURSHORDWE, C. J.   *Anesth. & Anal.*, 1937, July-Aug., p. 211.
43. BROWN, H. H.   *Brit. Med. Jour.*, 1938, Dec. 31, p. 1390.
44. HENSON, E. B.   *West Virginia Med. Jour.*, 1936, Feb., p. 83.
45. MACDONALD, N. M.   *Brit. Med. Jour.*, 1944, April 1, p. 470.
46. SINGH, I., and SHAH, M. J.   *Lancet*, 1940, May 18, p. 922.
47. TOVELL, R. M.   *Ann. Roy. Coll. Surg. Eng.*, 1951, Dec., p. 383.
48. { *Brit. Med. Jour.*, 1952, Aug. 9, p. 334 (Annotation).
     { *Lancet*, 1952, Aug. 9, p. 286 (Annotation).

CHAPTER XXVIII

ANÆSTHETIC CHARTS AND RECORDS

In previous chapters, there have been many references to blood pressure and pulse rate changes during anæsthesia, and charts are usually kept during all prolonged operations. The form of these charts differs in various hospitals according to the type of case commonly encountered and they incorporate a varying amount of miscellaneous information relative to the patient, the operation and the anæsthetic. As a general rule this amounts to the sum total of anæsthetic records which are afterwards available for study.

For some time past it has appeared to the writer that it is unlikely that any revolutionary discovery will change the course of anæsthesia, but that it is much more probable that progress will be achieved by a series of comparatively small improvements in technique. The main difficulty is to determine whether a certain change in method is an advance or a retrogression. The only logical way to do so is to compare a large number of cases in which the change has been made with an equal number in which it has not, all other factors being the same. Under existing conditions this is impossible, and unless a new drug or method is quite obviously good or bad, it takes a long time for anæsthetists generally to assess its value. Many instances could be cited of so-called advances which have gradually lapsed into oblivion in spite of enthusiastic " write ups " which were based more on wishful thinking than on hard facts. Commercial interests have been known to impart a more roseate hue to direct and indirect advertisements than has been subsequently found justifiable by the results obtained by the products concerned. It is true that individual anæsthetists have made careful records of cases done under new methods, but a long time must elapse before the number of administrations becomes really convincing, while it is very difficult to compare the results with those of older techniques owing to differences in other factors.

The only way out of this *impasse* is for anæsthetists to keep *standardized* records which can readily be sorted out afterwards. The necessity for some such system was recognized in America a few years ago and resulted in a modification of the " Hollerith " punch card system by the Committee of Records and Statistics of the American Association of Anæsthetists.[1] Unfortunately, this necessitated a complicated and rather fragile card, the learning of an arbitrary code and an expensive mechanical sorting machine. In spite of these drawbacks, the system made progress and was adopted in some sections of the U.S. Army Medical Corps.[2]

In Great Britain, a simpler type of combined chart and card index has been designed by Dr. M. D. Nosworthy,[3] and many teaching hospitals are now adopting it with a view to preventing the large mass of valuable data from being wasted as has occurred in the past. A second edition of this card has now been issued with minor modifications.[4]

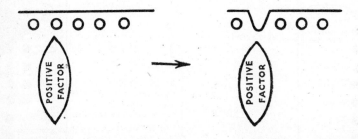

On referring to the illustrations, it will be seen that on one side of the card is a blood pressure and pulse chart specially adapted for operation records. The other side has a series of " positive factors " of all kinds each opposite a perforation near one edge of the card. At the time of operation, the anæsthetist encirlces the relevant positive factors, preferably in ink. This system eliminates all unnecessary writing. After operation the cards are completed and when the patient leaves hospital they are returned to the anæsthetic department, where each is issued with a serial number which, with the patient's name and operation performed, is entered in a card index. The holes opposite the encircled " positive factors " are then converted into V-shaped slots with two cuts of a pair of scissors or with a special nipping device. Finally, the corner of the card marked with the diagonal line is snipped off and all is ready for filing. It will be obvious by looking at the cut-off corners that the cards are in proper order and not either upside down or back to front. Sorting of a pack is done with great ease by means of a knitting needle. For example, suppose that it is desired to find the incidence of major pulmonary

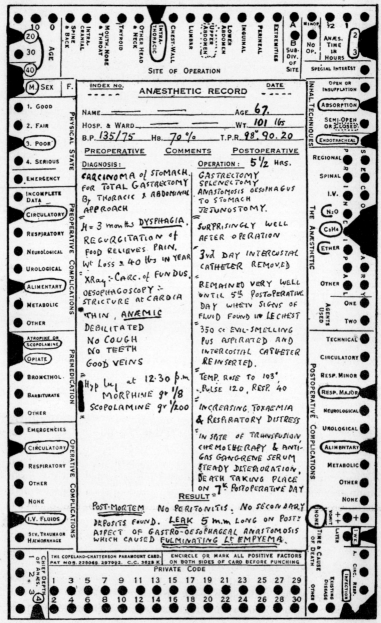

FIG. 168. Front of Record Card showing appropriate "positive factors" encircled and their holes converted into slots (M. D. Nosworthy).

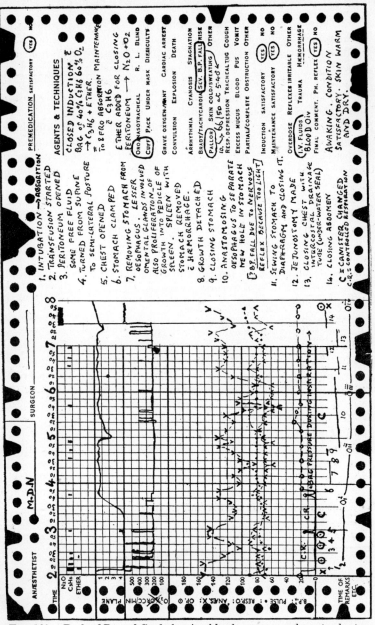

FIG. 169. Back of Record Card showing blood-pressure, pulse rate charts, etc. (M. D. Nosworthy).

complications after partial gastrectomy performed under (1) cyclopropane and (2) spinal block over a year's period. The needle is first inserted into the "upper laparotomy" hole and raised. All cards now remaining in the pack will refer to patients who have undergone an upper laparotomy. These can then be subdivided into "cyclopropane" and "spinal" cases by needling the appropriate holes and finally each of the subdivisions is needled for "major respiratory complications". The only hand sorting required is to separate partial gastrectomies from other upper laparotomies. It will readily be seen that the number of different investigations which can be carried out at any subsequent date is almost infinite.

Apart from facilitating research, the writer has found this system to be of great value for teaching purposes. If an anæsthetic clerk has filled in a card correctly, there is very little that he does not know about the administration of the anæsthetic and its immediate and remote effects upon the patient. The system also tends to focus attention upon the patient himself rather than upon anæsthetic apparatus and it is a certain prophylactic against the insidious disease of mind-wandering. Subsequently it may be found that the card will furnish more general information to an investigator than the patient's bulky dossier of hospital notes.

The cards can be adapted for special purposes comparatively easily. For example, at the Brompton Chest Hospital they have been modified by pasting a printed slip of the commoner thoracic operations over the general list which is standard. Alternatively special cards embodying the same principle of sorting have been evolved for particular (e.g. thoracic) cases.[5]

In America the "Nosworthy card" has been enlarged and elaborated into the "Chicago Anesthesia Record" which is also known as a "Keysort Card".[6]

In the opinion of the writer, the universal adoption of some such system by anæsthetists would constitute one of the most important "recent advances" in the specialty.

References

1. CHIVERS, E. M. *Brit. Jour. Anæsth.*, 1942, *xviii*, p. 69.
2. WANGEMAN, C. P. *Anesthesiology*, 1941, *ii*, p. 179.
3. NOSWORTHY, M. D. *Brit. Jour. Anæsth.*, 1943, *xviii*, No. 4.
4. NOSWORTHY, M. D. *Anesth. & Anal.*, 1945, Nov.-Dec., p. 221.
5. BALLANTINE, R. I. W. *Anæsthesia*, 1950, Jan., p. 44.
6. CONROY, W. A., *et al.* *Anesthesiology*, 1948, March, p. 121.

INDEX

Names of authorities mentioned in the text only are included. The remainder will be found in the list of references at the end of each chapter

Cardiazol (*see* Leptazol)
Cardiolysis, 350
Cardiospasm, 213, 239
Carotid sinus, 161
Carvell, E. M., 269
Cathelin, F., 218
Cauda equina lesions, 247
Caudal block, 221, 379
Cellulose acetate, 419
  nitrate, 419
Cephalin flocculation test, 6
Cerebellar operations, 287
Cerebellum, 13
Cerebral complications, 389
  cortex, 13, 47
Cerebrospinal fluid, 227
  pressure, 227, 246
Chaput's solution, 229
Charcoal, 143, 389
Charles's airway, 319
Charts, 424
Chemical sympathectomy, 210
Chevalier Jackson, 308
Childbirth, 365
Children, 26, 30, 36, 104, 182, 297, 311, 349, 362, 403
Chloral, 145, 376
Chlorbutanol, 170
Chlorethyl (*see* Ethyl chloride)
Chlorobenzene, 233
Chloroform, 2, 112, 261, 367
Chloryl (*see* Ethyl chloride)
Chlorylene (*see* Trichlorethylene)
Cholecystectomy, 235
Cholesterol, 2
Choline, 169
Cholinesterase, 169
Chorea, 33, 160
Christie's oxygen inhaler, 411
Cibalgin, 35
Ciliary action, 396
Cinchocaine, 191
Circle system of absorption, 80
Cisternal puncture, 227
Clausen's harness, 66, 328
Claustrophobia, 330, 419
Closed-circuit technique, 53, 77, 142
Clover's apparatus, 97
Coagulation time, 2, 52, 102
Cobb's adapter, 122
Cobefrin, 197
Cocaine, 123, 188
Colitis, 32
Collapse, 261
Coller, Carl, 188
Colles's fracture, 209
Colour codes, 87
Coloured fluids, 113, 114, 202

Congo red, 30
Conjunctivitis, 324, 389
Connell apparatus, 72
Continuous flow gas-oxygen machines, 68
  syringes, 205, 328
Continuous intravenous anæsthesia, 155
  spinal analgesia, 232
Controlled respiration, 21, 52, 338
Convulsions, 92, 103, 160, 161, 184
Cool flames, 137
Copper, 91, 95
Coramine (*see* Nikethamide)
Corbasil (*see* Cobefrin)
Corneal abrasions, 389
Corvotone (*see* Nikethamide)
Coughing, 85, 330, 347, 395
Coxeter's flowmeter, 69, 71
Crafoord's operation, 350
Crampton test, 8, 10
Cranial nerve palsies, 116
  surgery, 33, 286
Crico-thyroid membrane, 133, 309
Crile's theory, 13, 270
Critical gas flow, 74
Cross-infection, 86
Crush syndrome, 239, 271
Crutchfield caliper, 287
Cuffed tubes, 130, 320
Curare, 94, 161, 166
  after effects, 173
  antidotes, 169
  contra-indication, 171
Cushing, H., 286
Cut-offs, 75
Cyanosis, 45, 324, 329
  peripheral, 47
Cycliton, 278
Cyclobarbital, 35
Cyclobutane, 55
Cyclonal (*see* Hexobarbitone)
Cyclopropane, 50, 243, 332, 339, 370
Cyclopropyl-ethyl ether, 106
Cyclopropyl-methyl ether, 106
Cyclural (*see* Hexobarbitone)
Cypreth ether, 106
Cyprethylene ether, 106
Cyprome ether, 106
Cystitis, 161
Cystoscopy, 40, 160

Davis gag, 117, 314
Davy, Sir Humphry, 405
d'Arsonval experiment, 17
Decamethonium iodide, 176
Decicaine (*see* Amethocaine)
Dehydration, 58, 270